Emergency Telephone Numbers

Doctor _____

Doctor _____

Doctor _____

Poison Control Center _____

Hospital (Emergency) _____

Paramedics _____

Ambulance _____

Fire _____

Police _____

Parents' work number _____

Local pharmacy _____

24-Hour pharmacy _____

Electric company _____

Gas company _____

Neighbor _____

Relative _____

Editorial Consultants

The following distinguished physicians have provided valuable editorial suggestions and advice during the preparation of this book.

Stephen Epstein, MD, FACS
Clinical Associate Professor of Otolaryngology and Head and Neck Surgery
Georgetown University School of Medicine and George Washington School of Medicine

Lay Fox, MD, FACC
Associate Professor of Medicine (Cardiology)
Georgetown University School of Medicine

Robert Gordon, MD, FACS
Clinical Associate Professor of Orthopedic Surgery
Georgetown University School of Medicine

Jorge Kattah, MD
Associate Professor of Neurology
Georgetown University School of Medicine

Michael Keegan, MD
Associate Professor of Medicine (Gastroenterology)
Georgetown University School of Medicine

Jennifer Patterson, MD
Clinical Dermatologist
New York University

Robert Ralph, MD, FACS
Clinical Associate Professor of Opthalmology
Georgetown University School of Medicine

James Ramey, MD
Clinical Associate Professor of Medicine (Endocrinology)
Georgetown University School of Medicine

William Rogers, MD
Director of Emergency Medicine
Southampton Hospital, Southampton, Long Island, NY

Henry Yeager, MD
Professor of Medicine (Pulmonary Medicine)
Georgetown University School of Medicine

DOCTOR
—— *in the* ——
HOUSE

Your Best Guide to Effective Medical Self-Care

For Victor and Dee Dee Gerdin

John C. Harbert, MD

John Harbert, M.D.

✳ HUMANA PRESS • TOTOWA, NEW JERSEY

Acknowledgments

The author wishes to thank the following physicians for their thoughtful reviews of and suggestions for this book: Drs. Robert Ralph, James Ramey, Jorge Katah, Henry Yeager, Stephen Epstein, Michael Keegan, Lay Fox, Jennifer Patterson, James Ramey, Robert Ralph, William Rogers, and Robert Gordon.

The information and recommendations in *Doctor in the House* are firmly grounded in the medical literature, and/or the author's and his sources' clinical experience, and so are relevant and appropriate in most cases. For more specific information concerning your personal medical condition, it is suggested that you consult a physician. The names of organizations appearing in this book are given for informational purposes only.

Illustrations by Patricia Cleary

Printed in the United States of America. 9 8 7 6 5 4 3 2 1

Library of Congress Cataloging in Publication Data

Harbert, John Charles, 1937–
    Doctor in the House : the best guide to medical self-care / by John C.
    Harbert.
        p. cm.
    Includes index.
    ISBN 0-89603-219-1
        1. Medicine, Popular. I. Title.
    RC81.H32 1994
    610—dc20   93-33242
                                                      CIP

Contents

How to Use This Book

Doctor in the House is written to help you and your family take your health into your own hands by informing you about your body and its illnesses, and letting you know just what you can manage on your own and what you cannot. Essential to this purpose is an understanding of the signs and symptoms of common diseases and disorders, over 400 of which are covered in these pages.

Doctor in the House will tell you the most frequent, as well as many of the less common, causes of particular signs and symptoms of diseases, what simple remedies are likely to be effective in relieving them, and when you should seek professional medical attention—that is, when self-medication or everyday measures are unlikely to result in improvement or cure.

In simplest terms, a **symptom** is an unpleasant physical sensation that interferes with one's comfort or productivity. A **sign** is an alteration in the structure or function of an organ or part of the body that is caused by disease, and that the patient or doctor can detect by direct objective examination. For example, itching is a *symptom* that only those who itch experience. The doctor may see the person scratching (a *sign*), but cannot personally experience the itch that is so real to those who suffer it. The doctor can only infer the symptom from the signs he observes and, of course, from the history given by the patient: "Doctor, I itch!"

The topics discussed in *Doctor in the House* have generally been arranged along anatomical lines, beginning with the region of the body: for example, "Your Nervous System" or "Your Respiratory System." Within these body regions are listed the organs and structures found in that region. Beneath organ headings are listed disorders common to that organ along with the signs and symptoms associated with those disorders. Thus, if you are interested in reading about "nearsightedness," you will find that topic treated under "Your Eyes" as listed in the Table of Contents. Or, more easily, you can find it listed directly in the **index**.

The **index** is especially useful because most signs and symptoms are associated with more than one disorder or organ and will consequently be discussed separately in different parts of the book. Thus the heading for pain will list several subheadings that will direct you to discussions of the causes of "chest pain," "back pain," "abdominal pain," and so on.

The signs and symptoms of diseases discussed in this book are those commonly encountered in the western hemisphere, and more particularly, in the United States. The incidence of these diseases and the causes of the signs and symptoms vary throughout the world, and even within different regions of any country. Such regional differences are not generally discussed because the author is not an epidemiologist (an expert in regional differences in disease prevalence, effects, and causes). When doubt about the nature and cause of a symptom exists, you should consult your doctor, who is more likely to know the patterns of regional disease prevalence as well as "what is going around." And most importantly, your doctor knows you.

Please take the time right now to fill in the emergency care and names telephone numbers in the spaces provided on the first page of this book. In an emergency, you will then always immediately know exactly where to look for the number to call.

Psychiatric disorders are not covered here because they are not generally amenable to self-diagnosis and treatment. Neither are most pediatric and obstetrical problems, because they should almost always be addressed by your doctor. Exceptions, such as colds, flu, earache, and so on, are discussed.

John C. Harbert, MD

CHOICES

HEALTH INSURANCE

VACCINATIONS

SECOND OPINION

annual physical

outpatient

occupational exposures

HOSPITAL

prescriptions

CANCER SCREENING

diet

Taking Charge of Your Health

How to Get the Best Medical Care

Choosing Your Doctor

Do you have a personal physician? If you don't have one, you should! It is important that one specific doctor know your entire medical history and take responsibility for maintaining your medical file. If you suffer a serious problem, this personal physician is then ready to take charge of your care, making sure that you are sent to the best hospital or clinic, and receive the attention of the best specialists.

In an increasingly mobile society, most of us (doctors too) must sooner or later shop about for a personal physician, at the very least, when we or our physician moves. A so-called "primary-care physician" should be competent to handle most medical problems you will encounter. Although many people rely for their regular care on specialists they have seen, or perhaps go to an emergency room or walk-in clinic when they fall sick, *these options are mistakes.* Specialists are not likely to be interested in handling minor medical problems. Frequently, one reason they went to such great effort to learn a specialty in the first place was to avoid just that.

Emergency rooms do not have access to your personal medical records if you have not been previously treated there, and the doctors may not welcome you if your medical problem is not an emergency. They may even resent your misuse of their service, and they can seldom be expected to take the time to treat or advise you about other, unrelated conditions that may also need medical attention.

The "walk-in clinic" is a relatively new health care innovation found mostly in larger cities. This may be viewed as a hybrid between an emergency room and a health maintenance organization (HMO). Although walk-in clinics don't usually offer as extensive medical services as emergency rooms, and don't have hospital beds available, they are equipped to treat a wide variety of medical problems. However, and you may perceive my bias right here, the doctor you see will be whoever happens to be on duty at the time you walk in. The clinic may maintain a medical record for you, but there will be no single doctor, whom you call *"My Doctor"* who has "the big picture" of your health status and with whom you can develop an ongoing, confidential relationship. The same criticism can be made of HMO programs, although the quality of most HMO programs is higher than that found in walk-in clinics.

You not only need a primary-care physician, you need to make the choice while you are well and have the time to carefully consider such matters as qualifications, availability, hospital affiliation, and personality. When you are sick, you want help in a hurry. That is no time to be shopping for a doctor.

There are basically three types of doctors that you are likely to find in your community who qualify as personal physicians: general practitioners (GPs), family practitioners, and internists.

- GPs have usually had one year of post-medical school training after graduating instead of the three or four years that family practitioners and internists have. Nevertheless, they often have extensive experience, and most are able medical practitioners. GPs seldom deliver babies now, unless they practice in rural areas; malpractice insurance for delivery services has become prohibitive.
- Family practitioners complete a three-year residency program and pass a certifying examination (the "Board"). To *maintain* certification they must be reexamined every six years. Family practitioners study in six broad areas of medicine: pediatrics, surgery, internal medicine, obstetrics and gynecology, psychiatry, and community medicine. Their training is designed to produce comprehensive health care providers to all members of your family.
- Internists are not to be confused with "interns," who are doctors in their first postgraduate year of training, Rather, internists are specialists in "internal medicine," the broad field of medicine that deals with the internal organs of the body: heart, kidneys, intestines, etc. Their specialty training consists of three or four years of advanced training after medical school. With additional training, internists may subspecialize in specific areas such as diseases of the kidneys (nephrologists), heart (cardiologists), endocrine glands (endocrinologists), blood (hematologists), immune system (immunologists), or they may limit their practice to such special diseases as cancer (oncologists), arthritis (rheumatologists), or allergies (allergists).

Here are some questions to ask yourself *(and others!)* when selecting a doctor:

- *How is the doctor regarded by other doctors in the community?* Peer reputation is the biggest factor that doctors consider in selecting their own doctors. Seek the advice of nurses and other health care workers. They see doctors at work and are frequently well qualified to assess competence and judge professional manner. Of course ask friends whose opinion you trust.

   If you do not know local doctors from whom you can seek advice, call the Department of Internal Medicine or Family Practice at your nearest medical school. Another good source is the "doctor referral service" of your local hospital. If you are given several doctors' names, you may choose on the basis of convenience of location, whether the doctor participates in your medical insurance program, or how you feel about the doctor after a first visit.
- *Where does the doctor have hospital privileges?* If there is a university hospital in your area, admitting privilege there is a good indication of the doctor's competence and familiarity with current medical knowledge. In a medical school setting, doctors continuously interact with their peers, and their performance is regularly evaluated by other doctors of established qualifications.
- *Does the doctor participate in your health insurance program?* Can your insurance company be billed, or must you pay the doctor directly? This is important, because if your doctor does not participate in your insurance plan, you may have to pay the full difference between the amount billed and the insurance reimbursement. This means that your medical care could cost as much as 20% more. If you are a Medicare recipient and concerned about cost, learn whether the doctor accepts "assignment." If he does, this means that the doctor will accept Medicare reimbursements as payments in full with no additional charge to you. If you are a Medicaid recipient, make sure the doctor accepts Medicaid patients and will bill Medicaid directly.
- Finally, you should make an appointment to introduce yourself and learn whether you think you can have the confidence to tell your doctor everything that relates to your health. Sometimes there will be no charge for an introductory visit, but even if you are charged, the investment is worthwhile for your having established the beginning of an ongoing relationship. Your doctor will most likely appreciate that you are a careful and discriminating patient—the sort of which no doctor has too many.

During your first visit here are some things to look for:

- *Were you able to get a timely appointment?* If you had to wait longer than two weeks, it may be an indication that you will have difficulty seeing your doctor promptly in the future.
- *Does the doctor show sensitivity* by sitting and talking with you before you are asked to disrobe?
- *Will your doctor make your tests results available to you if you ask?* Many doctors now mail printouts from the laboratory and indicate whether the results are within the normal range. Ask for these and make them a part of your personal health record.
- *Is the waiting room crowded, or do you have to wait long before seeing the doctor?* Don't be reluctant to ask other patients who are waiting if such is usual. Doctors who habitually keep patients waiting more than 20 minutes haven't learned to schedule their (or your!) time effectively.

During later visits you will have an opportunity to assess your doctor's practice habits. Beware of a doctor who makes telephone diagnoses, or is quick to order expensive or elaborate tests for what seem to you to be minor problems. Be concerned if your doctor always gives you a prescription. Let's face it, frequently there are other options, such as diet, exercise, and behavior modification, that may be as, or more, effective than medication, especially for minor problems.

Getting a Second Opinion

When your doctor recommends that you have a major surgical procedure or a complicated treatment program, it is often a good idea to have a second expert's opinion beforehand. There is a good possibility that you may avoid unnecessary surgery or risky therapy. A second opinion will also improve your understanding of your medical condition and increase the likelihood that you will receive the best possible treatment.

Don't be concerned that you will offend your doctor by asking for a second opinion. Rather you should understand this to be a prudent and reasonable exercise of your responsibility for your own health. Medicare and most insurance plans will pay for second opinions. In fact many insurance companies require second opinions before paying for procedures that tend to be overused, e.g., coronary bypass surgery, hysterectomy, gall bladder removal, and tonsillectomy.

You will save time and expense by having all of your health records and results of recent medical tests sent to your second opinion doctor in advance of your appointment.

Make certain that such opinion is rendered by an entirely independent doctor. This may mean that you will have to travel, especially if you live in a rural area, but the time and effort are worthwhile. If you don't know an independent doctor, the Federal Government operates a program called Second Opinion Toll-Free Hotline, established by Congress in an effort to reduce health care costs, eliminate unnecessary surgery, and increase patients' medical awareness. The Hotline maintains local referral centers that distribute the names of physicians, osteopaths, and podiatrists willing to give second opinions.

In most cases the two specialists will agree with one another. However, in case of disagreement, you need to get a *third* opinion. This, too, may be covered by your insurance, but you should check with your carrier beforehand. Again, even if you have to pay for it personally, it may prove to be money well spent. By increasing your confidence in the correctness of your decision, you also become more likely to follow your doctor's advice. Good patients tend to get well sooner.

Second Opinion Toll-Free Hotline
1- 800-638-6833
Maryland residents call 1-800-492-6603

QUESTIONS YOU SHOULD ASK ABOUT ANY COURSE OF TREATMENT

Here are the questions you need answered about any course of treatment you may be considering, and particularly those you should have confirmed by the second opinion:

1. What does your doctor say is the matter with you?
2. What is involved in the treatment recommended?
3. What are the likely benefits to you of the treatment?
4. What are the associated risks and how likely are they to occur?
5. How long should the recovery period be and what is involved?
6. What are the anticipated costs of treatment? Will your insurance cover all of those costs?
7. What will happen if you don't have the treatment?
8. Are there other ways to treat your condition that could be tried first?

How to Choose a Hospital

For most of us, the decision about which hospital to use for any given hospitalization is made by the doctors we have chosen and where they have admitting privileges. There are times, however, when it might be appropriate to select your doctor based on where he or she practices. Such a decision requires that you know something about the hospitals in your area. For example, if there is a well-recognized birthing center, it may be appropriate to select an obstetrician who delivers there. Too, if your community is fortunate enough to have a university medical center, you may want to choose a member of the university medical staff, particularly if you have a complicated medical problem.

University hospitals have many advantages over community hospitals. The quality of the medical staff is often higher. The staff is usually familiar with the latest treatment techniques, and both treatment and diagnostic capabilities are extensive. Most patients are seen by more than one doctor, so it is less likely that errors will go undetected than if you are seen by a single doctor. True, you may find yourself surrounded by an entourage of white-jacketed students and residents at six o'clock in the morning, but remember: they are there to ask questions and learn the latest healing skills, not a bad environment if you have a complex medical problem. The more input into your medical problem, the better. Here are points to keep in mind:

- Many insurance companies and all federal insurance programs require that hospital care be rendered at an institution *accredited* by the Joint Commission on Accreditation of Hospitals (JCAH). Find out whether the hospital you are considering is accredited by calling the Medical Director's office. If it is not, be sure to find out if your insurance covers care there. You do not want to find yourself unwittingly responsible for expensive medical bills you would otherwise be insured for.
- If you or a member of your family is advised to have a complicated procedure—open heart surgery, say—it would seem reasonable to try to find out which hospitals in your area or in the country have the best success with this operation. Such data is kept by the Health Care Financing Administration (HCFA), and has recently been published in an abbreviated form by the Consumer's Checkbook organization. Their helpful publication, *The Consumers' Guide to Hospitals,* tabulates data for virtually all the nation's community

KEEPING HOSPITAL COSTS DOWN

If you must personally pay for your hospitalization, or even pay a portion of the costs not covered by your insurance program, you will be interested in learning some ways of reducing these costs without sacrificing quality of care. The *Consumers' Guide to Hospitals* referred to above offers some helpful suggestions:

- Ask your doctor whether you can have any needed tests, e.g., laboratory tests and X-rays, performed at an outside laboratory or as an outpatient before you are admitted. The outside tests may be less expensive and you may save yourself one or more days of hospitalization.
- Ask your doctor whether hospitalization is your only treatment option. For example, many surgical procedures that used to be performed only on hospitalized patients are now routinely performed in the outpatient surgery.
- If possible, check in late and check out early. Remember that hospitals operate like hotels; there is a time when each admission day begins and ends. Find out when these times are. Then check in after the previous day has ended, and check out before the next admission day begins. If possible, too, ask whether you may check in and out the same day as your procedure.
- Many insurance carriers, including Blue Cross/Blue Shield, require authorization before nonemergency hospitalization and shortly after emergency hospitalizations. Make sure these authorizations are obtained.
- Check whether your insurance requires a second opinion for your scheduled treatment.
- Check your bill carefully to see that you have not been charged for more days than you have been hospitalized or for procedures that were either canceled or never ordered. Remember too, that some insurance programs will not pay for routine hospital tests unless they have been ordered by your doctor. At the time of your first blood and urine tests in the hospital, ask whether these have been ordered by your doctor.

and university hospitals and lists the number of patients they see each year with stroke, heart disease, lung disease, acute gastrointestinal disorders, and metabolic diseases (e.g., diabetes). The tables also provide mortality statistics, i.e., the number of patients with each of these conditions who died in the hospital or within 30 days of discharge. Although these figures don't always tell you which hospital is "best," they do provide a means of comparing the patient outcomes from one hospital with others in the state or city and with an *expected* outcome. If the mortality figures for patients with your medical condition at your anticipated hospital are higher than average, you may want to ask your doctor to explain his reasons for this.

- If you have an uncommon disease and want to learn which hospitals specialize in its treatment, contact the National Health Information Center, 1-800-336-4797.

Selecting a Health Insurance Plan

The chances are that if you or your spouse works, you will be eligible for employer-provided family health insurance, also known as "group" health insurance. You should take advantage of such insurance whenever possible, because it is the least expensive coverage available.

But what if you are unemployed, self-employed, or your employer is too small to qualify for a company plan? Or what if the benefits provided by your group plan don't adequately provide for your health needs? These are some of the situations that can mandate the need for "individual" health insurance, coverage for the individual or family who belongs to no group and needs some kind of health insurance protection.

There are lots of individual health insurance plans. Usually they are expensive. They frequently do not cover all of your health needs and they may not cover such medical problems as cancer, diabetes, AIDS, pregnancy, or psychiatric illness. Such exclusions are called "waivers." You may not be covered at all for waivers, or else there may be a waiting period of 12 to 24 months of coverage in force before such benefits will be covered. Here are some ideas that may guide you in selecting an individual health plan:

- First of all, don't buy health insurance at all without trying to join some kind of trade, alumni, church-related, club, union, farm bureau, or other association's group plan for which you may be eligible. In many cases it is worthwhile joining such a group just to avail yourself of its insurance plan. In many cases, your premiums will be lower, benefits better and exclusions fewer, than an unnegotiated individual plan.

- If you are self-employed or belong to a group of up to 50 workers, you may join the Small Business Service Bureau of Worcester, MA, which groups its members to buy coverage at favorable rates and with as few exclusions as possible from among plans in the member's locality. Currently individual dues are $85 annually. For information and an application, phone 1-800-222-3434.
- If you have just left a job, federal law provides that you may keep your former employer's group plan for up to 18 months, provided you pay the entire cost of the premium. This will often give you enough time to shop around for another satisfactory plan, if you can afford the premium.
- If you smoke, stop, because some insurance providers charge non-smokers less.
- Consider consulting an insurance broker. They usually know the most reliable providers and what they should charge. They also know how well each provider reimburses and by how much premiums are likely to increase each year. You can find such brokers in the yellow pages of your phone directory under "Health" at the end of the "Insurance" listings.
- Before you begin shopping for insurance, decide how much you are able to spend. Many plans offer less expensive monthly premiums if you are able to make co-payments or select a higher deductible.
- Before subscribing to a plan, read the literature provided carefully for coverage and exclusions. Don't count on anything you don't find in writing.

How to Get the Best Cancer Treatment

First the good news: cancer can be cured, and every year more cancer victims survive who would have died just a few years ago. As evidence, consider that deaths from cancer of the uterus have decreased more than 70% since 1940. Similar advances have been made for bone cancer, Hodgkin's disease, and many other cancers. These are remarkable improvements and have largely been won through earlier diagnosis and new treatment strategies.

On the darker side, however, is the fact that many cancer victims still receive less than what is currently considered optimum care. In most cases, the mistakes made in cancer treatment are ones of omission, rather than the selection of a wrong treatment approach. For example, additional chemotherapy or radiation therapy to destroy traces of cancer that may have remained after primary surgery may not be prescribed. This omission is especially common after breast cancer surgery.

In some cases doctors are reluctant to use a highly toxic drug because of debilitating side effects. The result, however, is that in a few of these cases residual cancer remains to grow and spread, making subsequent treatment more difficult or impossible. In other cases doctors do not give the full recommended dosages of drug. As a consequence, not only do these patients still get sick from the drug, but their tumors may continue to grow.

Sometimes oncologists (cancer specialists) are not available locally. Or they may not have the necessary approvals to use the latest, but still experimental, drugs deemed most effective. All of these reasons point up the need for cancer patients to be aware of what treatment options they have. Here are some suggestions from the National Cancer Institute that will help you get up-to-date cancer care:

- Be certain to select a doctor who is board certified in the specialty required to treat your particular cancer. Cancer should almost never be entrusted to general practice or family practice doctors unless their care is monitored by an oncologist.
- Look for doctors who are involved in national clinical trials of new cancer treatments. They are usually the best informed specialists. Get a second opinion about the nature of the treatment proposed for you and then either call, or ask your doctor to check, the Physicians' Data Query (PDQ), the National Cancer Institute's central listing of cancer therapy programs (*see* box on next page). This service describes experimental programs in cancer treatment around the country and informs you which new treatment programs at the National Institutes of Health in Bethesda, MD, are open (free) for additional patients.
- Consider enrolling in university-sponsored or National Cancer Institute experimental treatment programs. Such programs, called *protocols*, are usually compared with state-of-the-art treatment. As a result you may receive better than the "best" treatment, and sometimes at no cost or reduced charge.
- Be very wary of anyone who promises you a "revolutionary" new treatment, or who says, "I'll cure you and there will be no side effects." Quacks abound in the cancer arena. If a recommended therapy program doesn't check out with one of the services listed below, be extremely careful in committing yourself to it.

SOURCES OF CANCER THERAPY INFORMATION

- Patients can get a National Cancer Institute PDQ cancer information printout free by phoning 1-800-4-CANCER; in Alaska, call 1-800-638-6070; in Hawaii, call 524-1234. This details cancer treatment programs for every type of cancer throughout the United States. All medical center libraries also supply this service.
- Information about cancer-related psychiatric and emotional counseling can be obtained through the Cancer Counseling Institute, 1-301-320-4925.
- The American Cancer Society has a wide-ranging cancer information service. They will send you data sheets describing in detail the latest treatment options for any cancer. Local chapters will also provide the names of cancer specialists nearest to you. Call 1-800-227-2345 or your local American Cancer Society telephone listing.
- The American Medical Center Cancer Research Center provides general counseling and information about causes of cancer, prevention, detection and diagnosis, treatment, treatment facilities and rehabilitation. Call 1-800-525-3777; in Alaska and Hawaii, call collect 1-303-233-6501.

What You Can Do to Prevent Cancer

First the bad news: this year almost half a million people will die of cancer. Twice that number will have cancer diagnosed, thus facing the prospect of anxiety, suffering, lost work, and great expense. Now the good news: nearly 80% of all those cancers can be prevented by practicing a more healthy lifestyle. The National Cancer Institute has identified seven areas of risk in our lives that deserve our most careful consideration in this regard: tobacco, diet, alcohol, radiation, work place, estrogens, and viruses.

Of these risk factors, tobacco and diet are by far the most important. It is estimated that 30% of cancer deaths are directly attributable to tobacco use, while 35% are related to diet, especially dietary fat. The remaining five factors are responsible for from 1 to 5% of cancers each.

Tobacco

In 1992 there were more than 200,000 tobacco-related cancer deaths, more than 130,000 from lung cancer alone. The remaining deaths were caused by cancers of the mouth, lip, esophagus, pharynx, larynx, bladder, kidney, and pancreas. People who smoke have from 10 to 25 times greater chance of getting cancer than people who don't smoke.

Although cutting down on the number of cigarets you smoke and switching to low-tar, low-nicotine cigarets may reduce slightly your risk of developing lung cancer, the only way to eliminate that life-threatening risk is to QUIT smoking. (*See* p. 492 for tips on quitting smoking).

Cigarets are not the only dangerous form of tobacco. Pipe and cigar smokers risk developing cancers of the mouth, tongue, and throat. Snuff and chewing tobacco, the so-called "smokeless" tobaccos, also increase the risk of mouth cancers.

Numerous studies have shown that "passive" smoking, i.e., breathing other people's smoke, can increase the risk of lung cancer. Furthermore, passive smoking contributes to the severity of such diseases as asthma and respiratory infections. Children raised in homes with smoking parents have significantly more respiratory diseases than their peers who have nonsmoking parents. Women who smoke during pregnancy are more likely to have children with low birth weight and possibly developmental abnormalities as well. The only gains from cigaret smoking belong to the manufacturer. And their future is not rosy.

Diet

Several large studies have shown that high-fat, low-fiber diets are associated with greater risk of cancers of the breast, colon, and prostate gland. Current evidence suggests that by choosing a well-balanced diet, your risk of cancer may be reduced by 35% or more. To adopt a well-balanced diet for yourself and your family:

1. Reduce your consumption of both saturated and unsaturated fats. Fat is strongly associated with breast and colon cancers. No more than 30% of your calories should come from fats (40% is the current average in the United States). Do the following:

- Choose lean red meats, fish, and poultry.
- Trim fat from steaks, roasts, and chops.
- Remove the skins from poultry after cooking.
- Broil, roast, and bake meats and fish, rather than frying them.

- Limit your use of butter, margarine, shortening, vegetable oils, and dairy products.
- Avoid hidden fats in salad dressings, sandwiches, and snack foods.
- Learn the joy of ripe, fresh fruits instead of high-fat desserts.

For more information on cholesterol, *see* p. 192.

2. Increase the amount of vegetables and whole grain cereals in your diet.

- Such fruits as oranges, grapefruit, peaches, strawberries, cantaloup, and honeydew melons are high in vitamins A and C. Vitamins C and E and beta carotene are *antioxidants* that prevent cancer by clearing *free radicals* that damage DNA.
- Choose leafy green and yellow-orange vegetables such as spinach, kale, sweet potatoes, carrots, cabbage, cauliflower, broccoli, and brussels sprouts.
- High-fiber foods include grain breads, cereals, raw fruits, and vegetables, especially if eaten with the skins on.

3. Reduce your consumption of salt-cured and smoked foods. Esophageal and stomach cancers are common in China, Japan, and Iceland, where these foods are frequently eaten.

In summary, choose your foods thoughtfully, eat a variety of foods daily, and maintain a healthy body weight for your height and sex (*see* p. 314). By reducing dietary cholesterol and sodium, you also do your heart a favor. For more information about diet, write for NIH Publication No. 87-2878 from the Superintendent of Documents, US Government Printing Office, Washington, DC 20402.

Alcohol

Heavy drinking is associated with cancers of the mouth, throat, esophagus, and liver. Those who drink alcohol *and* use tobacco increase their risk of oral cancers by as much as 15 times. A maximum of one or two drinks daily is a good limit to opt for. If you are pregnant, do not drink at all.

Radiation

Excessive X-radiation can increase your risks of such cancers as leukemia, breast, and thyroid cancers. Doctors are aware of this and do not order unnecessary studies, but it is always prudent to ask whether a suggested X-ray is essential, especially when suggested as a follow-up test after treatment.

Prolonged exposure to sunlight is definitely linked to skin cancer, the incidence of which is increasing in the United States. The fair-skinned are especially at risk. Avoid the strongest rays between 11 AM and 2 PM. Wear lightweight clothing, but select clothes with sleeves and long pants. Wear brimmed hats and use a sunscreen or sunblock (15 or higher) when prolonged exposure is unavoidable. Certainly you should shun tanning parlors and sunlamps. I predict that the peaches-and-cream skin of yesteryear is going to regain fashion among the fair-skinned. For more information about sun exposure *see* p. 467.

If you live in a region of the country known to have radon in the soil, or if you live in a basement apartment, or if you live in a new home that is tightly sealed, it is prudent to have your home tested for the presence of radon. For more information, write for the pamphlet: *A Citizen's Guide to Radon* (#OPA-86-004) from: Environmental Protection Agency, 841 Chestnut Street, Philadelphia PA 19107; or telephone the Radon Hotline at 1-215-597-8320.

Occupational Exposures

Although numerous industrial chemicals have been associated with cancer in laboratory animals, only about 30 have been found to cause cancer in humans. The most serious of these are asbestos, benzene, chromate, nickel, arsenic, uranium, aromatic amines, coal tars, vinyl chloride, chloromethyl ether, and acrylonitrile. Industries in which these substances are commonly found, other than those directly manufacturing them, include boot and shoe manufacture and repair, furniture manufacture, nickel refining, the rubber industry, and underground iron mining (radon exposure).

Estrogens

Estrogen therapy is now widely used as hormone replacement in postmenopausal women and in birth control pills. Long-term estrogen replacement in postmenopausal women reduces many menopausal symptoms (*see* p. 344) and also retards the development of osteoporosis. In high doses, estrogens are known to increase the risk of endometrial (uterine) cancer. However, in smaller doses and combined with the hormone progesterone, hormone replacement therapy is considered generally safe. Discuss hormone replacement with your doctor.

Most studies show no increase in cancer risk for those using oral contraceptives. They may even have some slight protective effect against the development of ovarian and endometrial cancers. Recent studies also offer no evidence to suggest that birth control pills increase the risk of breast cancer.

Viruses

The precise role of viruses in causing cancer is still not known. They are thought to *initiate* or *promote* about 2% of all cancers in the United States:

- Hepatitis B Virus is associated with the development of liver cancer (hepatoma). There is now a vaccine for hepatitis B. The high-risk individuals for whom vaccinations are recommeded are listed on p. 29.
- Epstein-Barr virus (EBV) is associated with some nose and throat cancers and with Burkitt's lymphoma. No vaccine exists for EBV.
- Human papilloma virus (HPV) is a sexually transmitted virus that causes genital warts and is associated with genital cancers (*see* p. 395).
- T-cell leukemia/lymphoma virus (HTLV-l) causes adult T-cell leukemia or lymphoma. This is a sexually transmitted disease. Condoms can reduce the risk of contracting this disease if you have more than one sexual partner.

Cancer Screening Tests

Because of the prevalence of cancer it is important that everyone have a rational approach to the detection of possible cancers in themselves as early as possible. Many cancers are curable. With the great medical advances made in recent years, nearly half of all cancers can now be completely eliminated. But early detection is essential because nearly all cancer treatments work better when the cancer is small, before it has spread.

Tumor Staging

The degree of development of most cancers is measured by assigning stages—usually numbered I to IV— at the time of diagnosis. The stage depends upon the size of the tumor, whether it has spread to nearby lymph nodes, and whether it has spread to distant organs, such as liver or bone. The staging system varies with each cancer, but generally Stage I is assigned to a small tumor that has not spread to regional lymph nodes. This stage carries the greatest probability of cure. Stage IV tumors have generally spread (metastasized) to other organs; the treatments available are always limited, and the probility of cure is greatly reduced for this stage. Thus screening programs that detect cancers early are essential.

Cancer Screening Recommendations for the General Public*

Cancer	Test	Age	Frequency
Breast	Self-exam	Over 20	Every month
	Physical exam	20–40	Every 3 years
		Over 40	Every year
	Mammogram	20–40	Baseline exam
		41–50	Every 1 to 2 yr
		Over 50	Every year
Cervical	Pap smear	20–65 or	Every 3 yr after
		under 20	2 negative
		if sexually	exams 1 year
		active	apart
Colon and	Test for occult blood	Over 50	Yearly
Rectum	Flexible	Over 50	Every 3 years
	sigmoidoscopy		

*Source: Cancer Screening, What You Can Do to Detect Cancer. American Council on Science and Health, 47 Maple Street, Summit, NJ 07901.

As of 1994, the recommended cancer screening tests are outlined in the table above. More information about the nature of each screening procedure listed in this table is given elsewhere in this book. See the index listing for each organ.

Other Cancers

1. Lung Cancer. Lung cancer can be detected by both chest X-rays and by examination of sputum specimens (sputum cytology). Unfortunately, even in individuals at high risk of developing lung cancer—cigaret smokers and those exposed to asbestos—no savings in lives have been demonstrated using these screening tests routinely.

The reason is that by the time the tumor is detected, it has usually already spread. A screening method to detect very early lung cancer would probably be of value. However, at this time, routine chest X-rays or sputum cytology tests are not recommended for lung cancer screening. In other words, these examinations do not reduce the risk of dying from lung cancer. On the other hand, if there is a suspicion of lung cancer or other lung disease because of specific symptoms (cough, bloody sputum), chest X-rays should be obtained. Ask your doctor whether you need a chest X-ray.

2. *Oral Cancer.* Approximately 30,000 cases of oral cancer are diagnosed each year. These occur principally in people who smoke, chew tobacco, take snuff, or drink alcohol in addition to tobacco use. Screening for oral cancer consists of a simple oral and neck examination and can be done as a part of the routine physical examination by your doctor or by your dentist. It adds no cost to your examination and should be done yearly (assuming you see either your doctor or dentist annually).

3. *Endometrial Cancer.* Endometrial cancer occurs in older women who have not had a hysterectomy. Endometrial cancer is detected by a procedure known as "dilatation and currettage" (D&C) in which the lining of the uterus is scraped and the tissue examined microscopically. The procedure is painful and must be done under anesthesia. Alternatively, salt water can be injected into the uterus and the recovered cells examined. This procedure is also painful and carries a small risk of infection. Neither of these procedures is currently recommended for *routine* screening because endometrial cancer is usually associated with postmenopausal bleeding (an absolute signal for a gynecologic examination!) at an early stage and has a cure rate of 60–80% without screening.

4. *Prostate Cancer.* Cancer of the prostate occurs in older men. Currently, the only useful screening test is the digital rectal examination that should be a part of every routine physical examination. If an irregularity is found, a biopsy is then obtained to determine whether a malignancy is present. *The recommendations for prostate cancer screening are currently being scrutinized and will probably be revised.* If you are an older man, ask you doctor's advice about the usefulness of rectal ultrasound examinations and about the value of measuring your blood level of PSA (prostate-specific antigen).

Your Periodic Physical Examination

I remember that when I was growing up in the 1950s and my parents were in their forties, they went to our family doctor every year for their Annual Physical. This was a program developed early in this century by the Metropolitan Life Insurance Company to promote better health among policyholders. Indeed this was a significant advance over the ancient notion that you only sought a doctor when you were ill. Periodic checkups and preventive health measures have already contributed greatly toward ensuring a healthier nation. But such procedures are costly and often not covered by insurance. Furthermore, it is now generally recognized that a complete physical examination, chest X-ray, electrocardiogram, and many blood and urine tests don't need to be done every year. On the other hand certain tests have come to be recognized as both cost-effective and sensitive in detecting diseases at an early stage when they are more easily treated. Thus, the timing of checkups and screening tests done should be tailored to each individual depending on age, sex, past medical illnesses, social habits, and family medical history.

Much more important than annual checkups are visits timed to coincide with such "health interventions" as vaccinations, testing for physical and behavioral development, and cancer screening procedures. In essence, it is the timing of these interventions and screening procedures that determines when you should see your doctor and what you can expect to have done.

After many years of examining these issues, the Preventive Services Task Force, a commission of the US Department of Health and Human Services, has come out with a nearly comprehensive set of recommendations for essential visits to your doctor. The population is divided into six age groups as shown in the tables on the following pages. Along with those procedures recommended for everyone, they provide a set of screening and preventive procedures that are recommended only for people in certain high-risk categories. For example, Pap smears are not recommended for women under age 18 unless early sexual activity places them at risk for cervical cancer. These risk categories are quite numerous and I have included only those that affect most people. If you believe you have a special health problem, ask your doctor what screening procedures you need.

What Is a Complete History and Physical?

The *medical history* is the most important part of your checkup. Almost half of all medical problems can be detected by your doctor's careful questioning about your past health problems, previous illnesses in your family, and about any symptoms you may now have. Your doctor should also question you about your eating and drinking habits, drug use, the medications you are taking, your occupation, leisure activities, and emotional, marital, and sexual problems if appropriate.

The *complete* physical consists of a thorough examination of those parts of the body that are accessible to your doctor through a series of

---

WHAT YOUR DOCTOR LOOKS FOR DURING A PHYSICAL

- *Eyes:* Looks for eye tumors and cataracts. The appearance of the retina is a clue to blood vessel disease in the rest of the body. Eyeball pressure is measured to rule out glaucoma.
- *Ears:* Looks for ear infection and obstruction. Hearing should also be tested, particularly as you grow older.
- *Mouth:* Looks at the tongue and throat to reveal oral cancer, throat infection, and vitamin deficiency.
- *Neck:* Feels for lymph nodes for possible infection or cancer, and for thyroid size and consistency.
- *Chest:* Taps the chest to detect pneumonia and heart size. Listens with stethoscope for lung and heart disease.
- *Breast:* Palpatates for breast cancer and cysts.
- *Abdomen:* Feels for enlarged organs and tumors.
- *Groin:* Probes for hernia, testicular tumor.
- *Arms and legs:* Hammer taps check reflexes for neurological disorders.
- *Rectal:* Palpates for tumors and prostate enlargement in men. Takes stool sample for occult blood (colon cancer).

---

thumping, poking, probing, listening, and peering into body orifices (*see* box above). You should be fully disrobed for the physical examination, so that your doctor can visually inspect all parts of your body. The physical examination will pick up about 20% of detectable health problems.

Your doctor will also order various screening tests that are listed below and are appropriate for your age and sex. Chest X-rays are no longer considered routine. They should be ordered only if you have signs and symptoms of lung or heart disease, such as a chronic cough, blood in your sputum, and so on.

Electrocardiograms are also ordered only if you have a high probability of having heart disease, because otherwise this is not a very sensitive test for detecting heart problems.

How Often Do You Need a Complete History and Physical?

It is not expected that you will have a complete history and physical every time you see your doctor for routine screening procedures. However, periodic complete examinations are important to pick up such nonsymptomatic conditions as skin cancer or glaucoma. The

Preventive Services Task Force does not provide a guideline about the frequency of complete examinations, leaving this up to your doctor's discretion. Therefore, in the tables below I have given the recommendations of the American Academy of Pediatrics and widely regarded family practice recommendations concerning the frequency of complete physical examinations. Your doctor may offer compelling reasons for a different schedule.

Behavior Modification as Prevention

One of the big changes in the way doctors look at disease prevention has been the recognition that health counseling to modify poor health practices is far more effective than all screening tests combined in promoting health and preventing disease. Most doctors now realize that getting their patients to:

STOP SMOKING • STOP ALCOHOL AND DRUG ABUSE
REDUCE DIETARY FAT • INCREASE EXERCISE
REPORT EPISODES OF PHYSICAL ABUSE

are a lot more effective in promoting general health than screening for the diseases that result from bad habits.

Birth to 18 Months*					
	Months				
Procedure	2	4	6	15	18
Complete physical examination	X	X	X	X	X
Blood hemoglobin and hematocrit			X		
Hearing test					X
Diphtheria-tetanus-pertussis (DTP) vaccine	X	X	X	X	
Oral poliovirus vaccination	X	X		X	
Influenza vaccination		X	X	X	
Measles-mumps-rubella vaccination				X	
Hepatitis B vaccination	X	X	X		

*You can see that visits to the doctor during infancy are timed according to recommended vaccination against infectious diseases. At these times the doctor has an opportunity to measure head circumference (to assess brain development) and monitor expected landmarks of physical and emotional development.

In addition to the procedures outlined above, your doctor may advise:

• Fluoride supplements to prevent tooth decay if you and your child live in an area with inadequate water fluoridation.

• A blood test for lead, if you live in housing built before 1950, or a parent works in a lead-related occupation.

Ages 2–12*								
Procedure	*Years*							
	2	3	4	5	6	8	10	12
Complete physical exam	X	X	X	X	X	X	X	X
Vision testing		X						
Urinalysis			X					
Diphtheria-tetanus-pertussis (DTP) vaccine			X					
Oral poliovirus vaccine				X				
Measles vaccine			X					X

*Additional procedures for children in high-risk categories include:

• A tuberculin skin test for children who live in a household that includes a person with active tuberculosis, or with a recent immigrant from a country with endemic tuberculosis.

• A hearing test before age 3 years, if not earlier, for children with: a family history of childhood hearing impairment; a personal history of congenital infection with such diseases as herpes, syphilis, or rubella; or a congenital malformation of the head or neck, e.g., cleft palate.

Ages 13–19			
Procedure	*Years*		
	14	16	18
Complete physical exam	X	X	X
Tetanus-diphtheria booster	X		

Specific procedures for teenagers in high-risk groups include:

• A complete skin exam for teens with increased recreational or occupational exposure to sunlight, a family history of skin cancer, or the presence of large congenital moles.

- A testicular exam for boys with a history of undescended or atrophied testicle. (Many pediatricians recommend that all males be taught to examine their own testicles for the presence of lumps every month to detect early testicular cancer.)
- A test for rubella antibodies in females of childbearing age who have not had childhood rubella vaccination in order to prevent congenital rubella syndrome (brain, kidney, and other malformations).
- Pap smears every 1–3 years for females who are sexually active to detect early changes of cervical cancer. Less frequent testing is appropriate after three consecutive negative tests.
- Tests for syphilis, chlamydia, and gonorrhea for persons who have multiple sexual partners, or who have had sexual contact with a person with diagnosed sexually transmitted disease.

Ages 19–39*	
Procedure	*Frequency*
Complete physical exam	Every 5 years
Height and Weight	Every 1–3 years
Blood pressure	Every 1–3 years
Teatanus-diphtheria booster	Every 10 years
Pap smear	Every 1–3 years
Breast physical examination	Every 3 years
Mammography	Baseline between ages 35 and 39

*Most of the tests recommended for teenagers in high-risk groups apply to young adults. Additional recommendations are:

- Periodic complete oral exam to detect early cancer in those who smoke, chew tobacco, or use excessive alcohol. This exam should be a part of your regular dental checkup.
- Periodic clinical breast exam and mammography to detect early breast cancer in women aged 35 and older with a family history of breast cancer in a first-degree relative (mother, grandmother, sister)
- Tests for blood and urine sugar to detect diabetes in persons who are obese, those with a family history of diabetes, or women who had diabetes during pregnancy.
- Colon test (sigmoidoscopy) to detect early colon cancer in persons with a family history of colon polyps.
- Heptitis B vaccine for homosexually active men, intravenous drug users, persons who receive blood products, or persons in health-related jobs with frequent exposure to blood products.

- Pneumococcal and influenza vaccines for persons with chronic heart, lung, or kidney diseases; with diabetes, no spleen, alcoholism, cirrhosis, multiple myeloma; and anyone with an immune deficiency.
- Measles–mumps–rubella vaccine for persons who were not vaccinated previously.

Ages 40–64*	
Procedure	*Frequency*
Complete physical exam	Every 5 years to age 60, then every year
Height and weight	Every 1–3 years
Blood pressure	Every 1–3 years
Tetanus-diptheria booster	Every 10 years
Blood cholesterol level	Every 1–3 years
Digital rectal examination	Every 1–3 years
Breast physical examination	Every year
Mammography	Age 40–49: every 2 years†
	Age 50 and over: every year
Pap smear and pelvic exam	Every 1–3 years

*All of the recommendations for high-risk groups that apply to young adults apply to this group of middle-aged adults, plus the recommendations listed below.

†There are ongoing debates about the usefulness of mammography before age 50, consult you doctor.

- Electrocardiogram for men with two or more cardiac risk factors (high blood cholesterol, high blood pressure, cigaret smoking, diabetes mellitus, family history of coronary artery disease, and sedentary males), planning to begin a vigorous exercise program.
- Annual tests for stool occult blood—or sigmoidoscopy— for all persons over 50 who have a first-degree relative with colon cancer; any person with endometrial, ovarian, or breast cancer; or a previous diagnosis of inflammatory bowel disease, polyps, or colorectal cancer. *Many doctors recommend annual tests for occult blood for all individuals, regardless of medical history.*
- Analysis of bone mineral content for women at increased risk for osteoporosis (e.g., Caucasian race, removal of the ovaries before menopause, slender build) *and* for whom estrogen replacement therapy would otherwise not be recommended.

Ages 65 and Above*	
Procedure	*Frequency*
Complete physical examination	Every 2 years to age 74, then every year
Height and weight	Every year
Blood pressure	Every year
Visual acuity and glaucoma test	Every year
Hearing test	Every year
Total blood cholesterol	Every year
Urinalysis for sugar and protein	Every year
Stool test for blood	Every year
Influenza vaccination	Every year
Pneumococus vaccination	Once at age 65
Tetanus-diphtheria booster	Every 10 years
Clinical breast examination	Every year to age 75
Mammography	Every 1–2 years to age 75
Pap smear and pelvic exam	Every 1–3 years

*During this period in life accurate and complete medical records are especially valuable, because it is much more likely that you will visit more than one doctor who will not be familiar with your past health record and therefore may order needless tests, or prescribe medications that may be inappropriate in light of your medical history. It is also a time when the likelihood of spending time in an extended care facility is greater. Remember that all of the recommendations for high-risk individuals in the early adult and middle-age adult groups (outlined above) apply to elderly individuals.

Remember, too, that this is not a complete list and your doctor may add some procedure or may recommend either more or less frequent exams and surveillance procedures for you, depending upon your medical background.

What You Should Know About Vaccinations

Vaccination (immunization) programs during this century have been responsible for saving millions of lives by eliminating the great epidemics of smallpox, influenza, diphtheria, polio, and whooping cough that periodically raced through populations, felling thousands in a season. These programs have been so successful that some people have the perception that vaccinations are no longer needed in many cases, or that they cause more harm from adverse vaccination reactions than the diseases themselves cause. This is a dangerous notion!

Vaccination programs cannot be ended until a disease is wiped out. Of all human infectious diseases, this victory has been attained with only one: smallpox.

The folly of relaxed vaccination programs can be cited in the examples of Great Britain and Japan, which some years ago abandoned routine vaccinations for whooping cough (pertussis). Within two years, over 100,000 cases were reported in Great Britain, including 28 deaths. In Japan 13,000 cases were reported, with 40 deaths. Even in the United States, more than 1000 cases of whooping cough are reported among the 10% of children who miss school vaccination programs. In contrast, the incidence of serious pertussis vaccine reactions is practically nil.

Infants and Children

The table below gives the vaccination schedule recommended by the American Academy of Pediatrics Committee on Infectious Diseases.

Recommended Infant and Child Vaccination Schedule								
Age	*DTP*	*Polio*	*Measles*	*Rubella*	*Mumps*	*T/D*	*H. flu*	*HBv*
2 months	X	X					X	X
4 months	X	X					X	X
6 months	X							
15 months	X	X	X	X	X		X	X
18 months								
4–6 years	X	X						
11–12 years			X					
14–16 years				X		X*		
Key: DTP = Diphtheria-Tetanus-Pertussis. Polio = Oral live poliovirus vaccine. T/D = Tateanus + Diphtheria. H. flu = Hemophilus influenza. HBv = Hepatitis B vaccine. *And every 10 years thereafter.								

In the extremely unlikely event of a serious vaccination reaction, no-fault insurance now provides compensation for those who can prove injury resulting from polio, DTP, or measles–mumps–rubella vaccines. Information about filing petitions can be obtained from the US Claims Court, 717 Madison Place NW, Washington, DC 20005.

Adults

It is widely believed that vaccinations are given during childhood, and that upon reaching adulthood, people are either fully immunized or they are no longer needed. Nothing could be further from the truth. Every year thousands of adults are felled by diseases they never would have contracted had they been properly vaccinated.

In this age of widespread childhood vaccination programs, diseases that children used to get routinely may not be widely circulated and unvaccinated individuals may not become exposed until much later than would otherwise be the case. Today, college campuses still experience outbreaks of measles because some students have not been vaccinated.

Recent recommendations for adult vaccinations were published by the US Center for Disease Control and the American College of Physicians. These cover routine vaccinations that everyone should have, as well as special categories that apply to certain lifestyles or professions.

Measles Vaccine

It is estimated that one young adult in 20 may be susceptible to measles. Adults born before 1957 most likely had naturally acquired measles as children, and therefore have permanent immunity. All adults born after 1957 should be vaccinated with live measles vaccine unless they have had physician-documented measles, or have other documentation of vaccination with live measles vaccine on or after their first birthday. A parental report of vaccination by itself is not considered adequate documentation. College students in particular should be vaccinated against measles, because they are exposed to widespread contact among a highly susceptible population.

Measles in adults is a serious disease. It causes brain inflammation (encephalitis) in one of every 2000 cases, and death in one of every 3000 cases. Measles acquired during pregnancy increases the risk of spontaneous abortion, premature labor, and low birth-weight babies.

Tetanus and Diphtheria Vaccines

It is estimated that 11% of adults aged 18–40, and fully half of those over 60 years of age, are not adequately immunized against tetanus (lockjaw). This is a disease usually caused by bacteria that enter deep cuts, wounds, and burns. Half of all those over 50 years of age who contract the disease die of it. The percentage of adults unprotected against diphtheria is even higher. The respiratory form of diphtheria can progress to inflammation of the nerves (polyneuritis) and lining of the heart (endocarditis), and can even be fatal.

All adults should receive a tetanus–diphtheria booster every 10 years. The mid-decades—ages 25, 35, 45, etc.—have been recommended as the best times for these boosters. If you have not had the primary series (administered as DTP) during childhood you should get it. When booster doses of tetanus vaccine are given in association with injuries, the standard recommendations are that clean and minor wounds do not require a booster dose if the patient either has completed a primary series (see chart above) or received a booster dose within the last 10 years.

Mumps Vaccine

Most Americans have had mumps, or have developed immunity by age 20. However, vaccination is recommended for adult males if they have no history of the disease. In adult males, there is a 20% chance of developing inflammation of the testes (orchitis) if mumps is contracted (*see* p. 375). In some cases this results in sterility. Mumps also causes deafness in one out of every 15,000 cases.

Rubella (German Measles) Vaccine

The primary reason to vaccinate adults against rubella is to prevent fetal infection. In up to 80% of fetuses, infection during the first trimester can lead to congenital rubella syndrome, characterized by heart, eye, and ear defects, and by mental retardation.

Routine immunization against rubella is recommended for all adults, particularly women and college students, unless they have had the disease or have been previously vaccinated. Women should not be vaccinated if they are pregnant and they are advised not to become pregnant for three months after vaccination. For susceptible adults, a combined measles–mumps–rubella (MMR) vaccine is available as a single shot.

Influenza (Flu) Vaccine

Everyone over 65 years of age should be vaccinated against viral influenza every year. From 60 to 80% of all influenza deaths occur in this age group. Recent reports from the US Center for Disease Control estimate that only 17% of Americans who need flu shots actually receive them. Vaccination is especially important for people in nursing homes and institutions, where crowded conditions increase the risk of contracting the disease.

Vaccination is recommended for people of all ages who have such chronic conditions as heart, lung, or kidney diseases, diabetes mellitus, anemia, asthma, or immune suppression (e.g., AIDS victims and patients on long-term steroid medication).

Because influenza viruses are continually changing, a flu shot made up of the latest vaccines must be obtained every year. The vaccines vary in effectiveness from year to year, because no one knows for certain which viruses will attack. The choice of vaccines is made each year by the US Food and Drug Administration. They estimate that immunization of just 70% of high-risk patients would prevent 20,000 deaths per year in the United States.

The best time to have a flu shot is during October or November, well in advance of the "flu season." Those with a history of allergy to eggs should not receive the vaccine, because the viruses are cultured in eggs. Such people should ask their doctors about the advisability of prophylaxis with the drug, amantadine.

Pneumococcal Vaccine

This vaccine is made from *Streptococcus pneumoniae*, the bacterium that causes pneumococcal pneumonia. Immunization is recommended for all persons more than two years of age if:

1. They have chronic cardiac or pulmonary disease.
2. They have an illness or condition known to predispose to pneumococcal infection (sickle cell disease, kidney diseases, Hodgkin's disease, absent spleen, cirrhosis, alcoholism, multiple myeloma, cerebrospinal fluid leak, and immunosuppression).
3. All adults over 65, because they are most likely to die from pneumococcal pneumonia and its complications. This vaccine should be given only once because of a risk of allergic reactions in revaccinated individuals.

Recent reports from the US Center for Disease Control estimate that only about 9% of Americans for whom pneumonia vaccinations are recommended are actually protected.

Hepatitis B Vaccine

Approximately 100,000 new cases of hepatitis B are reported each year in the US. The disease itself is often lengthy and debilitating. Worse, it can lead to chronic hepatitis, cirrhosis, and liver cancer. Each year 5000 people die of hepatitis B virus-related diseases. Hepatitis B virus is transmitted through blood, semen, and saliva. Health workers at risk for contracting this disease include surgeons, gynecologists, dentists, cardiologists, blood bank personnel, intravenous therapy nurses, and clinical laboratory staff who work directly with blood samples. Staff in prisons and institutions for the mentally retarded—including the residents—run an increased risk of hepatitis B infection from exposure to human bites, open skin lesions, and saliva.

Homosexually active men and intravenous drug abusers run a high risk of hepatitis B; 10–20% of both groups acquire the virus each year, and at any one time up to 80% show evidence of having been infected. Vaccination is also recommended for household contacts and sexual partners of hepatitis B carriers.

There is a probable link between hepatitis B and AIDS infection, because of the very high association between the two infections. It is possible that hepatitis B serves as a "cofactor" to initiate active AIDS infection. Therefore, it is advised that individuals who are not infected with AIDS, but who are in a high risk category (*see* p. 400), be vaccinated. See your doctor for further advice.

Currently the vaccine must be given in three doses over six months and is expensive. Therefore it is often recommended that recipients have a blood test for evidence of prior exposure, in which case there is no need for immunization.

Polio Vaccine

Routine polio vaccination is not recommended for adults in the United States, because most are already immune. There are exceptions. Health-care workers should be immunized, as should those traveling to underdeveloped countries (even despite childhood immunization, because immunity seems to wane). Also susceptible adults run a small risk of contracting polio when children in the household are given the oral polio vaccine. These individuals may consider being vaccinated before the child.*

Special Categories

- Vaccinations for tuberculosis should be given only to persons who are tuberculin-negative but in close contact with active cases of

---

*In a recent court case (*Johnson v. American Cyanamid Company;* 718 p.2d 1318 Kan Sup Ct, May 19, 1986), it was held that the vaccine manufacturer is not liable for such cross infections, because this is an unavoidable complication of a vaccine that has been otherwise proven overwhelmingly valuable to society.

pulmonary tuberculosis and where prophylaxis with oral isoniazid is not feasible.

- Veterinarians and animal handlers should receive rabies vaccination.
- People who work with imported animal hides, wool, and hair should be vaccinated for anthrax.
- Persons traveling abroad to certain endemic areas are advised, and in some cases, required to have vaccinations. This topic is discussed in detail on p. 42.
- As a rule, women should avoid vaccinations of any kind during pregnancy. In special or emergency cases, it is safe to administer vaccine, especially those made of inactivated microbes, by delaying administration until the second or third trimester. In any case, a doctor should always be consulted prior to vaccination.

How to Take Medicines

Your doctor writes a prescription, you have it filled, take the medicine, and promptly get well. That's the usual scenario, right? Well, in many cases, no. Unfortunately.

The US Food and Drug Administration (FDA) estimates that:

- Two-thirds of all patients who visit a doctor's office come out with a prescription, but as many as 20% never have it filled.
- About half of all prescriptions fail to produce the desired results because the medicines are taken improperly.
- From 12 to 20% of patients take other people's medicines.
- More than 10% of all hospital admissions are related to prescription drug misuse, either too much or not enough, or the wrong combination of medicines are taken. Among older people, this number is even higher.
- More than 20% of nursing home admissions are related to improper self-administration of medicine.
- 60% of all patients cannot identify their own medicines.

These are not encouraging statistics. Here are the five most common errors patients make with their medicines:

1. *Not having the prescription filled at all, and thus not taking any medicine.* Who knows why people with real complaints take the time and expense to consult their doctor, then ignore the advice? Maybe they went thinking they had cancer, and when they learn they *only*

have high blood pressure, thank their lucky stars and, confident they will live to see the morrow, toss the prescription.

2. *Taking doses that are too large or too small.* Many Americans grow up in a folk medicine culture unused to visiting doctors short of their death beds. They develop a sense that they know what remedy, and how much, is best for themselves. Indeed, most people are not good at following directions to the letter.

3. *Taking medication at the wrong intervals—too often or not often enough.*

4. *Forgetting to take one or more doses.*

5. *Discontinuing the medication too soon.* This error is especially prevalent with antibiotics, which are usually prescribed for 7–10 days. If patients feel well after three days, they are apt to stop the antibiotic, thus increasing the chances of having a residual infection that may be difficult to treat. Remember, if you didn't take your medicine as directed *and* have to see your doctor again for the same problem, be sure to say so, because your doctor may think you are not responding properly and may prescribe *another* (second choice) medicine.

Are we then a nation of dummies? I think not. Rather, I believe there are two general problems we must confront and overcome. The first is that most of us have an intuition that taking pills is somehow bad for us and should be avoided if at all possible. Certainly taking pills unnecessarily is to be avoided. But only the truly overconfident believe they know better than their doctor. The second problem is that taking medicines properly is more complex than many patients suspect. Some very serious consequences can result from taking drugs unwisely.

Adverse Drug Reactions

Not everyone reacts to drugs the same way. Almost every drug has one to several side effects or *adverse reactions*. These reactions range from mild (rash, headache, drowsiness) to severe (anemia, bleeding, shock). If you experience an undesirable symptom, ***stop the medication*** and call your doctor. Always ask your doctor what the medicine prescribed is supposed to do and whether it is associated with common side effects. In many cases your pharmacist can also help provide this information.

Drug–Drug Interactions

Many people take more than one drug at any given time. Occasionally these drugs interact so as to either increase or decrease the action of one of them. For example, antihistamines often serve to *potentiate*, or enhance, the sedative effects of tranquilizers and pain killers. Such an unwanted side effect could be disastrous for a train switchman, to name but one hazardous occupation. Antacids speed or slow the absorption of numerous drugs, e.g., propranolol, digitalis, antibiotics, and tranquilizers, sometimes rendering their drug effects unpredictable.

Several drugs are known to *reduce* the effectiveness of oral contraceptives. This includes some antibiotics, barbiturates, anticonvulsants, analgesics, and anti-inflammatory drugs. The list is long and complicated.

When your doctor prescribes a new drug, tell—or better, bring, your prescription bottles with you to show just what drugs you are currently taking. If you neglect to do this, take the list to your pharmacist when you have the new prescription filled and ask whether there is a possibility of a drug interaction with something you are already taking.

Drug–Alcohol Interactions

Chronic use of alcohol can cause changes in the liver that speed the metabolism (breakdown or elimination) of some drugs, thereby reducing their effectiveness. In other instances, alcoholic cirrhosis may reduce the liver's ability to metabolize drugs, thus increasing or prolonging their effect. For example, taking such depressant drugs as Valium and Darvon along with high quantities of alcohol can result in serious overdose and even death (the *ultimate* adverse reaction).

Of particular concern for alcoholics is the common analgesic acetaminophen (sold as Tylenol, Datril, and Panadol and contained in many combination drug products). Specific liver changes that occur in chronic alcoholics are responsible for changing acetaminophen into a substance that is highly toxic to the liver. Taken in large quantities or over prolonged periods, the result can be catastrophic liver failure. Most people who have several drinks each day do not think of themselves as *alcoholics*. But if you do, ask your doctor to advise you about *any* pain medications you take.

Drug–Food Interactions

Foods contain a variety of substances that may also speed, slow, or interfere with the absorption of drugs. A common example is the interference of milk or cheese with the absorption of tetracycline. The calcium in most dairy products binds to this antibiotic, preventing its absorption, and therefore decreasing its effectiveness.

One of the most serious drug–food interactions involves a class of tranquilizers know as "monoamine oxidase (MAO) inhibitors," used to treat depression and high blood pressure (Eutron, Nardil, and

Parnate). They react with *tyramine*, an amino acid found in such foods as Parmesan cheese, Chianti wine, chicken livers, and a host of other foods. As a result the blood pressure may rise to dangerously high levels. If you are prescribed an MAO inhibitor, your doctor will no doubt alert you to such interactions. But it is then up to you to avoid the foods on the danger list. *Make certain you know what they are.*

Several drugs have the potential for causing nutritional deficiencies and therefore require an adjustment in your diet to make up for vitamin or mineral losses. For example, the high blood pressure drug, hydralazine, and the antituberculosis drug, INH, can deplete your body's supply of vitamin B_6. Dilantin, a drug used to treat epilepsy, can lead to vitamin D and folic acid deficiencies. Several drugs, including colchicine, which is used to treat gout, and certain antidiabetic drugs can interfere with the absorption of vitamin B_{12}. Long-term use of diuretics, such as chlorothiazide (Diuril or HydroDiuril), can deplete your body of potassium, causing weakness and greatly increasing the danger of taking such drugs as digitalis. Potassium losses can be made up by increasing your dietary intake of such potassium-rich foods as bananas, nuts, oranges, tomatoes, potatoes, figs, and raisins, or your doctor may prescribe potassium supplements.

Drug Reactions to Sun and Heat

Several drugs can alter the body's resistance to heat and ultraviolet radiation, increasing the risk of heat stroke in hot weather and sunburn. If you take one of the drugs listed in the following table, you should avoid excessive heat and dehydration, or you should be carful to protect yourself from sunlight with sunscreens, and protective hats and clothing.

Drugs that Increase the Risk of Sunburn	Drugs that Increase the Risk of Heat Stroke
Oral contraceptives (estrogen, Progestin)	Atropine (an anticholinergic)
Amitriptyline (Elavil)	Diazepam (Valium)
Promethazine (phenergan)	Furosemide (Lasix)
Sulfamethoxazole (Bactrim, Gantanol, Septra)	Hydrochlorothiazide (Esidrix)
Tetracycline, Doxycycline	
Triamterene	

What You Can Do About Your Medicines

If the foregoing does nothing else, it should convince you that taking medicines is not as simple as it may seem. You, the patient (or parent or nurse, as the case may be) must be alert to the potential for problems. Here is what you should always do:

Tell your doctor—

- What medicines you are taking on a regular basis
- If you have had any allergic reactions to a drug
- If you are being treated by another doctor
- If you are pregnant or breast feeding
- If you have diabetes, liver or kidney disease
- If you are on a special diet
- If you use alcohol or tobacco

Ask your doctor—

- What is the name of the medicine he is prescribing? Write it down, lest you forget!
- What the medicine is supposed to do, and when can you anticipate a change in your symptoms or condition? Many studies have shown that some doctors are not very conscientious about explaining prescription medicines to their patients. But all doctors will do so if you insist.
- What side effects might occur? (*See* Drug Interaction sections)
- How should you take the medicine? Does "four times daily" mean "with meals and at bedtime," or every 6 hours? Should you take the medicine *with* meals, or *before* meals?
- How long should you take the medicine? Can you stop when you feel well?
- Are there foods or beverages (including alcohol) you should avoid?
- Are there other medicines you should avoid?
- Can your prescription be refilled automatically, or is another appointment necessary? Before having your prescription refilled, call your doctor to find out if you still need to be taking this drug.

Ask your pharmacist—

- To explain anything on the typed label you don't understand. Most people take their filled prescription out of the store without first reading the label. When you have the pharmacist in front of you is the time to ask questions.
- To maintain a medication profile for you and your family. If you move, take the profile with you.

- To supply your medicines in a container to suit you. If you have no small children at home and if childproof caps are difficult to open, ask for another kind of cap.

GOOD DRUG PRACTICES

- Never take other people's drugs or give them yours.
- Destroy leftover medicines by flushing them down the toilet. Keep your medicines out of the reach of children. *More than one-third of all cases of childhood poisoning from prescription drugs involve a grandparent's medication.*
- Unless otherwise instructed, take pills and capsules with plain water. It helps to take a swallow of water first to lubricate your esophagus. *Stand up* and *drink plenty of water* to get the medicine down into your stomach. An aspirin tablet lodged in your esophagus, for example, can cause a burn or ulcer in your mucous linings. If you think a tablet or capsule is stuck in your esophagus, eat a banana or other soft food to help propel the medicine along. *Do not take medicines lying down.*
- Never take medicines in the dark. Better to risk waking your sleeping partner than poisoning yourself!
- Never take powders in dry form; mix or dissolve them in plenty of water.
- Be especially careful of taking drugs if you are breastfeeding. Numerous prescription and nonprescription drugs are excreted in breast milk and can affect your baby, especially premature and newborn infants. These include caffeine (coffee, tea, soft drinks), alcohol, opiates, aspirin, barbiturates, tranquilizers (Valium, Librium), acetaminophen (Tylenol, Panadol), antihistamines, decongestants, bronchodilators, antibiotics, nicotine, cimetidine (Tagamet), and many others. Always ask your doctor if it is permissible to continue breastfeeding while taking a drug.

Over-the-Counter Drugs

By law, nonprescription drugs must be safe for general use without medical supervision. But "safe" does not mean that side effects may not be encountered, or that such drugs are entirely harmless. You should always read the labels and package inserts whenever you buy a nonprescription drug. Take the drug as recommended unless your doctor advises differently. Manufacturers can and do alter the strength of their products. They also change the instructions as new information is gained about usage and side effects. Even if you use a nonprescription drug regularly, check the instructions to make certain no changes have been made that you have not learned about.

Certain nonprescription drugs have a potential for habituation. Some commonly encountered examples are:

- *Laxatives.* Frequent use of laxatives may create a dependency so that you can't achieve regularity without them. The "stimulant" laxatives, such as Dulcolax, Ex-Lax, and Feen-A-Mint, have the greatest potential for dependency. Bulk laxatives, such as Metamucil, Fiberall, Serutan, and others, are less prone to cause dependency, but all laxatives have this potential. To kick the laxative habit, increase the fiber in your diet, especially fruits and vegetables, and drink at least two quarts of fluids (nonalcoholic) each day (dehydration is probably the most common cause of constipation). If you take diuretic drugs, or consume alcohol, you must increase your fluid intake to make up for increased urination.
- *Nasal sprays.* Do not use nasal sprays that contain a decongestant longer than 3 days. They often create a "rebound" effect that increases nasal stuffiness (*see* p. 231).
- *Eye drops.* Eye drops that contain a decongestant (e.g., tetrahydrazoline) are sometimes taken to reduce redness caused by engorged blood vessels in your eyes. The drug can have the same rebound effect as nasal sprays. Do not use eye drops longer than 48 hours. If redness persists, see your doctor.
- *Codeine cough syrups.* Codeine is an excellent drug for suppressing cough, but, like all narcotics, it is habit forming. Do not take such cough syrups as Naldecon CX or Ryna-C for a chronic cough. Children, pregnant women, and nursing mothers should not take codeine-containing drugs without the advice of a doctor.

A final word of caution: When using any over-the-counter drug, check the package for evidence of tampering before using the drug. Virtually all such drugs must now have tamper-resistant packaging and must bear a label telling you how to check the seal. This is a simple measure that will protect your health. Unfortunately, we live in an age when crazies stalk the aisles of drugstores. Few pernicious acts can guarantee such spectacular media attention as placing a little cyanide inside a bottle on a shelf.

Generic vs Brand-Name Drugs

There is widespread belief that brand-name drugs are "better" than generic drugs. This is understandable in a society whose values are largely formed by the media and the media are also the paid agents of the brand-name drug industry. This notion has unfortunately been reinforced recently by isolated, but much-publicized examples of the scandalous practices of a few generic drug manufacturers.

What Are Generic Drugs?

When a new drug is discovered, it is patented and given a brand or trade name. For example, Motrin is Upjohn Company's brand name for ibuprofen, the generic name for this common analgesic and anti-inflammatory drug. The patent gives the drug company exclusive manufacturing rights for 17 years, and the right to charge for the drug whatever the market (and public sentiment) will bear. When the patent expires, as it has for Motrin, other companies can then manufacture the same drug under the common or 'generic' name (or some new brand name—like Advil—if they desire). The manufacturer of the generic brand must meet the same FDA standards required of the original patent holder, although the long and expensive testing in patients for drug efficacy does not have to be repeated.

In most instances the drugs are chemically the same. In most instances also, the *bioavailabilities* of the drugs are the same (or sometimes better). Bioavailability is a measure of the active ingredient in the medicine that is actually absorbed by the body in a form necessary to fulfill its intended pharmaceutical function. This concept is important; for example, some calcium products intended for treatment or prevention of osteoporosis, such as calcium from oyster shells, are only partially absorbed because of their physical or chemical form.

Nevertheless, controls by the FDA are generally sufficient that a brand-name drug can be replaced in most cases by a generic product of equal strength with little change in drug efficacy. In fact some large drug companies buy their brand-name drugs from a smaller company and relabel them.

Small differences between one manufacturer's product and another's nonetheless may be sufficient to make a difference if the drug is taken over a long period of time. Therefore, you should ask your pharmacist to fill your prescription with the 'same' generic brand each time.

In some cases, it is probably unwise to substitute brand name for generic drugs without monitoring by your doctor. Most of these cases involve drugs in which the *therapeutic dose,* the amount of drug needed to have an effect on your medical problem, and the *toxic dose,* i.e., the amount of drug taken that will produce unwanted side effects, are very close to one another. Some medicines with which this occurs are: drugs used to prevent blood clotting, such as warfarin; drugs used to prevent seizures in epileptics, such as phenytoin (Dilantin); drugs used to ease breathing for asthmatics, such as theophylline; various hormone preparations, such as thyroid medications; and topical corticosteroids used for different skin diseases.

If you are taking any of these drugs, check with your doctor before asking your pharmacist for a substitution.

Does all this mean that the generic drug will be less expensive? Not necessarily. Even though the generic product is sold to the pharmacy for less than the brand name, the markup may be so great that the generic brand costs the same or even more than the brand name. At this writing only 18 states require pharmacies to pass on to customers the full savings available through generic drugs. Thus you should ask your pharmacist the difference in price between brand-name and generic. If it is negligible, you should shop around. For many, particularly the elderly, drug costs represent a significant item in their budgets.

How to Save on Prescription Drug Costs

Here are some suggestions that will help you reduce your prescription drug costs:

- *Shop around for the best prices on prescription drugs.* The product is largely standardized and the quality of pharmacy service is relatively easy to judge. It is only ignorance that allows the differences in drug prices to vary so widely, often by 100% or more in many communities.
- *Consider mail-order pharmacies.* Their prices are often one-half to one-third regular pharmacy charges for prescription drugs. Ordinarily you must send the prescription to the mail-order firm with payment. The delay may be a week or more, so you must plan ahead. It is often worth it. For a list of mail-order pharmacies, see your telephone directory Yellow Pages or write or call: American Association of Retired Persons (AARP), 601 E St. NW, Washington, DC

20049, 1-202-728-4413. Or the: National Council of Senior Citizens, 1331 F St., NW, Washington, DC 20004, 1-202-347-8800.

- *Ask your doctor for free samples.* If you need only a small supply of a drug, ask your doctor for a few of the free samples that are often distributed by drug manufacturers to practicing physicians.
- *If your doctor approves, buy in quantity.* The cost per pill is often less if bought in units of 100 or 1000, rather than smaller quantities.
- *If you qualify, be sure to ask for a senior discount from your pharmacy.*
- *Seek reimbursement from your insurance company.* Many insurance programs pay for all or a part of prescription drug costs. Call your carrier to learn what your coverage is. In other cases, your insurance program will participate in a plan that allows you to purchase drugs at discount. Ask your carrier about such programs.
- *Don't feel that you have to buy prescription drugs from your doctor if such is suggested.* Doctors who dispense drugs seldom do so at the most competitive prices.

The Home Medicine Chest

Every family (of one or more) should have a medicine chest. You should keep your medicine chest relatively simple and periodically go through it and throw out old prescription medicines and any preparation that has changed appearance. Here are the basics:

- For fever and pain you should have both acetaminophen (Tylenol, Panadol) and aspirin. Acetaminophen is preferable for those with easily upset stomach, and for children, because of the link between aspirin and Reye's syndrome. People who drink heavily should avoid acetaminophen because of the potential for liver damage.
- For menstrual pain and as an anti-inflammatory drug (e.g., joint pain), ibuprofen (Motrin, Advil, Nuprin) is recommended.
- Calamine lotion for itching.
- For an antibiotic ointment: Polysporin (contains polymyxin and bacitracin)
- For rashes, a hydrocortisone cream such as Cortaid (1/2% hydrocortisone).
- For colds and hay fever, an antihistamine, such as chlortrimeton and a decongestant, such as Actifed or Dimetapp.
- An antacid, such as Maalox or Gelucil.
- For constipation, Metamucil or Colace. For the elderly, milk of magnesia may be more gentle.
- For diarrhea, Kaopectate or Pepto-Bismol.

- An oral thermometer. If you have a child under three years of age, a rectal thermometer.
- A first-aid kit containing Band-Aids, adhesive tape, sterile gauze squares, a two-inch and a four-inch Ace bandage, scissors, cotton, a tourniquet, burn ointment, eyewash, Vaseline, or petrolatum, and an antiseptic such as Betadine.
- A bulb syringe is useful for irrigating ears and some wounds.
- If you have small children, syrup of ipecac and activated charcoal are essential in case of poisoning. But always call your local Poison Control Center before administering.

Your medicine chest should be out of reach for children, and many experts suggest that a cool, dry closet is better that the bathroom, where warm, moist air speeds the deterioration of many medicines.

Donating Blood for Yourself

If you are anticipating elective surgery, i.e., planned, nonemergency surgery such as a hip repacement or plastic surgery, you may wish to consider donating your own blood for later transfusion during surgery, should the need arise. So-called *autologous* blood transfusion is the safest blood you can receive because the chance of your having a transfusion reaction or contracting a disease transmitted by transfusions of your own blood is practically nil.

What Are the Risks of Blood Bank Transfusions?

Despite testing of all blood donated to blood banks for the presence of human immunodeficiency virus (HIV) that causes AIDS, a few blood recipients in the United States become infected every year from banked blood. Standard HIV tests fail to detect the presence of virus in those (rare) cases when the blood had been drawn in the earliest stages of the disease before HIV antibodies become detectable. Still the risk of contracting AIDS from banked blood is only 1 in 40,000 to 1 in 250,000 (the risk of serious mishap from general anesthesia is about 1 in 1600).

The risk of contracting hepatitis from banked donor blood is much higher, about 1 in 200. Of these, about 10%, or 1 in 2000, will go on to develop cirrhosis of the liver because no reliable test exists yet to detect all the different forms of hepatitis virus.

Despite careful typing and crossmatching your blood with that from a banked donor, a serious transfusion reaction (for example, an allergic reaction or clumping of blood cells that damage your lungs) can occasionally occur. Thus donating your own blood, which eliminates all of these mishaps, makes great sense whenever it is possible.

What You Must Do

You should ask your doctor whether your elective surgery may require a blood transfusion. If so, your doctor will make the necessary arrangements with the nearest blood bank. At the appointed time, you will be screened by the blood bank personnel by means of a short medical history and brief examination and blood test to make sure you are not anemic. If your doctor, in consultation with the medical director of the blood bank, determines that you are an acceptable donor (the criteria for autologous donations are very liberal), you may donate up to 1 unit (about a pint) of blood per week for up to 6 weeks, depending on the anticipated need. The last donation must be at least 3 days before surgery to allow time to replace that donation. The cost of autologous blood varies from about 20% more to 20% less than donor blood, depending upon individual blood bank policies.

What About Stored Frozen Blood?

As interest in autologous blood donation has grown, some clever entrepreneurs have entered the market to collect, freeze, and store your blood in anticipation of either an elective or emergency need. The frozen blood can be stored for up to three years at various of these companies' locations around the country. However, neither the American Red Cross nor the National Institutes of Health endorses this expensive service. The prevailing experience indicates it is unrealistic to expect that such frozen reserves can be thawed, processed, tested, and delivered in time to be useful in an emergency. For elective surgery, the procedures described above are adequate and much less expensive.

Medical Advice for Travelers

Planning a trip to the Rwanda highlands? Staying with the Sultan of Brunei? If so, you may need to consult more than your travel agent. Most travelers give little thought to their possible medical needs when abroad. And for the majority of those voyaging to Canada, Europe, or Antarctica, there is little need to think about more than packing a journey's worth of aspirin and an extra pair of glasses. But for many folks, and for all travelers to countries with prevalent pestilence, careful forethought will help you avoid the Miseries.

Vaccinations

Persons traveling to countries in which communicable diseases are endemic are advised, and in some cases required, to have certain vaccinations. Typhoid fever is common in Africa, Asia, and Central and South America. Cholera occurs throughout much of Asia, the Middle East, Africa, and some parts of Europe. Yellow fever occurs in equatorial Africa and South America, and vaccinations can be obtained only at approved yellow fever vaccination centers. Travelers to Nepal and India may be advised to be vaccinated for meningitis. People staying in Asia longer than three weeks should be vaccinated for Japanese-B encephalitis, a mosquito-borne virus that is *always* fatal if the brain is affected.

Polio virus is common in many developing countries; vaccination may be advised, despite childhood immunization, because immunity seems to decline with age. Some experts recommend that persons traveling to China receive an immunoglobulin shot for protection against hepatitis-A infection. Shanghai in particular has experienced recent epidemic outbreaks of this disease.

If you were born after 1956, consult your doctor about the advisability of revaccination for measles–mumps–rubella.

For information about other vaccination requirements, contact your local health department, travel agency, or international travel line well in advance of departure. Further information can be obtained by sending $4.25 for the booklet, "Health Information for International Travel" to Superintendent of Documents, Government Printing Office, Washington, DC 20402. This publication also lists agencies providing information about emergency medical aid for international travelers.

Malaria

Malaria is caused by mosquito-borne parasites and is a serious public health problem in many parts of Africa, Central and South America, India, and the Pacific Islands. There is currently no effective immunization for malaria; however, the antibiotic chloroquine often protects against this disease. It is recommended that prophylaxis begin two weeks before travel, that it be taken weekly during your stay in endemic regions, and that it be continued for eight weeks after leaving.

In some regions malaria has become resistant to chloroquine, in which case you will be advised to add the antibiotic Mefloquine or substitute it for doxycycline. In other cases, your travel doctor may provide you with a prescription for Fansidar to be taken if you develop symptoms of malaria (flu-like symptoms such as headache, chills, fever, nausea, vomiting, dizziness). All of these drugs must be given to children in doses proportionate to their body weight. Use of these drugs in patients with liver disease must be reviewed by your doctor, and all individuals on long-term prophylaxis should be monitored periodically. If you take other medications regularly, you must check with your doctor about possible drug interactions with antimalarial drugs. Make sure that the exact dosage and schedule are written out and that you understand the instructions. Keep them with the drug container.

Antimalarial drugs are generally contraindicated during pregnancy. It is recommended that women of childbearing age not become pregnant while taking these drugs and that they delay travel to endemic regions until after pregnancy whenever possible.

It is a good idea to take along insect repellent. If you are planning to camp outdoors in endemic regions, take mosquito netting (sporting goods stores that cater to hikers are the best source). Do not expect to buy these items locally; an aversion to insects seems to be largely a Western trait.

Traveler's Diarrhea

About one-third of all Westerners traveling to developing and underdeveloped countries will contract diarrhea (the "turista"), usually lasting 3–5 days and often accompanied by nausea and cramps, and occasionally by fever. The most common causes are viruses and certain strains of *E. coli* bacteria that are particularly prevalent in Africa, Central and South America, the Mediterranean and Middle Eastern countries, and Southeast Asia.

The best way to avoid diarrhea is to be prudent in what you eat and drink. Follow these guidelines to reduce your risks:

- Choose restaurants with a reputation for safety (use your travel guide book liberally).
- Avoid foods from street vendors.
- Eat cooked foods and fruits that can be peeled.
- Do not drink or brush your teeth with tap water or use ice cubes.
- Drink bottled carbonated beverages; the carbonation creates an acidic environment unfavorable to the growth of microorganisms.

The most serious consequences of diarrhea are dehydration and loss of body salts. For mild cases, take lots of clear liquids, such as fruit juices, soda pop, tea, and purified water. To purify your own water, boil it for 10 minutes, or use iodine or hypochlorite tablets (available at hiker's stores), according to directions.

For more severe cases of diarrhea, the US Public Health Service recommends the "two-glass" approach.

Make up two glasses, adding to the first glass eight ounces (a waterglass full) of fruit juices, 1/2 teaspoon of honey or sugar, and a pinch of salt. In the second glass, add eight ounces of carbonated or purified water with 1/2 teaspoon of baking soda. Drink alternately from each glass until your thirst is quenched. In addition to this regimen, take two ounces of Pepto-Bismol four times daily until your symptoms clear.

In severe diarrhea, you lose a lot of potassium, which can make you tire easily. Good sources of potassium are bananas, orange juice, bouillon (yes, the cubes), and that good old American favorite the world over, Coca Cola. You will find, particularly if nausea or cramping is present, a bland diet most satisfying. If you have an antibiotic prescription, take it as directed, or see a local doctor. Do not take Iodochlorhydroxyquin, sold in many countries as *Vioform* or *Enterovioform*. It can cause severe neurologic damage and blindness.

The occurrence of high fever or of blood in your stools is an ominous sign that tells you to see a doctor at once. The need for antibiotics is almost assured.

The most frequently prescribed antidiarrheal medications are Pepto-Bismol, which can be bought over-the-counter, and Lomotil, which is a prescription drug that slows intestinal motility. The adult dosage of Pepto-Bismol is two tablets (or two tablespoons of the fluid) repeated every 4 hours as needed up to 8 doses in a 24-hour period. See the manufacturer's label for children's dosages. *Do not take* Pepto-Bismol if you are allergic to aspirin.

Lomotil is just as effective, although it is a narcotic and may cause more serious side effects, such as sedation and dry mouth. The recommended adult dosage is two tablets four times daily. Do not give Lomotil to children under 2 years of age. If improvement doesn't follow in 1–2 days, an antibiotic, such as trimethoprim-sulfamethoxazole (Bactrim) can be taken. The most popular medications taken to prevent diarrhea are Pepto-Bismol, Lomotil, and Bactrim. Most authorities, however, do not recommend prophylactic antibiotics, because of their side effects. Pepto-Bismol, to be effective, must be taken in two-ounce doses four times daily, which is inconvenient to say the least. Preventive medications should probably be limited to those travelers who cannot afford to be sick—those engaged in business, athletics, and affairs of state. For the rest of us, prudence.

Prescription Medicines

You will naturally take your usual prescription medicines with you when traveling. Take extra prescriptions along just in case you run out or lose your medicines. Try to have these written for generic equivalents (*see* p. 487) because many brand drugs are unavailable abroad. Be aware that some European states will not honor foreign prescriptions; England is one such country.

If you have special medical needs for which you will require monitoring, the International Association for Medical Assistance to Travelers, 447 Center St, Lewiston, NY 14092, 1-716-754-4883, can provide a list of medical specialists able to provide assistance in most countries of the world.

If you will be traveling to cities at high altitude (Kathmandu, Cuzco, La Paz, for example), and you have a heart or lung problem, it may be useful to request from your doctor a prescription for acetazolamide (Diamox). This drug increases ventilation and oxygen transport to the blood. It also halts *periodic breathing* (almost universal during sleep at altitude). *See* Altitude Sickness, p. 59.

All of this sounds complicated and a lot to bear in mind. However, if you are the average tourist you will be fully immunized for wherever it is you intend to go. You will also be in reasonably good health to ignore most of these precautions. But travel to the world's exotic spots is wonderfully tempting and rewarding. I highly recommend it. Every year more and more travelers are Lars Linbladding to the nethermost planetary reaches. And they take these measures seriously or wish they had. The medical annals are filled with the case histories of those who didn't.

Living Wills

A Living Will, unlike a traditional will, provides for actions to be undertaken in your behalf while you are still alive, but no longer able to manage your own affairs. Such situations occur with increasing frequency as our population ages and as modern technology allows doctors to sustain life well past the cessation of competent mental functioning. If you feel strongly that you would not want extraordinary medical measures to be taken to sustain your life when your doctor and other consultants hold no hope of cure, you ought to have a living will.

Living wills essentially provide a guideline directing those who will be caring for you on the extent of life support you desire. The requirements for living wills vary from state to state. You can obtain sample documents that satisfy your state's requirements by writing to the: Choice in Dying, 250 West 57 Street, New York, NY 10107; 1-212-246-6973.

A sample living will prepared for the US Senate Special Committee on Aging is presented below.

It is generally recommended that you also prepare and execute a *Medical Directive* and *Durable Power of Attorney*. These are merely instruments to provide for another person, a spouse, friend, relative, priest, and so on, to act in your behalf when you are unable to do so, in order to carry out your wishes regarding life support. Sample documents are provided on the pages following.

LIVING WILL

DECLARATION

Declaration made this _____ day of _____ 19_____

I, _____ , being of sound mind, willfully and voluntarily make known my desires that my dying shall not be artificially prolonged under the circumstances set forth below, and do declare:

If at any time I should have an incurable injury, disease, or illness certified to be a terminal condition by two (2) physicians who have personally examined me, one of whom shall be my attending physician, and the physicians have determined that my death will occur whether or not life-sustaining procedures are utilized and where the application of life-sustaining procedures would serve only to artificially prolong the dying process, I direct that such procedures be withheld or withdrawn, and that I be permitted to die naturally with only the administration of medication or the performance of any medical procedure deemed necessary to provide me with comfort, care or to alleviate pain.

In the absence of my ability to give directions regarding the use of such life-sustaining procedures, it is my intention that this declaration shall be honored by my family and physician(s) as the final expression of my legal right to refuse any medical or surgical treatment and accept the consequences from such refusal.

I understand the full import of this declaration and I am emotionally and mentally competent to make this declaration.

Signed_____

Address_____

I believe the declarant to be of sound mind. I did not sign the declarant's signature above for or at the direction of the declarant. I am at least 18-years of age and am not related to the declarant by blood or marriage, entitled to any portion of the estate of the declarant according to the laws of intestate succession of the _____ or under any will of the declarant or codicil thereto, or directly financially responsible for declarant's medical care. I am not the declarant's attending physician, an employee of the attending physician, or an employee of the health facility in which the declarant is a patient.

Witness_____ Address_____

Witness_____ Address_____
ss:

Before me the undersigned authority, on this _____ day of _____ 19____, personally appeared _____, _____ , and _____, known to me as the Declarant and the witnesses, respectively, whose names are signed to the foregoing instrument, and who, in the presence of each other, did subscribe their names to the attached Declaration (Living Will) on this date, and that said declarant at the time of execution of said declaration was over the age of eighteen (18) years and of sound mind.

[Seal]
My commission expires: _____
                                          Notary Public

Note: Check requirements of individual state statute.

*The Medical Directive**

Introduction

As part of a person's right to self-determination, every adult may accept or refuse any recommended medical treatment. This is relatively easy when people are well and can speak. Unfortunately, during severe illness people are often unconscious or otherwise unable to communicate their wishes—at the very time when many critical decisions need to be made.

*Copyright 1989 by the American Medical Association. All rights reserved. Adapted with permission from L. L. Emanuel and E. J. Emanuel, "The Medical Directive: A New Comprehensive Advance Care Document," *JAMA* 261:3288–3293, June 9, 1989.

The Medical Directive states your wishes regarding various types of medical treatment in several representative situations so that your desires can be respected. It comes into effect only if you become incompetent (unable to make decisions or to express your wishes), and you can change it at any time until then. As long as you are competent, you should discuss your care directly with your physician.

The Medical Directive also lets you appoint someone to make medical decisions for you if you should become unable to make your own; this is a proxy or durable power of attorney. Additionally, it contains a statement of your wishes concerning organ donation.

Pages 50–53 contain Medical Directive forms on which you can record your own desires. Since such wishes usually reflect personal, philosophical, and religious views, you may want to discuss the issues with your family, friends, or religious mentor before completing the form.

Completing the Form

First you will be asked to consider four different situations that involve mental incompetence: an irreversible coma or a persistent vegetative state (situation A); a coma with very slight and uncertain chance of recovery (situation B); irreversible brain damage or brain disease together with a terminal illness (situation C); and irreversible brain damage or disease but with no terminal illness (situation D). For each of these situations, you will be asked to indicate your wishes concerning possible medical interventions ranging from pain medications to resuscitation. You can refuse a certain treatment or request that it definitely be used, should it be medically appropriate. Alternatively, you can state that you are unsure about your preference for the treatment, or that you would like it tried for a while but discontinued if it does not result in definite improvement. This phase of completing the Medical Directive is best done in consultation with your physician.

Next you will be given the opportunity to designate a proxy decision-maker. This person would be asked to make decisions under circumstances in which your wishes are unclear—for example, if your situation is not covered in this document or if your preference is undecided. (It is expected, in the former case, that the proxy would be significantly guided whenever possible by your choices in situations A–D.) You can indicate whether the proxy's decisions should override (or be overridden by) your wishes. And, should you name more than one proxy, you can state who is to have the final say if there is disagreement.

Then you will be able to express your preference concerning organ donation. Do you wish to donate your body or some or all of your organs after your death? If so, for what purpose(s) and to which physician or institution?

Before recording a personal statement in the Medical Directive, you may find it helpful to consider the following question. What kind of medical condition, if any, would make life hard enough that you would find attempts to prolong it undesirable? None? Intractable pain? Permanent dependence on others? Irreversible mental damage? Another condition you would regard as intolerable? Under circumstances such as these, medical intervention may include only securing comfort; it may involve using ordinary treatments while avoiding more invasive ones; or employing those that offer improved function; or trying anything appropriate to prolonging life—regardless of quality. You should record here anything you feel is necessary to clarify your personal values concerning the limits of life and the goals of medical intervention.

What to Do with the Form

Finally, to make the Medical Directive effective you will need to sign and date it in the presence of two witnesses. They must sign and date the form as well. You don't need to have it notarized. States vary in the details of legislation covering documents of this sort. If you wish to know the laws in your state, you should call the office of its attorney general or consult a lawyer privately. If your state has a statutory document, you may want to complete the Medical Directive and append it to this form.

You should give a copy of the completed document to your personal physician, as well as to a family member or a friend, to ensure that it will be available if it is needed. Your physician should have a copy of it placed in your medical records and should flag it so that anyone who might be involved in your care can be aware of its presence.

My Medical Directive

This Medical Directive expresses, and shall stand for, my wishes regarding medical treatments in the event that illness should make me unable to communicate them directly. I make this Directive, being 18 years or more of age, of sound mind, and appreciating the consequences of my decisions.

Situation A

If I am in a coma or a persistent vegetative state, and in the opinion of my physician and several consultants, have no known hope of regaining awareness and higher mental functions no matter what is done, then my wishes regarding use of the following, if considered medically reasonable, would be:

	I want	I want treatment tried. If no clear improvement, stop.	I am undecided	I do not want
Cardiopulmonary Resuscitation: if at the point of death, using drugs and electric shock to keep the heart beating; artificial breathing.		Not applicable		
Mechanical Breathing: breathing by machine.				
Artificial Nutrition and Hydration: giving nutrition and fluid through a tube in the veins, nose, or stomach.				
Major Surgery, such as removing the gall bladder or part of the intestines.		Not applicable		
Kidney Dialysis: cleaning the blood by machine or by fluid passed through the belly.				
Chemotherapy: using drugs to fight cancer.				
Minor Surgery, such as removing some tissue from an infected toe.		Not applicable		
Invasive Diagnostic Tests, such as using a flexible tube to look into the stomach.		Not applicable		
Blood or Blood Products, such as giving transfusions.				
Antibiotics: using drugs to fight infection.				
Simple Diagnostic Tests, such as performing blood tests or x-rays.		Not applicable		
Pain Medications, even if they dull consciousness and indirectly shorten my life.		Not applicable		

My Medical Directive

This Medical Directive expresses, and shall stand for, my wishes regarding medical treatments in the event that illness should make me unable to communicate them directly. I make this Directive, being 18 years or more of age, of sound mind, and appreciating the consequences of my decisions.

Situation B

If I am in a coma and, in the opinion of my physician and several consultants, have a small likelihood of recovering fully, a slightly larger likelihood of surviving with permanent brain damage, and a much larger likelihood of dying, then my wishes regarding use of the following, if considered medically reasonable, would be:

	I want	I want treatment tried. If no clear improvement, stop.	I am undecided	I do not want
Cardiopulmonary Resuscitation: if at the point of death, using drugs and electric shock to keep the heart beating; artificial breathing.		Not applicable		
Mechanical Breathing: breathing by machine.				
Artificial Nutrition and Hydration: giving nutrition and fluid through a tube in the veins, nose, or stomach.				
Major Surgery, such as removing the gall bladder or part of the intestines.		Not applicable		
Kidney Dialysis: cleaning the blood by machine or by fluid passed through the belly.				
Chemotherapy: using drugs to fight cancer.				
Minor Surgery, such as removing some tissue from an infected toe.		Not applicable		
Invasive Diagnostic Tests, such as using a flexible tube to look into the stomach.		Not applicable		
Blood or Blood Products, such as giving transfusions.				
Antibiotics: using drugs to fight infection.				
Simple Diagnostic Tests, such as performing blood tests or x-rays.		Not applicable		
Pain Medications, even if they dull consciousness and indirectly shorten my life.		Not applicable		

My Medical Directive

This Medical Directive expresses, and shall stand for, my wishes regarding medical treatments in the event that illness should make me unable to communicate them directly. I make this Directive, being 18 years or more of age, of sound mind, and appreciating the consequences of my decisions.

Situation C

If I have brain damage or some brain disease that in the opinion of my physician and several consultants cannot be reversed and that makes me unable to recognize people or to speak understandably, *and I also have a terminal illness,* such as incurable cancer, that will likely be the cause of my death, then my wishes regarding use of the following, if considered medically reasonable, would be:

	I want	I want treatment tried. If no clear improvement, stop.	I am undecided	I do not want
Cardiopulmonary Resuscitation: if at the point of death, using drugs and electric shock to keep the heart beating; artificial breathing.		Not applicable		
Mechanical Breathing: breathing by machine.				
Artificial Nutrition and Hydration: giving nutrition and fluid through a tube in the veins, nose, or stomach.				
Major Surgery, such as removing the gall bladder or part of the intestines.		Not applicable		
Kidney Dialysis: cleaning the blood by machine or by fluid passed through the belly.				
Chemotherapy: using drugs to fight cancer.				
Minor Surgery, such as removing some tissue from an infected toe.		Not applicable		
Invasive Diagnostic Tests, such as using a flexible tube to look into the stomach.		Not applicable		
Blood or Blood Products, such as giving transfusions.				
Antibiotics: using drugs to fight infection.				
Simple Diagnostic Tests, such as performing blood tests or x-rays.		Not applicable		
Pain Medications, even if they dull consciousness and indirectly shorten my life.				

My Medical Directive

This Medical Directive expresses, and shall stand for, my wishes regarding medical treatments in the event that illness should make me unable to communicate them directly. I make this Directive, being 18 years or more of age, of sound mind, and appreciating the consequences of my decisions.

Situation D

If I have brain damage or some brain disease that in the opinion of my physician and several consultants cannot be reversed and that makes me unable to recognize people or to speak understandably, *but I have no terminal illness*, and I can live in this condition for a long time, then my wishes regarding use of the following, if considered medically reasonable, would be:

	I want	I want treatment tried. If no clear improvement, stop.	I am undecided	I do not want
Cardiopulmonary Resuscitation: if at the point of death, using drugs and electric shock to keep the heart beating; artificial breathing.		Not applicable		
Mechanical Breathing: breathing by machine.				
Artificial Nutrition and Hydration: giving nutrition and fluid through a tube in the veins, nose, or stomach.				
Major Surgery, such as removing the gall bladder or part of the intestines.		Not applicable		
Kidney Dialysis: cleaning the blood by machine or by fluid passed through the belly.				
Chemotherapy: using drugs to fight cancer.				
Minor Surgery, such as removing some tissue from an infected toe.		Not applicable		
Invasive Diagnostic Tests, such as using a flexible tube to look into the stomach.		Not applicable		
Blood or Blood Products, such as giving transfusions.				
Antibiotics: using drugs to fight infection.				
Simple Diagnostic Tests, such as performing blood tests or x-rays.		Not applicable		
Pain Medications, even if they dull consciousness and indirectly shorten my life.				

DURABLE POWER OF ATTORNEY

I understand that my wishes expressed in these four cases may not cover all possible aspects of my care if I become incompetent. I also may be undecided about whether I want a particular treatment or not. Consequently, there may be a need for someone to accept or refuse medical interventions for me in consultation with my physicians. I authorize

_____

_____

as my proxy(s) to make the decision for me whenever my wishes, as expressed in this document, are insufficient or undecided.

Should there be any disagreement between the wishes I have indicated in this document and the decision favored by my above-named proxy(s),

(Please delete one of the following two lines.)

I wish my proxy(s) to have authority over my Medical Directive

(or)

I wish my Medical Directive to have authority over my proxy(s).

Should there be any disagreement between the wishes of my proxies,

_____ shall have final authority.

ORGAN DONATION

I hereby make this anatomical gift to take effect upon my death.

(Please check boxes and fill in blanks where appropriate.)

I give
- ☐ my body;   ☐ any needed organs or parts;
- ☐ the following organs or parts _____

_____

to
- ☐ the following person or institution: _____

_____

- ☐ the physician in attendance at my death;
- ☐ the hospital in which I die;
- ☐ the following named physician hospital, storage bank, or other medical institution:

_____ ;

for the following purposes:
- ☐ any purpose authorized by law;   ☐ transplantation;
- ☐ therapy of another person;   ☐ research;
- ☐ medical education.

MY PERSONAL STATEMENT (use another page if necessary)

_____

_____

Signed: _____ Date _____

Witness: _____ Date _____

Witness: _____ Date _____

FIRST AID

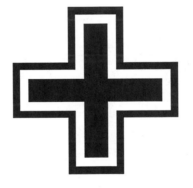

First Aid
and Emergency Medical Procedures

Getting Medical Help Fast

When you are confronted with a medical emergency, quick action and a cool head will spare injury and save lives. Here are the general principles that should guide your approach:

- Render whatever emergency first aid procedures you can. If you are unsure of what to do, don't do anything. Some victims are injured by unskillful first-aid measures aggressively applied. To avoid being caught in such embarrassment, it is a good idea to take a course in First Aid and to become familiar with cardio-pulmonary resuscitation (CPR). Call your local American Red Cross for information about courses offered in your area. And whatever you do, read the rest of this chapter!
- First Aid and CPR. While one person gives emergency care to a sick or injured person, another must seek medical help.
- Dial 911—or the Emergency Number for your area. Be ready to give the following information:
  1. Location of the emergency, including cross streets, floor and room numbers, and the number of the phone you are calling from.
  2. What happened? Relate as much as possible about the accident, injury, or illness.
  3. How many people need help?
  4. Is anyone bleeding, unconscious, or without a pulse? What first aid is being given? Take down any instructions.
  5. Don't hang up first! Be sure you have given all the information that is needed.

Who Needs Emergency Medical Help?

True medical emergencies include the following:

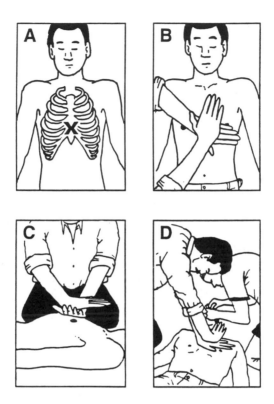

Figure 1. *Cardiopulmonary Resuscitation* (CPR). This procedure requires proper training for safe and effective use. **(A)** Apply pressure only at the base of the breastbone, placing the palms of the hands one atop the other, as shown in **(B)**. Press firmly and rhythmically at a rate of 80–100 per minute for 10 seconds. Then give two breaths mouth to mouth. Continue until renewed signs of life emerge, or it becomes clear that nothing further can be done.

- Major injuries, such as broken legs, chest wounds, or penetrating injuries. Do not try to remove an object that is impaled in the body.
- Brisk bleeding that can't be stopped by applying pressure to the wound. *See* p. 71.
- Unconsciousness, stupor, or disorientation. *See* p. 76.
- Shortness of breath or difficulty breathing. *See* p. 74.
- Severe pain
- Severe burns. *See* p. 75.
- Knocked out teeth. *See* p. 277.
- Amputated finger or limb. *See* p. 71.
- Poisonous snake bite. *See* p. 68.

- Anyone in shock. Shock is recognized by pale sweaty skin; rapid, weak pulse; and rapid, shallow breathing. The blood pressure is low, and the patient may be thirsty and in pain. *See* p. 89.

In Case of Multiple Emergency Problems

It is not unusual in cases of trauma, especially those arising from automobile accidents where drastic forces may batter the body, that multiple injuries are sustained, requiring some decision about the order of emergency attention. In general, the order of importance is to: (1) restore breathing and heartbeat, (2) stop bleeding, and (3) treat shock, in that sequence .

While Waiting For the Ambulance

While the victim receives first aid, have someone:

- Remove jewelry and loosen clothing that might impair circulation.
- Collect any medicine that the victim takes regularly or is found on the person.
- Collect any pertinent medical records that may be useful to the emergency room doctors.
- Gather any insurance information that may be needed at the hospital.
- Leave valuables at home or secure them for the victim.

Altitude Sickness

Acute Mountain Sickness; High-Altitude Pulmonary Edema; High-Altitude Cerebral Edema

As you ascend and the atmospheric pressure decreases, the total volume of oxygen per liter of air breathed also decreases. This causes you to breathe more rapidly and your heart to beat faster in order to supply the body with the oxygen it needs. You lose water when rapidly breathing dry air, but at the same time the tissue cells tend to retain water. People react differently to high altitudes. Children and premenstrual women are especially vulnerable. People who have had one attack of altitude sickness are more likely to experience the problem the next time they return to high altitudes.

Acute Mountain Sickness

This is the most common form of altitude sickness and may occur as low as 6500 feet. The symptoms include headache, a feeling of fatigue, nausea, shortness of breath, rapid heart rate, and difficulty sleeping. The symptoms worsen with exertion and usually disappear within a few days as you accommodate to higher altitudes.

First Aid

Measures include drinking extra water to counteract dehydration; analgesics (e.g., aspirin or acetaminophen) for headache, a light diet, oxygen if available, and mild exercise. Returning to lower altitude immediately relieves these symptoms. Acetazolamide, a prescription drug (e.g., Diamox), 250 mg daily is both curative and often prevents the onset of symptoms. Ask your doctor whether you need this or the drug verapamil if you are contemplating going to a high elevation.

High-Altitude Pulmonary Edema

This is a less common manifestation of altitude sickness, usually brought on within 24 to 48 hours of rapid ascent above 9000 feet. In addition to the symptoms of acute mountain sickness, shortness of breath becomes severe and is accompanied by cough and occasionally bloody sputum. If untreated, weakness and coma may follow.

First Aid

Measures include bed rest and oxygen, but immediate descent to lower altitudes is more effective. If acetazolamide or other diuretics are administered, vigorous fluid replacement is essential because the victim is already dehydrated. Drink a glass of water every hour for several hours.

High-Altitude Cerebral Edema

Brain swelling is probably present to some extent in all forms of altitude sickness, but in some the symptoms may be severe: headache, mental confusion, staggering, clumsiness, double vision, hallucinations, and coma. These symptoms demand that the individual return to lower altitude as soon as possible. Diuretics and corticosteroids are helpful if a doctor is available.

Prevention

People known to be sensitive to high altitudes should ascend slowly —if possible, no more than 1000 feet per day above 6000 feet. Physical fitness and climbing experience do not prevent any form of altitude sickness. Avoid strenuous effort until you accommodate to the altitude. If you tire easily, reduce your activity. Drink lots of water to replace that lost through respiration in dry air. Avoid alcoholic beverages, and avoid excess salt.

Your doctor may prescribe acetazolamide, 250 mg daily by mouth, before, during, and a day after ascent. Ask your doctor about the value of phenytoin (e.g., Dilantin) or verapamil to prevent altitude sickness.

Ankle Sprain

Any joint can be sprained, but the ankle is probably the most common, resulting in stretching or tearing of ligaments, tendons, muscles, and blood vessels. The joint swells, may become discolored, and hurts with any movement or weight bearing.

Treatment

Remove the shoe and elevate the leg. Apply ice in a bag or towel. Since it is almost impossible to distinguish a sprain from a fracture, it is wise to have it examined and X-rayed unless the swelling is very slight. In the latter case, remember the acronym RICE: Rest the injury; apply Ice; apply Compresses (e.g., elastic bandages); and Elevate above the level of the heart to reduce swelling. Once swelling has subsided, applying heat to the injury will speed healing by increasing blood flow. Remember too, that severe sprains may be slower to heal than fractures and an improperly treated ankle sprain can result in a chronically unstable and painful joint.

Prevention

Wearing firm shoes that come slightly above the ankles and prevent lateral motion is the best means of preventing sprained ankle. If you have had more than one sprained ankle, or an unstable ankle, consult an orthopedic supply house for advice about proper shoes.

Bites

Dog Bites

If you are bitten by a dog, rinse the wound thoroughly with water to remove dirt and saliva. Then wash the wound with soap and warm water for 5 minutes. Rinse, dry, and apply a sterile gauze dressing.

If the bite is deep, you should consult your doctor who may then prescribe antibiotics. Most states require that dog bites be reported to local health authorities. The animal must then be kept under observation for signs of rabies: agitation, viciousness, paralysis, and eventually death of the animal. Because of required rabies vaccinations, rabid pet dogs are very rare. If the dog has been vaccinated in the last

two years, you probably don't need to be concerned about contracting rabies. Check with your doctor about the need for rabies shots.

Tetanus infection is also possible, although uncommon. If you have
not had a tetanus shot within the last five years, you should consider
asking for a booster shot.

Wild Animal Bites

The principal reservoir of rabies in wild animals is in racoons,
skunks, foxes, and bats. The most obvious signs of a rabid animal are
daytime activity of a normally nocturnal animal and loss of the usual
fear of humans. If you are bitten, thoroughly wash the wound with
soap and warm water for five minutes. Thorough cleansing of the
wound is thought to be the best prophylaxis against rabies. Then go
to your doctor or to an emergency room for treatment.

Rabies is caused by a virus that is present in the saliva of infected
animals and attacks the nervous system. The symptoms of rabies
in humans appear from 10 days to two years after exposure; the
average is about one month. The earliest symptoms are mental
depression, restlessness, fever, and often flu-like symptoms. These
symptoms give way to uncontrollable excitement, excessive salivation, and intense pain on swallowing. Although very thirsty,
the victim cannot swallow, hence the name "hydrophobia." Death
is the usual outcome; however, modern vaccination renders the
development of rabies very rare.

Human Bites

Human bites are very serious because the numerous bacteria in
saliva can cause serious and disabling infections, particularly if the
tendons or joints of the hand are involved. There is also the potential
for tranmission of hepatitis B and even HIV infection. The potential
is especially serious with "fight bites' acquired in the act of striking
another person. First aid consists of washing the wound thoroughly
with soap and water. The victim should then be taken to an emergency room where the wound will be evaluated, damaged tissue
removed, and possibly antibiotic prescribed.

Insect Stings

The most common insects that sting are bees, wasps, yellow jack-
ets, hornets, and fire ants. Their venom produces sudden, intense
burning, and sometimes welts and itching around the sting. Wash
the sting with soap and water. Applying an ice pack will bring con-

siderable relief. Several home remedies have their advocates, mostly untested: meat tenderizer, baking soda, calamine lotion, powdered aspirin, all applied gently with a small cloth pad for 10–20 minutes.

Bees may leave their stinger in the skin. Don't pull out a stinger with your fingers, because the venom sack may still be attached. Squeezing the venom sack only injects more venom under the skin. Scrape the sack away at the skin with a knife. Then remove the stinger with fingernails or tweezers.

Anyone who has been stung several times should be taken to an emergency room. Because insect venom can act much like snake venom, the more injected, the more profound the symptoms (*see* Shock, p. 89). Children are especially vulnerable because of their small size.

The most dangerous aspect of insect stings is the possibility of a severe allergic reaction. This subject is discussed in detail on p. 243. People who are allergic to insect stings should obtain an epinephrine (adrenalin) kit from their doctors *and be thoroughly instructed in its use.*

Prevention

Some evidence suggests that stinging insects are attracted to bright colors and strong scents from perfumes and scented soaps. Wear drab clothing and avoid perfumes while outdoors. Do not walk barefoot in the grass. Yellowjackets and some other insects nest in or near the ground. At picnics, cover food well to avoid attracting stinging insects. If an insect annoys you, don't swat at it. Ignore it or walk away. If attacked by a swarm of bees, lie face down and cover your head.

Spider Bites

Nearly all spiders are venomous, but only a few have fangs rigid enough and long enough to penetrate your skin. In the United States, two spiders are of concern: the black widow and the brown recluse. An attempt should be made to catch and identify the spider once it has bitten you because the identity may affect treatment.

Black Widow Bites

The bite usually is felt as a sharp pinprick, followed by a dull, numbing pain in the bitten extremity. This is followed frequently by cramping and muscular rigidity in the stomach, shoulders, and chest. Generalized symptoms include anxiety, sweating, headache, dizziness, skin rash and itching, nausea, and vomiting. Children may experience difficulty breathing. Fatalities, while rare, do occur.

No first aid measures are of real value. An ice cube placed over the bite may partially relieve pain. It is recommended that victims under 16 and over 60 years of age, or anyone with high blood pressure or heart disease, be hospitalized because of possible respiratory and cardiovascular distress. There is a specific black widow antivenin that can be administered.

Brown Recluse Bites

There is usually little immediate pain, but localized pain often develops within an hour. The bite area becomes reddened and then discolored as the poison breaks down blood vessels that bleed into the area. A bleb forms, creating a *bull's eye* appearance. Later an ulcer forms, covered by a blackened scab. Pain can be severe. Generalized symptoms include nausea and vomiting, anemia, and kidney failure.

Again, an ice cube placed on the bite may help relieve pain. If an ulcer develops at the site within 12 hours and enlarges during the subsequent 12 hours, see your doctor, who may recommend medications to lessen the development of generalized symptoms.

Tick Bites

Ticks transmit a host of serious diseases, including Rocky Mountain spotted fever, Q fever, tularemia, Colorado tick fever, encephalomyelitis, Lyme disease, and tick paralysis.

If a tick embeds itself in your skin, it may be removed intact by anesthetizing it with ether, or suffocating it with gasoline, oil, glycerin, kerosene, or charcoal lighter fluid on a piece of cotton. Most ticks will dislodge themselves if touched with a hot (not lighted) match, or with tweezers that have been heated over a match flame. If the tick is pulled out by force, leaving the head and mouthparts anchored in the skin, the wound may fester for several days.

If you are bitten by a tick, call your doctor for instructions regarding the necessity for observation or prophylactic antibiotics. These vary greatly from region to region. It is also helpful to *save the tick* for identification, because not all species in any area carry disease.

Prevention

When in tick-infested countryside, it is prudent to examine yourself at frequent intervals, especially around your head and neck. Almost all diseases carried by ticks are prevented if the tick is removed within 2 to 3 hours. Tick bites are painless, so only a careful search of your body will reveal their presence.

Scorpion Stings

Most North American scorpions are relatively harmless and are best treated by an ice cube over the sting site to relieve pain. One species, *Centruroides exilicauda*, has a more potent venom. This scorpion is found only in Arizona, New Mexico, and the California side of the Colorado River. The sting results in immediate pain, with possible numbness and tingling. Generalized symptoms include rapid heart rate, high blood pressure, weakness, and partial paralysis. Children and older adults may experience difficulty breathing.

If you are stung by a scorpion outside the above area, no specific treatment is required. If you are stung within the range of *C. exilicauda*, get to a doctor or emergency room for supportive care. Information about a specific antivenin can be obtained from the Arizona Poison Control System, Tucson, AZ, 1-602-626-6016.

Chigger Bites

Chiggers are the annoying little larvae of the mite *Trombicula*. In the North they come out in April or May (year-around in Southern regions), climb the nearest plant, and wait for the first animal to come along to scavenge a meal. If you brush against the chigger's perch, it will drop on you and attach itself to your skin. The chigger feeds by secreting enzymes that dissolve the skin. These enzymes are irritating and produce an intense, itching dermatitis that lasts for a week or more, even though the mites remain on the skin only a few days.

First Aid

For itching you may try starch or oatmeal baths (Aveeno is a commercial oatmeal preparation for bathing) or apply calamine lotion. In severe cases your doctor may prescribe an antihistamine or topical steroid preparation. Relief of itching is important to avoid secondary infections from scratching.

Prevention

Chiggers do not suck blood, burrow into the skin, or transmit diseases. They are best avoided by wearing long sleeves and trousers. You may also use insect repellent (*see* Insect Repellents on the following page) on exposed skin and outer clothing. If you are hiking in chigger country, examine yourself afterward. Look for tiny red flecks and scrape them off with a knife or your fingernail. You can rid yourself of the mites by applying gamma-benzene lotion (Kwell) or the prescription drug, Crotamiton, which also relieves itching.

Centipede and Millipede Bites

Some larger centipedes can inflict a painful bite that produces local redness and swelling. Swelling of regional lymph nodes (lymphangitis) is common. Rarely, headache, fever, and vomiting may result. An ice cube placed over the bite will reduce pain. In case of fever and headache, bed rest is advised. No other treatment is usually necessary.

Millipedes do not bite, but may secrete a toxin that is irritating to the skin. Washing the affected area with soap and water is effective. Do not use alcohol pads. If irritation persists, a topical steroid ointment, such as Cortaid may be applied.

Other Biting Beasties

Among the more common arthropods that use our bodies for dinner are mosquitoes, fleas, lice, bedbugs, kissing bugs, and the sand, horse, and deer flies. For the most part, it is the saliva of these biting brigands that irritates and even causes allergic reactions.

For most bites an ice cube offers satisfactory relief. In case of an extensive local reaction, a topical corticosteroid, such as Cortaid, may be necessary in addition to an analgesic.

INSECT REPELLANTS

The safest and most effective insect repellents contain the substance DET or deet (Off, Cutters, etc.). Sprayed on outer clothing and exposed skin, it is quite effective for chiggers, ticks, biting flies, and mosquitoes, but not against bees. Avoid preparations that contain 100% deet, since they may be too strong and have been known to cause allergic and toxic reactions in some people. Do not spray on cuts or scratches, and be very sparing in their use on children. Do not use repellants on infants. *Never Spray An Insecticide* on yourself or others to repel insects. Severe neurological reactions are common, and death may result.

Marine Animal Stings and Bites

Stingrays have a venomous spine located in their tails. Victims are usually stung while wading on beaches, bays, and tidal estuaries and unwarily tread on the backs of the creatures, which lie partially buried in the sand. The tail is thrust upward and the spine is jabbed into your foot or leg. The spine is covered by a protective sheath. When the spine is driven into the flesh, the sheath ruptures, releasing the venom into the wound. The result is instant pain, the like of which you are unlikely to forget. If the ray is large and the wound deep, systemic symptoms may develop: weakness, nausea, vomiting, sweating, cramps, anxiety, and even difficulty breathing.

The victim should be taken to a doctor or to an emergency room. While these arrangements are being made, an attempt should be made to remove the thin, membranous spine sheath if it is seen in the wound. Other first aid measures include soaking the limb in hot water for 30–60 min. Either table salt or magnesium sulfate (Epsom salts) can be added to the water. If the wound is large and jagged, it may require suturing to promote healing.

Octopus bites may be sustained by those who try to pick them up. North American octopus bites are seldom serious and can be simply cleansed and bandaged.

Sea Cones are a type of univalve mollusc. Only one variety in North American water is dangerous, the *Conus californicus*, which has a venomous stinger. The venom of a large cone may be serious to a child, to the elderly, or to those with heart disease. Such individuals should be taken to an emergency room if stung to provide cardiac and respiratory support measures if required.

Jellyfish have thousands of tiny stinging cells called "nematocysts" within their trailing tentacles. The venomous barbs are the means whereby the animal subdues its prey. These barbs can also penetrate the skin, producing small reddish welts that cause pain and itching. Severe stings, especially by the large Portuguese man-of-war (which is actually a colony of tiny animals known as hydroids) are uncommon. Contact with the tentacles may, however, be severe enough to produce such systemic symptoms as weakness, nausea, sweating, muscle pain, headache, and cardiac irregularity.

First Aid

For minor jellyfish stings no treatment is usually required. For painful stings, wash the area with seawater, but do not rub, since this will stimulate discharge of the remaining nematocysts. To deactivate these stinging cells, apply rubbing alcohol, vinegar, or a paste of baking soda. In the United States it is popular to sprinkle powdered meat tenderizer (containing papain) on the affected skin. For more serious stings, wet the area and cover with baking soda for 20 minutes. Then add more baking soda, and after a while carefully scrape away the soda with a knife to remove the stingers. Rinse, dry, and apply a hydrocortisone ointment (e.g., Cortaid).

If the systemic symptoms described above develop, or if pain is especially severe, the victim should be taken to an emergency room where narcotics, oxygen, and epinephrine may be given along with cardiac and respiratory support measures.

Sea Urchins are covered with sharp spines that become embedded in the skin and break off on contact. The result is a sharp pain that will persist, and the wound will then fester unless the spines are removed. This can be accomplished by someone skillful with a sewing needle if the spines are embedded in the hands or feet. If deeply embedded you should consult your doctor.

For stings from coral and sea anemones, follow the same instructions as for jellyfish.

Snakebites

A bite from a poisonous snake is a serious medical emergency. Poisonous snakes are found in virtually every state in the United States except Hawaii. Of the 8000 venomous snakebites each year, 99% are inflicted by the pit vipers, namely, rattlesnakes, cottonmouths, and copperheads; less than 1% of bites are inflicted by coral snakes or exotic pet snakes. Of all bites, only 10–15 people in the US die each year as a result; most are children and elderly. Almost one-fourth of all bites by poisonous snakes fail to inject venom into the wound—the fangs strike a bone or can't sufficiently penetrate outer clothing.

Most of our current thinking about snakebite—which is still controversial—comes from a report of the National Research Council of the National Academy of Sciences. This report divides the symptoms of snakebite into two categories, which largely determine the recommended first-aid treatment:

1. *Mild-to-moderate symptoms.* Mild swelling or discoloration, mild-to-moderate pain at the site of the bite, usually within a few minutes; tingling sensations; rapid pulse; weakness; dimness of vision; nausea; vomiting; and shortness of breath.
2. *Severe symptoms.* Rapid swelling and numbness, followed by severe pain at the site of bite. There may also be pinpoint pupils, twitching, slurred speech, shock, convulsions, paralysis, unconsciousness, and loss of breathing or pulse.

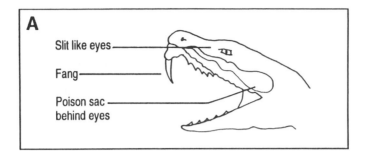

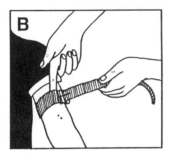

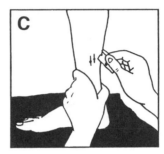

Figure 2. *Deadly Snake Bites.* Our native deadly snakes are almost always rattlesnakes, cottonmouths, copperheads, or coral snakes. Unlike most other snakes, the deadly varieties all have long fangs through which their venoms are delivered **(A)**. Anyone bitten by a coral snake must immediately be immobilized and rushed to medical care. Those bitten by the other deadly snakes are treated as shown in panels **B** and **C** above. **B.** A moderately tight cinch (some circulation must be maintained) is placed an inch or two above the bite, which is then washed with soap and water. Where possible the bite should be kept below heart level, and neither hot nor cold compresses should be applied. **C.** Using a razor blade or other sharp instrument, cut each fang mark a quarter-inch deep along the limb's length, and suck out the venom (spit it out immediately!). Medical assistance must always be sought after initial first-aid treatment for snakebite.

First Aid for All Snakebites

- The most important step is to get a snakebite victim to a hospital as soon as possible, even if you are not certain of the type of snake.
- Keep the victim as calm as possible and prevent moving about.
- Have the victim lie down and immobilize the bitten extremity. If possible, place the area of the wound below the level of the heart to slow the return of venous blood.

- Do not give the victim alcohol, sedatives, aspirin, or any medicine containing aspirin. Aspirin interferes with coagulation and hence may augment the effects of the snake venom.
- If the victim can reach a hospital within 4–5 hours and if no symptoms develop, no further first aid measure are necessary. Most people can get to a hospital within an hour, even from rural areas.

If it can be done safely and without delay in rescue time, kill the snake and take it to the hospital for identification.

Mild-to-Moderate Snakebite Symptoms

If the mild-to-moderate symptoms listed above develop, apply a constricting band 2–4 inches above the bite, but not around a joint—elbow, knee, wrist, or ankle—*and never around the head, neck, or trunk.* The band should be 1–2 inches wide, not thin like a string or rope. It should be snug, but loose enough for a finger to be slipped underneath. Loosen the band if it becomes too tight, but do not remove it. Check the pulse beyond the band to make sure that blood is getting to the extremity. The idea here is to restrict *venous* blood return, but not to cut off the oxygen-rich arterial blood supply to the extremity.

Severe Symptoms

Keep the victim lying down and cover with a blanket to help maintain body temperature. If breathing or pulse stops, administer CPR if you have been trained to do so.

Make an incision over each fang mark with a knife or razor blade just through the skin and about 1/2-inch long. Make the incision parallel to the limb, not crosswise, to avoid transecting larger blood vessels. Apply suction over a 30-minute period. Use your mouth if you do not have a suction cup from a snake-bite kit. Using an extractor cup you can remove up to 30% of the venom. Using your mouth you may remove 10–15%—not much, but better than none. Don't worry about the venom getting in your mouth; it won't hurt you, but don't swallow it either. Do not make incisions on the head, neck, or trunk.

CORAL SNAKES

Most experts agree that constricting bands and suction techniques do little good in the case of the rare coral snake bites. Their venom is quickly absorbed directly into the blood stream. Rather it is best to take no food or drink and get medical care as fast as possible.

If You Are Alone

First aid for a snakebite is difficult if you are the victim and you are alone. You cannot immobilize your leg because you must get to help. If there is immediate pain following the bite, use the cut-and-suck method if the bite can be reached. As quickly as possible, start walking for help, but keep a moderate pace. Rest every five minutes. If the bite is to your arm or hand, keep your arm down and use a constricting band. *And always keep in mind that the chances are good you will make it to help.*

Bleeding

Bright red and "spurting" blood indicate a severed artery. Dark red, oozing blood indicate a severed vein. To stop bleeding:

- Place a large piece of the cleanest cloth or clothing available directly over the wound.
- Apply direct pressure with your hand for several minutes, or until bleeding stops.
- Raise a bleeding arm or leg if there is no other injury. Have the patient lie down to prevent fainting.
- Get medical attention immediately. If bleeding is severe, treat for shock, p. 89.
- If a limb, finger, or toe has been amputated, wrap the amputated part in gauze or a clean cloth, seal it in a plastic bag and put it in ice water or on ice. With proper care the part may be able to be sewn back on.
- DO NOT use a tourniquet or bind the wound so tightly as to cut off circultion to a limb.
- DO NOT remove an impaled object; you may make the bleeding worse.

To treat a nosebleed, *see* p. 246.

Bone Injuries

Bone fractures and sprains (torn ligaments) are characterized by intense pain, often very localized; swelling; discoloration; loss of motion; and, if severe, a deformity, such as a lump or abnormal bend.

First Aid

- Control bleeding, if any, using pressure bandages as described above.
- If a fracture of the neck or back is suspected, *Do Not Move the Patient* without medical supervision unless failure to do so (a burning car; victim in the water) would result in grave harm.

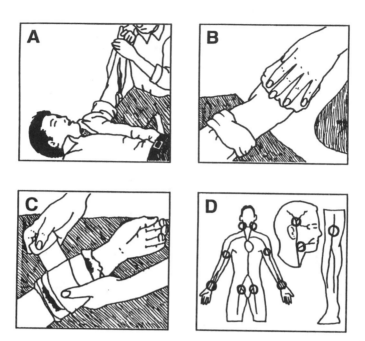

Figure 3. *How to Treat Severe Bleeding.* Measures for the treatment of severe bleeding are temporary, and additional medical help is not only advisable, but often necessary. **A.** To reduce blood flow, have the injured person lie down, and where feasible, elevate the wounded body part and remove or wash out foreign material. **B.** Stop the bleeding by holding the wound's edges together tightly and pressing a sterile pad securely over it. **C.** If necessary, use more pads until blood seepage stops, bandaging them so as to maintain firm pressure. When bleeding cannot be stopped by these efforts, the nearest major artery should be pressed firmly to its underlying bone. **D.** Key arterial pressure points on the head, body, and limbs are illustrated here.

- In such dire emergency, try to keep the victim's head, neck and body in a straight line, preventing the back from being twisted or bent during movement, and thus averting permanent paralysis. Use a board or length of rigid plywood to support the body if these are at hand.
- For other fractures and sprains, apply splints long enough to extend beyond the joints above and below the fracture. Any firm material can be used: a board, heavy or folded cardboard, umbrellas, metal rods, even magazines or a pillow wrapped around the injured area. You should pad hard splints with cloth or paper to prevent skin injury. Secure the splint(s) with ties placed at the injury and just beyond the joints above and below the injury.

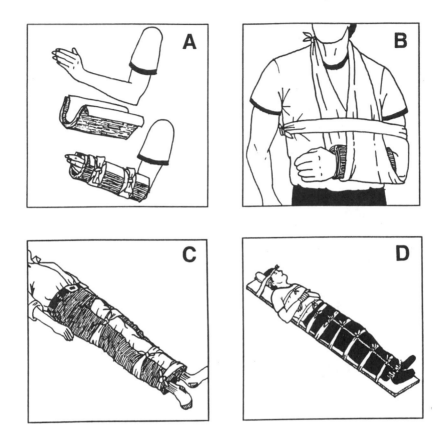

Figure 4. *How to Treat Injuries to Limbs and Bones.* These emergency measures should be used only while additional medical help is being obtained. **A.** Broken arms are placed in splints of wood, rolled paper, or other firm materials. After delicate straightening, ties are placed firmly above and below the break. **B.** A fabric sling that moderately elevates the hand above the elbow is then used to restrict movement of the damaged limb. Use a horizontal fabric strip to further restrict movement where this will be helpful. **C.** For broken legs, a full-length board or other firm, straight material is placed between the limbs; if padding is available, use it generously to cushion the limb. The broken limb is then gingerly aligned, and the board is tied in several places, though not near the break, in a manner that immobilizes both legs. **D.** Injuries to the neck or back are extremely dangerous, and can rapidly result in paralysis or death if treated improperly; thus, whenever possible, proper medical help should be obtained before any first-aid measures are attempted. If help is not available, immobilize the injured party's head, neck, and spine by tying them firmly to a board, bench, or other full-length hard object, and then padding and strapping them to it in several places, as shown here.

- In the event of a "compound fracture" (in which the skin is broken by bone fragments), keep the area as clean as possible. Cover with sterile dressing if available. Do not attempt to push the bone back under the skin.
- Apply a cold pack (e.g., ice cubes in a towel) around the splinted injury to minimize internal bleeding and swelling. Remember that swelling is the principal cause of pain.
- Get medical attention.

Breathing Problems

If breathing stops, the victim needs mouth-to-mouth resuscitation. While someone is calling for an ambulance, you should:

- Lift the neck gently and tilt the head back. Put your cheek and ear close to the victim's mouth and nose. Look, listen, and feel for breathing.
- If you cannot detect breathing, pinch the nostrils shut while continuing to support the neck with the other hand. Place your mouth over the victim's mouth and give two quick, full breaths.
- Be sure air is getting to the victim's lungs. You must see the chest rise and fall with your breaths. If the chest does not rise and fall, check the victim's position and check for airway obstruction (p. 76).
- Check again for breathing, and check for a pulse on the side of the neck.
- If there is a pulse, but no breathing, give one full breath every 5 seconds for adults (one puff every 3 seconds for infants). Remove your mouth between breaths so the victim can exhale.
- If there is no pulse and no breathing, give CPR if trained to do so.
- If the victim does not breath, death or permanent brain damage may occur in 4–6 minutes without CPR.

Burns

Minor Burns

- Flush the burned area with cold water for several minutes until pain is relieved.
- Apply sterile dressing. Do not break blisters; they seal out infection.
- Do not apply butter, ointments or other household remedies. They only retard healing.

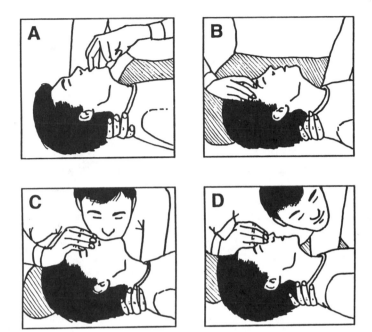

Figure 5. *How to Give Mouth-to-Mouth Resuscitation.* **A.** When a person's breath becomes extremely labored or ceases, quickly remove all foreign material from the oral and nasal passages, and lay the victim flat on a hard surface. **B.** Incline the head backward to raise the mouth and neck so that the air passages are as open as possible. **C.** Squeeze the nostrils shut with one hand, maintaining the other under the neck. Breathe deeply, then place your mouth tightly over the victim's and exhale strongly. **D.** When the nonbreather's chest is expanded, place your ear near the mouth and listen for sounds of air moving, observing whether the chest falls. Repeat this procedure several times per minute until breathing is restored or it is clear that nothing further can be done.

Major Burns

If the burn covers a large area or extends through the entire layer of skin (a third-degree burn), or if any burn occurs on the face, eyes, hands, feet, or genitalia:

- Rinse the burned area to remove as much dirt as possible. Do not remove dry clothing that adheres to the burn.
- Cover the burn with a sterile dressing or clean, dry clothing
- Call an ambulance.
- *Do not apply salves, ointments or other burn "remedies."*

Chest Pain

Sudden onset of chest pain, especially during or after exercise or strong emotion, may signal a heart attack. However, only a doctor can make this diagnosis. You should:

- Keep the patient calm.
- Call for an ambulance immediately. Remember that the victim's denial that a heart attack is in progress is to be expected, but procrastination can be fatal. Drive the victim to a hospital ONLY IF you cannot get an ambulance. If the patient gets worse while you are driving, there is nothing you can do to help. The ambulance crew is trained to render life support.
- If the victim is or becomes unconscious, check for pulse and breathing. If absent, begin CPR, if trained to do so.

Choking

If the victim can cough, speak, or breathe, DO NOT interfere with the victim's own efforts to rid whatever is blocking the airway.

If the Victim is Conscious

If the victim is *conscious* and cannot cough, speak, or breathe, administer abdominal thrusts (the Heimlich maneuver) as follows:

- Stand behind the victim, encircling the abdomen with your arms. Place one clenched fist just below the ribs, and your other hand on top of your fist.
- Give six to ten quick thrusts upward and inward.
- DO NOT use abdominal thrusts on pregnant women, infants or very small children *(see below)*.
- Since conscious people have gag reflexes and may also vomit into their lungs, do not use *finger sweeps* to remove foreign objects.

If the Victim is Unconscious

If the victim is unconscious, have someone call an ambulance immediately. Place victim with the back down, turn the head to one side, open the mouth and look for and remove any obstructing object.

Attempt mouth-to-mouth resuscitation (*See* Breathing Problems, p. 74). If successful, continue breaths every 5 seconds until the victim begins to breathe.

If you are unable to blow air into the victim's mouth, place the heel of your hand on the victim's upper abdomen and give a forceful push.

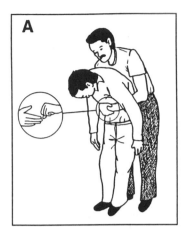 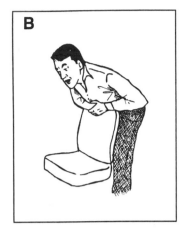

Figure 6. *The Heimlich Maneuver.* **A.** When the choking victim is standing or sitting, hold them from behind, as shown. Place one fist at the top of the abdomen, with the clenched thumb joint just below the breastbone. Grasp the clenched fist tightly with your other hand, and then force it sharply up and in. Repeat this movement until the food or foreign object is dislodged and breathing returns. **B.** If you ever find yourself alone and choking to death, you can perform the Heimlich maneuver on yourself. Simply stand over the back of a chair, or some other similarly hard and nonmoving object, place the chairback under your breastbone, where the clenched fist would otherwise be, and pull yourself sharply down onto the chair until the choking is relieved. *Everyone should learn the simple Heimlich procedure since it may one day save your own life, or that of someone you know or love!*

This should force the object into the mouth from which it can be removed manually.

Infants

For *infants* under one year of age: place the infant face down, supported by your hand and your arm. Rest your forearm on one thigh and deliver four brisk blows with the heel of your other hand between the infant's shoulder blades. If breathing is not restored, roll the infant over on the back and administer four rapid chest thrusts with two fingers over the breastbone (sternum) between the nipples.

If breathing is still not restored, open the victim's mouth by grasping both the tongue and the lower jaw between thumb and finger and lifting upward. This maneuver draws the tongue away from the back of the throat and may help dislodge an obstruction. If the object is seen, it may be manually extracted by a *finger sweep* using the index finger. Blind sweeps may cause further obstruction and should be avoided. If breathing is still not restored attempt ventilation with two breaths by mouth-to-mouth breathing. If necessary, repeat all of the above steps while someone is seeking emergency medical help.

Children

For *children* over one year of age who are choking and who cannot breathe: immediately place the child with back down. Place the heel of your hand on the child's abdominal midline between the navel and the rib cage. Give 6 to 10 abdominal thrusts using an upward motion until the object is expelled. If breathing is not restored, open the child's mouth and try the lift-jaw technique described above. If an object can be seen, sweep the obstructing object out with your index finger. If necessary, attempt mouth-to-mouth breathing and repeat the above steps.

Note: *Abdominal thrusts can cause internal injury.* They should be practiced in a CPR course. If used, the victim must have medical attention after breathing has been restored to check for possible injury.

Prevention

Choking is especially common in children because of their small-diameter airways and poorly developed habits of chewing. You can do much to prevent choking in small children by observing the following precautions:

- Avoid giving small children nuts, grapes, hard candies, and hot dogs. Almost half of all their choking incidents involve these foods.
- Always be present when children are eating. Encourage them to chew their food well.
- Never allow children to eat or drink while lying down.
- Cut up food into small pieces and give small amounts at a time
- Don't let children toss food into their or others' mouths. This is not only rude behavior; it is dangerous.

Cuts, Bruises, and Blisters

Cuts

For small cuts, rinse with running water, then clean the cut with soap and water. Apply a sterile gauze dressing or band-aid. Change the bandage if it gets wet or dirty. Two to three days is usually long enough for healing to close a shallow cut. A white, wrinkled skin beneath a bandage is a sign that the bandage has been too wet or has been on too long. Antiseptic solutions such as iodine and merthiolate are not necessary.

For large or deep cuts, apply a dressing and press firmly to stop bleeding. Use a tourniquet only if bleeding can't be stopped using pressure. Wrap with a bandage and see your doctor for suturing, tetanus shot, and evaluation.

Puncture Wounds

A puncture wound caused by a nail or sharp penetrating object may not bleed enough to wash out bacteria. Bleeding may be encouraged by pressing gently around the wound. Then wash with soap and water and apply a gauze dressing. If the wound is deep, keep the wound open by washing daily and changing the dressing. If you have not had a tetanus shot within five years or you don't know when you had your last tetanus shot, consult your doctor. If infection develops, the wound will become red, swollen and tender. See your doctor who may recommend antibiotics.

Puncture wounds of the hand are especially serious because infection may spread rapidly through many layers of tissue. See your doctor at once. Any puncture wound to your head, chest, or abdomen needs prompt medical attention because of possible internal injury.

Bruises

Apply a cold compress (e.g., ice cubes wrapped in a towel) for half an hour to relieve pain and minimize swelling. If the skin is broken, treat as a cut or scrape. For wringer injuries and bicycle spoke injuries, see your doctor.

Blisters

Blisters are caused by excessive friction on warm, moist skin. By far the majority of blisters in a lifetime occur on your hands and feet. Blisters form when the friction finally separates the upper layer, the epidermis, from the dermis below and fluid fills the space between.

The best treatment for an unbroken blister is to gently cleanse it with soap and water, cover it with a bandage, and apply additional padding (gloves, socks) to prevent further injury. Most blisters should not be broken because the fluid will reabsorb naturally and the intact skin prevents infection. If a blister develops on your foot, or an area that cannot be protected from further chafing, wash it gently but thoroughly with soap and water, sterilize a needle over an open flame, and puncture the blister on the side, just above the junction with normal skin. DO NOT remove the overlying skin. The upper and lower layers will adhere and heal faster. If the top layer comes off by itself, wash the area with soap and water, and then bandage the blister. It is advisable, but not necessary, to apply an antibiotic ointment to an open blister. Consult your doctor if you develop tenderness, pus, swelling, and red streaks around the blister, fever, or swollen lymph nodes, that signal deep, spreading infection.

Eye Injuries

Foreign Objects

- If you get something in your eye, do not rub the eye. Grasp the upper lid with your thumb and index finger and pull it down and over the lower eyelid; then roll your eye in all directions. Often the object will adhere to the dry outside of your lower lid, bringing instant relief.
- If this fails, look into a mirror. If you can see a speck over the white part of your eye, try to wick it out with the corner of a clean paper tissure. If the speck is over the colored part of your eye, *don't touch it*, you may scratch the cornea.
- If this fails, run plain water gently over your open eye. Dry your eyes and repeat the above.
- If the object cannot be washed out, it may mean that you have scratched your cornea, which gives the same sensation as having something in your eye. Cover your eye with a bandage. If, 12 hours later, it still feels like something is in your eye, get medical help promptly.

Wounds

A blow that wounds the eyelid or eyeball is potentially quite serious. Apply a loose sterile dressing over both eyes. Get medical attention at once.

- For a bruise, or "black eye," apply a cold compress or ice pack to relieve pain and reduce swelling during the first 24 hours. The next day, hot compresses may be applied to hasten absorption of the subcutaneous blood (hematoma). If you experience blurring, double vision, flashing lights, or floating specks, get medical attention at once—you may have a detached retina (*see* p. 135).

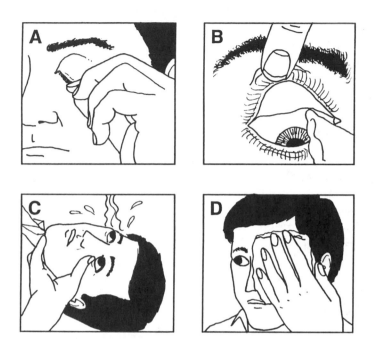

Figure 7. *Treating Eye Injuries.* **A.** When you feel that something is in your eye, but you cannot see it, try pulling your eyelid down and away to loosen the foreign object, which may then be swept away as the lid retracts. **B.** If there is a visible foreign object, do not rub your eye. Instead, try (or have a friend try) to remove it with a damp tissue corner. **C.** If that fails, or seems inappropriate for any reason, try washing your eye with a stream of water while you or a friend holds the lid open. The object can then often be readily removed by wiping the area where it is lodged gently with a damp cloth. **D.** If all these measures fail, cover the eye with a soft bandage and seek appropriate medical help.

Chemical Contamination

Wash the affected eye with copious amounts of cool, fresh water for 15 minutes. Do not rub your eyes. Call for an ambulance to an emergency room at once. Do not instill medications into your eye without a doctor's advice.

Fainting

Fainting (known medically as *syncope*) results from a sudden reduction of blood flow to the brain, usually as a result of temporary fall in cardiac output. Usually, this loss of consciousness is only momentary; as soon as the individual lies or falls down, normal blood flow returns to the heart, and blood flow to the brain is restored. There are many causes of fainting in otherwise healthy individuals: emotional stress, pain, fear, and hunger. There may be serious underlying causes, such as heart disease, inner ear problems, diabetes, or drug reactions, but usually the cause is benign.

- If someone faints in your presence, help them lie down and try to keep them from injuring themselves in falling.
- Turn the victim's head to the side and keep the mouth clear, in case of vomiting.
- Loosen constricting clothing and elevate the legs. Smelling salts probably won't be available and do not offer any advantage over waiting return of consciousness.
- Check pulse and respiration to make certain they are present. If not, begin CPR if you are trained to do so.
- Do not throw water in the victim's face. Although this is admittedly dramatic, it is not pleasant for the one who has fainted and it is not an effective reviving technique.
- After the person has revived, do not get them up quickly. Time for recovery is needed.
- If the person is very slow to revive or if fainting has been recurrent, call a doctor.
- If *you* feel faint or dizzy, lie down immediately to keep from falling down. Do not succumb to embarrassment and so hurry to resume normal activity. Check your pulse for regularity. If it is irregular or if you are uncertain why you became "giddy," see your doctor.

Frostbite

Frostbite is an insidious injury because the victim is already cold and may be entirely unaware of the numbness caused by frostbite. The first phase of frostbite is *frostnip*, which occurs before the tissues actually freeze. Frostnip is characterized by blanched skin, usually over the nose, ears, hands, or feet. First aid for frostnip consists of placing a warm hand over the affected area, or placing the frostnipped hands against the abdomen until color returns and numbness disappears. Do not rub the area; this only risks inducing trauma.

Frostbite is caused by exposure to dry cold air several degrees below freezing which results in actual freezing of a layer of exposed skin. Usually this layer is relatively thin, while healthy tissue lies below. The area is numb and the overlying skin is stiff and white. Prompt attention is needed to prevent further injury that may require amputation. The victim should be gotten indoors as quickly as possible. Immersion of the frostbitten area in warm (not hot) water is the most effective way to rapidly warm frozen skin. Be careful not to expose frostbite to a fire or a heater, because sensation in the frozen skin will have been lost and burning cannot be felt. Medical attention should then be sought, expecially if pain and swelling occur. Frozen feet should not be warmed if the victim must walk some distance for help, because trauma to the thawed tissue only increases the injury.

Frostbite is more easily prevented than treated. Remember the important "heat robbers":

- Wet skin and clothing. Moist skin and wet clothing efficiently conduct heat *away* from the body. Contact with metal or other cold objects does the same. Clothing should be loose to trap warm air.
- Exposed hands, feet, and head can account for up to 70% of body heat losses. Wind, especially on the head and extremities, magnifies these losses.
- Alcohol. Contrary to the popular belief in the "warming" effects of alcohol, it actually dilates surface blood vessels, thus promoting heat loss.
- Smoking. Nicotine constricts blood vessels in the extremities, thus increasing the liklihood of frostbite.

Head Injury

A blow to the head always carries the possibility of intracranial bleeding. You should seek immediate medical attention if:

- The victim is or was unconscious at any time.
- There is blood or fluid coming from the ears, nose, or mouth.
- The victim appears to be confused, disoriented, or staggers.
- The victim vomits.
- There are complaints of dizziness, nausea, double vision, or headache lasting longer than a few minutes.
- Pale skin color that does not return to normal in a short time
- The pupils are of unequal size.

In the meantime, cover open wounds lightly with a sterile dressing. Keep the victim warm and lying down, and give reassurance that help is on its way.

DO NOT apply pressure to head wounds nor try to stop blood or clear fluid (a possible skull fracture with spinal fluid leak) coming from the ears or nose.

Heat Cramps, Heat Stroke, and Heat Exhaustion
How the Body Regulates Heat

The human body conserves heat in cold weather by constricting blood vessels and by increasing its rate of metabolism through shivering. In hot weather, the body dissipates excess heat by dilating blood vessels, increasing heart rate, sweating, and to a small extent by increasing breathing rate. All of these adaptations are quite limited so that we live comfortably only within a very narrow range of temperature variation. The skin handles about 90% of the body's heat dissipation capacity by increasing blood flow to the skin and by sweating to increase skin moisture evaporation.

Sweating by itself does nothing to cool the body. It is the evaporation of sweat that removes heat from the skin, which in turn lowers the core body temperature. In hot weather the skin may lose as much as 2–3 gallons of water per day through sweating. Since high humidity retards evaporation, the heat dissipation capacity of sweating is reduced as air humidity rises. Sunburn causes skin changes that interfere with sweating, thus compromising this important temperature-regulating mechanism. Chronic diseases and alcoholism reduce the ability to regulate temperature, as do numerous drugs, including antihistamines, anticholinergics, sedatives, tranquilizers, diuretics, and antihypertensive and anti-Parkinsonism drugs.

Two other factors affect the body's temperature regulation: age and acclimatization. As we grow older, we lose our ability to quickly regulate temperature. By far the majority of all people who die each year of heat disorders (more than all deaths from lightning, hurricanes, tornadoes, floods, and earthquakes), are over 50 years of age. Very small children are also subject to heat disorders. Their small size allows them to take on heat much faster than adults. They also cannot indicate their thirst, except through irritability. They are completely dependent upon adults to make certain they get enough fluids.

On the other hand, acclimatization has to do with the ability to adjust the concentration of salt in the sweat to minimize body salt imbalance. As you become acclimatized to higher outside temperatures, you reduce the salt in the your sweat to conserve the total body supply.

Too Much Heat

When heat gain exceeds the body's ability to lose it, or the body cannot compensate for salt and fluid losses, the body's temperature begins to rise. This in turn results in heat disorders, which, ranked by increasing severity are: heat cramps, heat exhaustion, and heat stroke.

Heat Cramps

These are muscular pains and spasms caused largely by loss of salt through sweating or by inadequate salt intake. These symptoms signal that unless something is done, heat exhaustion and heat stroke will follow.

FIRST AID MEASURES

- Give the victim sips of salt water (1 tsp of salt per 8-oz glass) giving a glass every 15 minutes for one hour.
- The cramps can be relieved by firm pressure on the cramping muscles, or gentle massage, until muscles are relaxed.
- Minimize all physical activity and get the victim into the shade, or better, into an air-conditioned room.

Heat Exhaustion

As salt and water losses continue, the signs of heat exhaustion (or "heat prostration") set in: a pale, *cool*, clammy skin. The victim may complain of fatigue, weakness, anxiety, nausea, dizziness, and possibly cramps. The temperature may be normal, but the pulse is usually slow and relatively weak (termed a "thready" pulse).

FIRST AID MEASURES

- Get the victim out of the sun and into an air-conditioned room.
- Loosen clothing and apply cool, wet cloths.
- Give sips of salt water (1 tsp of salt per 8-oz. glass), giving a glass every 15 minutes for one hour.
- If the victim vomits or is difficult to revive, seek medical attention at once.

Heat Stroke

Also known as sunstroke, this is a life-threatening emergency with a high mortality, even among the young. Heat stroke may follow quickly after heat exhaustion and represents a complete failure of heat regulation. This occurs as the hypothalamus (the brain's function control center) directs blood flow to the brain and away from the skin. Consequently, sweating ceases and the body temperature rises rapidly to 105–108°F. The victim's skin is hot, flushed, and dry, the pulse rapid and strong. The victim is usually unconscious. If body temperature is not lowered at once, convulsions and death result.

Heroic first aid measures are essential. Every effort must be made to lower the victim's temperature as quickly as possible:

- Place the victim in a tub of cold water, a lake or stream, or use snow or ice packs, whatever is available while awaiting transportation to a hospital. *Warning:* If possible, measure rectal temperature every 10 minutes and do not lower body temperature below 101°F (38.3°C) to avoid circulatory collapse due to *hypothermia*.
- Do not give the victim stimulants.

How to Avoid Heat Disorders

For the most part, common sense is the best preventative:

- When it is hot, slow down. Strenuous activity in a hot environment with poor ventilation and high humidity is a prescription for disaster unless high intakes of salt and water are maintained.
- Dress for summer. Wear loose, light clothing. Outside wear a hat or take a parasol for portable shade.
- Drink plenty of fluids and do not allow yourself to get thirsty. Persons with chronic diseases or fluid-restricted diets should consult their doctors about fluid intake during hot weather.
- Avoid alcohol; it is a potent diuretic, causing increased fluid loss.
- Stay out of the sun if possible. Seek air-conditioned places such as malls, theaters, libraries, and museums if your home is not air conditioned. Use fans to circulate air and increase evaporation.
- Take cool baths or showers. Cool water removes body heat 30 times faster than cool air.
- Do not add to your inner fuel by heavy, high-protein meals. Digestion adds metabolic heat to your body and protein digestion increases water losses.

In some cases increased body temperature causes bizarre behavior that may be mistaken for a psychotic disorder, especially among the elderly ("summer madness"). Taking the person's temperature immediately points to the problem. Get medical help promptly.

Poisoning and Drug Overdosage

Poisoning by Mouth

The most difficult problem in treating poisoning is knowing whether or not the victim has been poisoned, and if so, what the poison is. It is rare that you will be told, "I just swallowed cyanide." If there is an empty container and the pills are still in the mouth, the question is quickly solved, but this too is rare.

You should suspect poisoning if you observe:

- An empty poison or pill bottle that you know was full.
- Fragments of pills, powder or poisonous plants evident.
- Burns around the mouth.
- Chemical odor on the breath.
- Victim is unconscious or drowsy.
- Pupils are dilated or contracted.
- Victim is convulsing or twitching.

First Aid

- Call the local Poison Control Center. If advised to induce vomiting, give Syrup of Ipecac from your medicine chest.
- Children under 1 year: obtain medical advice
- Children 1–10 years of age: 1 tablespoon (1/2 oz.) followed by 4–8 oz. water (1/2–1 glass). If no vomiting in 20 minutes, repeat *one* dose.
- Children over 10 years of age: 2 tablespoons (1 oz.) followed by 8 oz. water.
- Get the victim to an emergency room as soon as possible. Take any vomit and the poison container with you.

DO NOT induce vomiting if:

- Victim is unconscious, drowsy, or having convulsions. There is a danger of aspirating fluids into the lungs.
- Poison is corrosive (acid, lye, oven cleaner) or a petroleum product, unless otherwise directed by the Poison Control Center. These substances can often do more harm coming up than staying down.
- If the victim is unconscious. Maintain an open airway. Give CPR if needed and you are trained to do so.
- If the victim is having convulsions, DO NOT restrain. DO NOT insert your fingers, or hard objects, between the victim's teeth.
- If the airways become obstructed, tilt the victims head to correct it.
- After a convulsion, place the victim on the side so that fluids drain from the mouth.

Fumes and Gases

Fuel gases, auto exhaust, smoke from fires and fumes from poisonous chemicals can quickly overcome a victim. They can also quickly overwhelm you; do not enter a building you suspect of containing noxious gases to rescue someone if it will take longer than you can hold your breath.

If you can do so safely, get the victim into fresh air. Administer CPR if necessary and if you are trained to do so. Do not stop until the victim is breathing. Send someone for emergency help, but do not leave the victim.

Drug Overdoses

Activated charcoal is very effective in absorbing drugs still in the stomach. It can be purchased from a drugstore in the form of a slurry of activated charcoal and water. If you have small children, you should always have on hand Syrup of Ipecac (sold in 1-oz. bottles) and activated charcoal (sold in 25-, 30-, and 50-gram bottles) for use upon the advice of the Poison Control Center. The recommended dose of activated charcoal for children under 5 years of age is 30 grams.

Prevention

Most people are well aware of the importance of keeping poisons out of childrens' reach. Nevertheless, child poisonings occur with a surprising frequency in the United States: 3 million cases each year. Here are some facts to be aware of:

- In the majority of instances, parents were at home or nearby at the time of the poisoning.
- Many of the medicine overdosages in children occur because drugs have been put in the refrigerator within the child's easy reach. Very few medicines require refrigeration. They should be kept in a locked drawer or high medicine cabinet.
- A large percentage of accidental drug ingestions occur with child-resistant caps. They fail largely because repeated use causes wearing, which reduces their safety function. Always discard old medicine bottles. Do not reuse.
- A periodic home hunt to discard old medicines and poisons is a good practice to adopt. Old-fashioned remedies of little value (and which are unusually poisonous) include: oil of wintergreen, boric acid, ammoniated mercury, oil of turpentine, and camphorated oil.
- Children mimic adults. Do not take medicines within view of your small children.

- Nearly half of all accidental poisonings in the United States are caused by a small group of substances:

aspirin	cosmetics	vitamins	lye
Tylenol	insecticides	disinfectants	kerosene
bleach	soaps	deodorizers	laxatives
detergents	furniture polish		

Shock

There are numerous causes of shock, but most of the symptoms are caused by reduced blood flow to the brain. The person in shock is usually pale, clammy, and sweaty with a rapid, weak pulse. Confusion, drowsiness, thirst, and anxiousness are also common.

First Aid

- Lay the victim down, face up with the legs somewhat elevated to increase blood return to the heart.
- Loosen tight clothing and prevent heat loss by wrapping the person in a coat or blanket.
- Call for medical assistance.
- Do not give food or liquids unless help will be a long time arriving. Then, give only occasional sips of water to prevent dehydration.

Shoulder Dislocation

Falling on the outstretched arm can result in a painful dislocation in which the ball of the humerus comes out of the shoulder socket. You can recognize a dislocation by the obvious deformity of the shoulder as the skin is stretched over the joint.

First Aid

Do not attempt to reduce the dislocation yourself. Place a pillow under the arm and secure arm and pillow to the body by a strap or length of cloth. Place ice over the shoulder to reduce pain and swelling during the trip to the emergency room.

Stroke

Stroke occurs when one of the brain blood vessels becomes occluded or ruptures. The symptoms depend greatly upon how large the vessel involved is and where it is located. The usual symptoms include

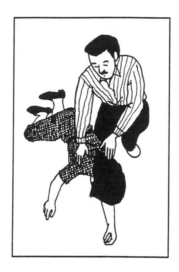

Figure 8. *Treatment of Seizures.* When the agitated movements of epileptic or other sufferers of seizures cease, the victims should immediately and
gently be placed in the recovery position (a basic sleep posture) illustrated
above. This curbs choking, and encourages restful sleep. During the seizure
itself, a victim's limbs should never be tightly constrained nor forcibly wrenched
to a supposedly proper position. Likewise, no effort should be made to force
open the mouths of seizure victims; they will not bite off or choke on their
tongues, but may well break a tooth, or even a jaw, when a foreign object is
forced into their mouths.

one or more of the following: loss of consciousness, paralysis, weakness, difficulty with speech, blurred vision, headache.
    If you suspect a stroke you should:

- Call an ambulance.
- Reassure the victim that help is on its way.
- If the victim is unconscious, tilt the head back and continue to check
  pulse and respiration.
- Stay with the victim.
- Avoid giving anything to eat or drink. *See* p. 93 for more discus-
  sion of stroke.

Seizures

    Seizures (convulsions) are most commonly associated with high
fever, head injury, poisoning, and epilepsy. A full-blown seizure is a
rather dramatic event with uncontrolled jerking movements and usu-

ally loss of consciousness. Remain calm. Do not attempt to restrain the victim during the seizure, but remove nearby objects that might be harmful if struck. Try to lay the victim flat with the head to one side to allow saliva or vomit to drain from the mouth.

Never put a solid object—especially your fingers—between the victim's teeth. Allow the victim to rest after the attack, but do not give anything to eat or drink. Seek immediate medical help.

Cross-section of the brain

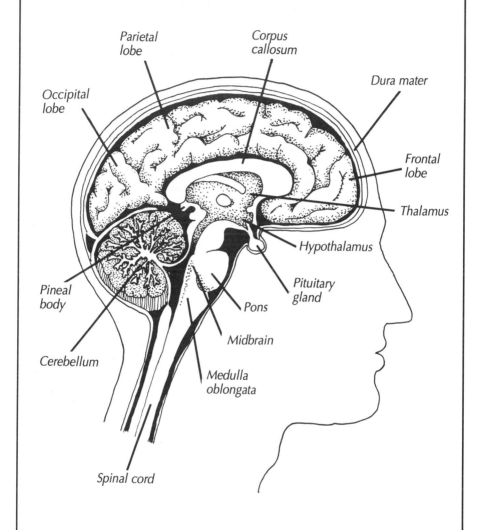

Parietal lobe

Corpus callosum

Dura mater

Occipital lobe

Frontal lobe

Thalamus

Hypothalamus

Pineal body

Pituitary gland

Pons

Cerebellum

Midbrain

Medulla oblongata

Spinal cord

Your Nervous System and Its Disorders

There are two principal parts to your nervous system: the *central nervous system* and the *peripheral nervous system*. The central nervous system includes the brain and spinal cord, whereas the peripheral nervous system includes all of the nerves and ganglia that supply the body. The peripheral nervous system also has two separate parts: the *somatic system* that controls all conscious activities, such as movement, and the *autonomic system* that controls such unconscious activities as heart rate, lung function, blood vessel tone, and intestinal motility.

The nervous system is subject to many types of disorders, including degeneration, vascular abnormalities, toxic effects, infections, trauma, and tumors.

Vascular Disorders of the Nervous System

Stroke

A stroke occurs when a part of the brain's blood supply is interrupted, resulting in death (*necrosis*) of a region of the brain. Strokes have three main causes:

Thrombosis. If an artery supplying part of the brain has been narrowed, usually by atherosclerosis (*see* p. 175), a blood clot (*thrombus*) may form at the point of narrowing and eventually block the flow of blood to that portion of the brain. About two thirds of all strokes occur in this way, with atherosclerosis as the underlying cause.

Embolism. A blood clot that forms in the heart or one of the larger arteries may break off to form a *thromboembolus*. This embolus will flow through the blood vessels until it becomes lodged in a smaller distant artery. If this narrower blood vessel happens to be in the brain, a stoke results. The likelihood of a brain vessel being thus blocked is high because the brain receives approximately one-fifth of the blood pumped by the heart.

Hemorrhage. In cerebral hemorrhage, one of the brain's blood vessels becomes weakened and eventually ruptures. When this occurs, blood seeps into and compresses the brain tissue, thus interrupting oxygen delivery to the brain. About half of such strokes prove fatal.

In rare cases, strokes result from a drastic fall in blood pressure (circulatory collapse), from carbon monoxide poisoning, from severe anemia, from acute blood loss, or from heart attack, all of which reduce the supply of oxygen to the brain.

Brain cells die within several minutes of being deprived of their blood supply. The region of brain tissue death is called a *cerebral infarction*. Once brain tissue dies, it is not able to regenerate. Functions can often be recovered, at least in part, but only when other parts of the brain are able to assume control of them.

Symptoms

Strokes that are caused by cerebral hemorrhage and embolism have a sudden onset. On the other hand, strokes caused by cerebral thrombosis may have a more gradual onset. The symptoms of a stroke depend of course on which brain vessel(s) are involved and the amount of brain tissue affected. Common symptoms include loss of consciousness, paralysis on one side of the body, numbness, blurred or double vision, slurred speech, confusion, and dizziness. Many strokes are first noticed upon rising in the morning, having occurred during the night when blood flow to the brain was diminished. The presence of severe headache is more suggestive of cerebral hemorrhage than thrombosis.

In about 10% of strokes, there is an advance warning in the form of one or more *transient ischemic attacks* (TIAs). These are in effect "ministrokes," signaling that a part of the brain is not getting enough oxygen, or that a very small cerebral embolism or thrombosis has occurred. Symptoms include temporary blindness in one eye, difficulty in speaking or writing, and transient numbness or weakness on one side of the body. These usually last only a few minutes with complete return to normal. TIAs should not be ignored because almost one-third of those who suffer such an attack will go on to have a full-blown stroke within five years.

DIAGNOSIS

If you think you, or someone you know, may have had a stroke, you should seek medical help at once. Usually, a CT (computerized tomography) scan of the brain will be performed to help distinguish an *ischemic* stroke (one that has no intracranial bleeding) from a hemorrhagic stroke, since their treatments are different. The CT scan is also

---

RISK FACTORS FOR STROKE

You are more likely to have a stroke if you:

- Are diabetic, especially if your blood sugar is difficult to control.
- Have high blood pressure that is not controlled by diet or medications.
- Have elevated blood cholesterol.
- Have suffered a heart attack, or shown evidence of coronary artery disease, since the same disease affects the blood vessels in the brain.
- Smoke. Smokers of 10 or more cigarets per day are twice as likely to suffer a stroke as those who do not smoke. The chances increase as the number of cigarets smoked increases. People who drink *and* smoke are even more likely to suffer a stroke.
- Are older, male, or black. Eighty percent of strokes occur in persons 65 or older. Men have a greater chance of suffering a stroke than women. The incidence of strokes is higher among blacks, probably because the incidence of high blood pressure is higher among blacks than whites.

---

useful in determining whether there are other causes of stroke-like symptoms, such as a brain tumor or aneurysm.

In the diagnosis of TIAs, Doppler ultrasound scans of the neck arteries are useful in detecting changes in the caliber of the vessels, as well as changes in the blood flow rate that signal the presence of narrowing. These scans are often accompanied by tests that measure pressure within the eye. Small differences in eye pressure suggest differences in blood flow rates, and therefore the presence of vascular disease. If doubt remains, cerebral angiography may be performed: dye is injected into the suspected arteries so that X-rays can distinctly outline the blood vessels in the head and neck. This test is not without risks of its own, including the possibility of worsening a stroke or, in rare instances, of hastening death.

Treatment. Since little can be done to aid recovery of brain tissue that has died, the principal aim of medical treatment is to prevent additional strokes. Anticoagulant drugs are given to prevent the formation of new clots. In some cases *thrombolytic* drugs that dissolve clots may be administered. In cases of bleeding, surgery may be necessary to relieve pressure within the skull.

Although the loss of function immediately following a stroke may be drastic, recovery of function through rehabilitation and retraining can also be dramatic. Other, uninvolved parts of the brain can take over a remarkable degree of the function lost by the damaged brain. Recovery is usually complete by six months, after which any remaining deficits are likely to persist.

In the case of TIAs, aspirin or dipyridamole (Persantine) is often prescribed to prevent blood clots from forming. When dangerous narrowing of blood vessels in the neck can be demonstrated, surgery may be recommended. The procedure chosen is usually a *carotid endarterectomy*, in which the diseased blood vessel is opened and cleaned out to relieve the obstruction. Before you consent to any such surgery, remember that both the endarterectomy and the angiogram that must be done beforehand have risks. Ask what these risks are in the hands of your doctor and the proposed hospital. If your doctor tells you that the risks are "very low," ask "How low?" If the combined risks of serious complications are greater than four percent, you are likely to be better off with more conservative treatment.

Intracranial Bleeding

The brain is covered by three membranous layers called the meninges. The outer layer, the *dura mater,* adheres closely to the inner side of the skull. The *pia mater* adheres closely to the brain, and the *arachnoid membrane* lies between. Between the pia and the arachnoid is a space, known as the *subarachnoid space*, which is normally filled with fluid. Bleeding can occur on the inside or outside of all of these layers, although their causes are usually different.

Bleeding outside the dura mater is called *extradural hemorrhage,* whereas bleeding on the inside of the dura mater is called *subdural hemorrhage.* Both types of bleeding are usually caused by head injuries that cause torn blood vessels. The symptoms appear within 24 hours of injury and include headache, confusion, drowsiness, nausea, and vomiting, and can result in coma and death.

Bleeding inside the pia mater is the same as hemorrhagic stroke described above.

Bleeding beneath the arachnoid membrane, *subarachnoid hemorrhage,* is more often the result of a stroke or rupture of a brain blood vessels. Often rupture is through an *aneurysm,* a localized dilatation of a weakened blood vessel, or an *arteriovenous malformation* (an abnormal mass of dilated blood vessels that tend to bleed). Symptoms of subarach-

---

PREVENTION OF STROKE

An examination of the risk factors for stroke listed above points to obvious things you can do to lessen the likelihood of a stroke:

- Lowering your blood pressure to normal is the single most effective means of preventing strokes.
- Do not smoke. Smoking increases the likelihood of having a stroke. A group that is at particularly high risk includes women who have migraine headaches, take contraceptive pills, and smoke. If you fit into this group, just stopping smoking can greatly reduce your risk of stroke.
- Reduce your blood cholesterol if it is elevated (*see* p. 193).
- Ask your doctor whether you should take daily aspirin to prevent stroke and heart attacks (*see* p. 182).

---

noid hemorrhage are similar to those of subdural hemorrhage and may include stiff neck and sensitivity to bright light (photophobia). Headaches may be particularly severe.

If you develop any of these symptoms, particularly after head injury, get medical help at once. Diagnostic CT scans will be taken to determine the site and probable cause of the bleeding.

Treatment. Extradural and subdural bleeding are usually treated surgically to repair the damaged blood vessels and remove any clotted blood (*hematoma*). If an aneurysm or arteriovenous malformation is discovered, the surgeons may either "clip" or remove it. When surgery is undertaken early, the chances of full recovery are often good.

First aid for the treatment of head injuries is discussed on p. 83.

Infections

Infections of the brain and meninges may be caused by either bacteria or viruses. Early recognition and treatment of these serious infections can be life-saving.

Meningitis

Meningitis is an inflammation or infection of the membranous layers covering the brain and spinal cord. Infections may be either bacterial or viral. Microorganisms can reach the meninges through the bloodstream, by way of infected ears, through infected sinuses in the skull, and through skull fractures following head injury. Meningitis is most common during childhood, but may occur at any age.

The symptoms of meningitis are fever, headache, stiff neck, nausea and vomiting, and intolerance of bright lights (*photophobia*). The onset of these symptoms is usually more rapid in bacterial than in viral meningitis. In rare cases, a deep red skin rash may be present.

Treatment. Meningitis is a serious infection that must be treated in the hospital. The type of meningitis is determined by examination of the spinal fluid. Bacterial meningitis is treated with intravenous antibiotics, often for as long as two weeks. Viral meningitis does not respond to antibiotics, but usually resolves by itself in 2–3 weeks. Supportive measures include bed rest, plenty of liquids, and drugs to manage fever, headache, and increased intracranial pressure.

Encephalitis

Encephalitis is an inflammation of the brain cells that is most often caused by viruses. Encephalitis may be either primary or secondary to other diseases. Examples of primary viral encephalitis include both *herpes encephalitis* and the *equine encephalitis* that is caused by a mosquito-borne virus. Secondary encephalitis may occur 5–10 days after bouts of measles, chicken pox, rubella, smallpox, and even following vaccinations. In secondary encephalitis, the virus probably does not attack the brain directly, but instead affects it by means of an immune reaction. A rare encephalitis, caused by a "slow" virus, is Creutzfeldt-Jakob disease, which takes years to manifest itself in adults as a dementia.

The symptoms of viral encephalitis may be very mild, with only a low fever and muscle aches and pains, thus resembling the flu. In more severe cases, there is restlessness and irritability, drowsiness, confusion, muscular weakness, and impaired speech and hearing. Rarely, seizures, coma, and death result. Some patients also exhibit all the symptoms of meningitis—fever, headache, vomiting, and stiff neck.

The diagnosis of encephalitis is made after examinations of the spinal fluid, electroencephalograms, and demonstration of rising levels of antibodies to the virus.

Treatment. In severe cases there are some antiviral drugs, such as acyclovir and interferon, that limit the severity of encephalitis and help prevent permanent nerve damage. Most patients recover completely in a few weeks. Children and the elderly are at greatest risk of death and serious disability from the disease.

Brain Abscess

A *brain abscess* is a collection of pus within the brain, or between the skull and the dura mater. Bacterial infections are the most common cause of abscesses, arising from the same mechanisms that cause meningitis (*see above*)—head injury, sinus and ear infections, tooth extractions, or the presence of infected emboli from the heart (*see* Endocarditis, p. 200). The expansion of walled-off pus can dangerously compress the brain and may prove fatal if left untreated.

The symptoms include headache, nausea, vomiting, drowsiness, seizures, and muscular weakness. The diagnosis is made by CT scanning and by examination of the spinal fluid.

Treatment. Brain abscesses are treated by long-term intravenous antibiotics and by surgical drainage if antibiotics do not relieve the swelling.

Polio *(Poliomyelitis)*

Poliomyelitis is a viral disease that attacks the brain and spinal cord, particularly the nerves that control muscle movements. The virus is highly contagious and is frequently epidemic in unvaccinated populations. Transmission occurs through personal contact with others who have become infected. The disease begins typically with fever, headache, sore throat, and general aches and pains. In severe cases polio leads to muscular weakness and permanent paralysis.

There is no specific treatment for polio. Symptomatic care involves bed rest and analgesics for pain. Every child should be immunized according to the schedule shown on p. 25. *Adults traveling to countries with endemic polio should also be reimmunized.*

Brain Tumors

Brain tumors may arise from any of the tissues within the skull, including the skull itself, the meninges, the cranial nerves, the brain-supporting tissues (gliomas), blood vessels, the pituitary, and the pineal body. Of course, secondary tumors that spread (metastasize) from tumors outside the skull can also affect brain structures. All brain tumors are serious, whether they are benign or malignant, because of the many vital structures within the brain whose function they may compromise, and the fact that the skull does not permit the expansion of growing tumors without compressing the brain, which also impairs its functionality.

The symptoms of brain tumors depend to a great extent on the structures in and around the areas in which they arise. However, there are symptoms associated with increased intracranial pressure that apply to many brain tumors. The latter include headaches that are more painful when you are lying down. Later these headaches may be accompanied by nausea and vomiting. Seizures, either generalized or confined to one limb, may occur. Drowsiness, lethargy, personality changes, and other impairment of mental functions are common. Dizziness, paralysis, loss of smell, behavioral disorders (psychoses), and visual distortions all depend on the location of the tumor.

Tumors of the pituitary gland can produce a variety of syndromes, caused by the uncontrolled production of one or more of the various pituitary hormones. For example, pituitary adenomas that secrete growth hormone may cause either dwarfism or gigantism (*see* p. 161). Tumors that produce excess ACTH cause Cushing's syndrome (*see* p. 167). Other pituitary tumors may cause visual and sexual behavior disturbances in both men and women.

The diagnosis of brain tumors has become quite sophisticated in recent years. Tests to locate the tumor and determine secondary effects, such as swelling and hemorrhage, include CT scanning, magnetic resonance imaging (MRI) radioisotope scans, electroencephalography, and arteriography.

Degenerative Disorders and Dementias

This group of disorders is characterized by selective destruction of nerve cells in the brain or spinal cord. The cause of nerve degeneration is still unknown, but recent advances in medicine have improved and prolonged life in many cases.

Parkinson's Disease

Parkinson's disease is caused by the slow degeneration of nerve cells that produce the chemical, dopamine, within the brain. Dopamine is essential for the regulation of fine and slow movements throughout the body. The supply of dopamine gradually decreases in all of us as we grow older, but in victims of Parkinson's disease, the loss is so great that it interferes with essential muscle functions.

Parkinson's disease is predominantly characterized by three symptoms: muscle rigidity, resting tremor of the hands and feet, and reduced movement (hypokinesia). Rigidity is caused by increased muscular tone, and is most evident in the arms, legs, and facial muscles. The face becomes an expressionless mask, suggesting a depressed personality. Fine movement in the hands and arms is impaired, leading to awkward movements and smaller and smaller handwriting. Postural control is affected, leading to frequent falls. In advanced cases, the walking gait may become a series of minced little steps with the body bent forward as though it were trying to catch up with its own center of gravity, which indeed it is. As the disease progresses, slowed or slurred speech may develop and the victim may drool as control of the facial muscles becomes increasingly impaired. Eventually, memory loss and impaired mental function (dementia) occur in about half of all those affected.

Some victims of Parkinson's disease develop a "resting tremor," that is, a rhythmic movement of the arms or legs that is most pronounced at rest and decreases when the limb is moved. In some individuals the tremor may involve the jaw, tongue, forehead, and eyelids. The tremor usually increases when the individual becomes nervous or tired, hence the other name for this disease, *paralysis agitans.* As the disease advances, it becomes increasingly difficult to initiate new movements. For example, it may be difficult to turn over in bed. Taking the first step may require great effort, or it may be difficult to get up from of a chair.

Parkinson's disease occurs most often in the elderly or in late middle age, and is somewhat more common in men. The cause of the degeneration of dopamine-producing cells is not known, although a virus may be responsible.

Secondary *parkinsonism* can be caused by toxins or drugs that block dopamine receptors in the nerves. Drugs such as reserpine and haloperidol are especially prone to produce parkinsonism as a side effect.

Treatment. Several drugs are effective in reducing the tremor and rigidity of Parkinson's disease, although no treatment will reverse or halt progression of the nerve degeneration. Currently, the most effective drug is levodopa (L-dopa), which is a building block of dopamine. Dopamine itself cannot be administered because it will not enter the brain from the bloodstream. However, L-dopa readily enters the brain, where it is then converted to dopamine. Unfortunately, the effectiveness of L-dopa decreases with time.

A new drug, deprenyl, acts by blocking the breakdown of dopamine. Preliminary studies have shown that this drug effectively delays onset of the more serious symptoms of Parkinson's disease.

An experimental surgical operation developed in Mexico is now being investigated in which parts of the adrenal gland are transplanted into the brain. The adrenal gland is the endocrine organ that rests atop the kidneys and produces dopamine, among other hormones. Thus far, the results of such transplants have been disappointing, and research has been stalled by the unfortunate ban on fetal tissue use.

As practical measures, patients with Parkinson's disease should develop personal programs for maintaining good general health, combined with regular exercise and rest. Physical therapy programs may also be useful. It is important to remember that prescribed medications be taken exactly as directed and never varied unless ordered by your doctor. Suddenly to stop taking some of the drugs used to treat Parkinson's disease may well lead to total immobilization.

Parkinson's disease patients need a great deal of emotional support to help meet the stresses of the illness and to carry on courageously in spite of increasing disability. A supportive and sympathetic family is often their greatest gift.

It should be borne in mind that many people develop minor tremors as they grow older, so that their onset need not cause undue alarm. If other symptoms of Parkinson's disease develop at the same time, your doctor will be able to make the diagnosis and begin treatment.

For more information contact the Parkinson's Disease Foundation at 1-800-475-6676 or 1-212-923-4700.

Familial Tremor

Familial tremor, also known as fast-frequency "action tremor," is much more common than parkinsonism, and has a hereditary basis. Action tremors are made worse by purposeful motion and disappear at rest—just the opposite of the tremor that occurs in parkinsonism. Action tremors are lessened by alcohol and other sedating substances. Familial tremor usually begins after adolescence. When it occurs in the elderly it is referred to as senile tremor. Usually no treatment is necessary; however, if it becomes severe or impedes useful activity, it can be treated effectively by such beta-blocking drugs as propranolol.

Huntington's Chorea

Huntington's chorea is a rare hereditary disease characterized by bizarre, uncontrollable movements, grimacing, slurred speech, and eventual mental deterioration (*dementia*). The term "chorea" means a dance, and derives from the walking gait in these patients, which sometimes seems to resemble a strange sort of dancing. The onset of symptoms usually occurs in middle age and is *always* associated with a family history of the disease. There is no cure for Huntington's chorea, although the abnormal movements can be partially suppressed by appropriate drugs, such as chlorpromazine or haloperidol. Genetic counseling is important, since half the offspring of an affected parent are at risk of developing the disease. Currently there is no absolute test to determine which offspring will become affected, although genetic testing can determine those who have a high or low risk for developing the disease. Such testing should always be undertaken in conjunction with counseling for psychological support.

Multiple Sclerosis

Multiple sclerosis (MS) is a disease of *myelin*, the whitish covering of nerve fibers that insulates them from each other, somewhat like electrical wire insulation. In MS the myelin sheath degenerates across many areas of the brain and spinal cord. The cause of the degeneration is not known, although it may possibly be a virus. The onset usually occurs between the ages of 20 and 40, and is more common in women.

The symptoms of multiple sclerosis are highly variable and depend upon the areas of nerve sheath degeneration. Classic symptoms include impaired vision, slurred speech, tremor, unsteadiness, numbness or weakness of arms or legs, difficulty urinating, fatigue, and emotional changes. The duration of symptoms may be brief, or last several weeks. The course of this disease is also highly variable. In some, only a single episode may occur, but more commonly, the symptoms occur repeatedly over 20–30 years, becoming more severe with each occurrence. In many cases these episodes are precipitated by infections, emotional trauma, injury, or pregnancy.

Treatment. Severe and debilitating symptoms are usually treated with steroid injections and bed rest until the symptoms subside. Numerous other drugs have been tried in those with serious debility. The frequency of recurrent episodes may be decreased by avoiding infection, trauma, and stress. In many instances the prognosis may be benign and consistent with a relatively normal life style.

For more information, contact the National Multiple Sclerosis Society. To receive a free packet of information, call 1-800-624-8236. To ask specific questions of the staff, call 1-800-227-3166.

Amyotrophic Lateral Sclerosis

Amyotrophic lateral sclerosis (ALS) is a degeneration of the nerve cells in the brain and spinal cord that control voluntary muscles. It is commonly referred to as Lou Gehrig's disease, after the famous baseball player who died of ALS in 1939. The cause of ALS is unknown.

The onset of ALS is gradual, beginning usually as a weakness in one limb, often a hand. Later, other limbs are affected as the nerves supplying those muscles shrink and disappear. Ultimately, complete paralysis may result. As the muscles of swallowing are affected, it becomes difficult to control eating and swallowing, and inhalation of food and drink becomes a risk. Death usually occurs within five years of diagnosis.

There is no cure for ALS, and no effective treatment, except learning to cope with the progressive disability. Emotional support from family and friends is crucial to help maintain a positive attitude.

Alzheimer's Disease and Other Dementias

The various dementias are more or less similar in that they are associated with an overall decline in mental functions, particularly in memory and reasoning. Dementias may be "static" or progressive. Static dementia is fixed in the level of impairment and often follows brain surgery or a head injury in which a certain amount of brain tissue is destroyed.

Progressive dementias start gradually, and the degree of mental impairment becomes increasingly more pronounced. Examples include the dementias associated with drug and alcohol abuse, malnourishment, brain tumors, Huntington's disease, Creutzfeldt-Jakob disease, multiple sclerosis, multiple small strokes, and Alzheimer's disease. Progressive dementias are much more common than static dementias.

Alzheimer's Disease

Alzheimer's disease is a progressive dementia in which a particular region of the brain degenerates—specifically, the group of cells lying under the frontal lobes that produce the neurotransmitter substance, acetylcholine. These cells first lose their capacity to secrete acetylcholine and then degenerate still further. This region of the brain is critical to higher brain functioning and the formation of memories.

What triggers the degenerative process is not known. For some time it was theorized that a toxic effect of aluminum might be responsible because large quantities of aluminum were found in degenerated areas of the brain. A popular notion emerged that overexposure to aluminum cooking pots and pans, or that the absorption of the aluminum contained in antacids and antiperspirants was the mechanism responsible. However, there is little to support this notion. Aluminum is plentiful in nature—it is poorly absorbed, and is readily excreted from the body.

It is possible that a "slow" virus may be responsible for Alzheimer's disease, although the only reason for believing so is that such viruses are known to cause other brain degenerative diseases in both humans and in animals. It is also thought that a genetic component must be present that renders certain individuals susceptible to the disease, although the responsible gene has not yet been identified.

Whatever the cause, Alzheimer's disease is common. Currently about 7% of the population over 65 is affected, and this figure will increase substantially as our population ages. Although it seems that Alzheimer's disease is more prevalent than formerly, there is no evidence to suggest so; there are merely many more older people living today, and Alzheimer's is predominantly a disease of the elderly.

Symptoms. Short-term memory loss may be the first noticeable sign of a dementia. Gradually over months or years, powers of reasoning and understanding decline. This may be accompanied by a loss of interest in family and routine activities, social withdrawal, neglect of personal cleanliness, and disintegration of the personality.

Treatment of Dementias. Your approach to someone in whom you suspect the onset of dementia should be one of gentle persuasion to see a doctor. The doctor will most likely perform a battery of tests to exclude one of the treatable forms of dementia, such as depression, hypothyroidism, a brain tumor, syphilis, drug overdosage (especially tranquilizers, antihypertensive medications, barbiturates, and bromides), and vitamin B_{12} deficiency. Bear in mind that CT scans may demonstrate cerebral atrophy (a loss of gray matter), in normal individuals, where it is often simply a result of aging, and does not necessarily indicate an irreversible cause of dementia.

A loving and protective attitude toward patients with dementia will do a great deal to relieve anxiety and prevent depression—emotional complications that only make treatment more difficult and the patient miserable. Friends and relatives should be encouraged to visit, and the maintenance of a bright, stimulating environment will help prevent social withdrawal. In the same way, providing memory aids helps people help themselves in day-to-day living. Such aids can include a large, visible calendar; a list of daily activities; written notes about simple safety measures; and directions for using, as well as labeling of, commonly used items. Occasionally, mild sedatives, anti-depressants, and antipsychotic drugs may be useful in controling behavior. The new drug, tacrine, may be helpful in mild cases.

For more information about Alzheimer's disease, dementias, and their self-help groups in your area contact:

Public Affairs Officer, National Institute on Aging, Federal Bldg. 31, Room SC-27, 9000 Rockville Pike, Bethesda, MD 20892; 1-301-496-1752.
Alzheimer' Disease and Related Disorders Association, 1-800-272-3900.

Finally, there is a worthwhile book entitled *The 36-Hour Day* by Nancy L. Mace and Peter V. Rabins, Johns Hopkins University Press, 1981.

Epilepsy

Most people associate epilepsy with seizures that start with the epileptic falling down, and then frothing at the mouth and biting the tongue while convulsing rhythmically. In fact, epileptic seizures come in a variety of forms, from episodes of slightly altered consciousness to generalized spasmodic seizures of the body and limbs. In about one-fourth of victims, the cause is recognizable as a focus of brain injury, tumor, or other physical stimulus, such as a drug, low blood sugar, or other agent. In most cases, no physical abnormality can be found. Presumably, an altered electric discharge in the brain spreads to other brain areas for yet unknown reasons.

Epileptic seizures may be *partial*, that is, they may involve only a limited area of the body, producing such limited effects as localized twitching of the muscles, chewing movements, smacking of the lips, smelling a strong odor, or visual hallucinations. Seizures may also be *generalized*, that is, they may involve total-body spasmodic shaking (*grand mal*), or merely absence of awareness or consciousness (*petit mal*). In the latter case, the seizure may appear as though the individual were "tuning out" or exhibiting sudden, but momentary loss of attention. Petit mal seizures are especially common in children. Such children are often mistaken as "day dreamers." Seizures may last from a few seconds to several minutes. After a seizure, there may be no awareness that anything has happened, or else there may be a prolonged period of slowness and fatigue as the brain "recovers."

Most epileptic seizures occur spontaneously, with or without an *aura* or warning. However, in *reflex epilepsy*, seizures occur under special circumstances, such as being exposed to flickering lights, passing from darkness to light, or being startled by a loud noise. In some cases, seizures may be initiated by drugs or by the withdrawal of alcohol in severely addicted individuals. Seizures are also associated with several systemic diseases, including water intoxication, thyroid storm, low blood sodium, low blood sugar, and kidney failure.

The diagnosis of epilepsy is often made by demonstrating characteristic patterns of electrical brain waves on the electroencephalogram. Laboratory tests and CT scans will also be ordered to rule out a treatable physical cause of the seizures.

Treatment. Children with petit mal seizures may grow out of their epilepsy as they grow older. In most cases, however, there is no cure, although anticonvulsant drugs are often effective in diminishing or preventing seizures. There are numerous anticonvulsant drugs, such as phenobarbital and dilantin, but none is effective for all types of seizures and many individuals must take several different drugs to suppress seizure activity effectively.

General principles of managing seizures include getting plenty of safe exercise, avoiding stressful situations and fatigue, and particularly avoiding alcohol and other drugs of abuse. All epileptics should be encouraged to live a normal life. Most state licensing agencies permit driving after seizures have stopped for one year.

The first-aid management of seizures is discussed on p. 90.

Tourette Syndrome

Tourette syndrome is a fairly common neurological disorder that affects about 100,000 Americans in its fully developed form and up to one in 200 people may have a mild form.

In Tourette syndrome, certain nerve impulses in the brain get jumbled and trigger a variety of unusual behaviors known as *tics*. These are involuntrary movements that have no purposeful reason and may be repeated over and over again. Such behaviors include exaggerated blinking, grimacing, jerking the head or shoulders, or smacking the lips. More complicated maneuvers are also possible, including kicking, striking out at others, throwing things, or repeatedly touching one's body or that of others. In its simplest form, the tic may involve clicking sounds with the tongue, or repeatedly clearing one's throat.

Of course, not all tics are signs of Tourette syndrome. Some people may habitually repeat such actions as straightening their hair or clothing out of nervous habit. The difference between such patterns and Tourette's is that the former is under conscious control and can be stopped with concentration.

Tourette syndrome begins in childhood and often lasts for life. The tics may come and go, and they may also change over time. Generally, they are worse when you are tired or anxious and improve with relaxation.

There is no specific test for Tourette syndrome; the diagnosis is made by the individual history. This syndrome is associated with learning disabilities, attention deficit disorder, and sleeping difficulties. The syndrome runs in families, so that more than one member of a family may be affected.

There is no cure for Tourette syndrome, although such medicines as haloperidol or clonidine can relieve symptoms. In many individuals, the tics are not so disabling that medicine is required.

For more information, contact the Tourette Syndrome Association, 42-40 Bell Blvd., Bayside, NY 11361 (1-800-237-1717). Many cities have local support groups.

Tardive Dyskinesia

Tardive dyskinesia is a disorder that resembles Tourette syndrome in some respects, but is, in fact, a side effect of certain antipsychotic drugs such as Haldol, Loxitane, Stelazine, Prolixin, Navane, Thorazine, Trilafon, and Mellaril. Tardive means "late" and dyskinesia means "abnormal movement."

Tardive dyskinesia most often affects the muscles of the face, hands, and feet. It usually begins with uncontrollable fine movements of the tongue and lips that may eventually lead to more exaggerated tic-like movements, such as puckering and smacking the lips, sticking the tongue out, chewing behavior, grimacing, and frowning. Uncontrollable movements of the hands, arms, and legs, such as neck twisting and body jerking, may also occur.

The development of these side effects is related to the dose and the length of time a person continues to take one of the causative drugs. Once these motions develop, they may be irreversible, though fortunately, the movements often disappear or lessen when the medicine is stopped. To decrease the chance of developing tardive dyskinesia, antipsychotic drugs should be taken only as needed and in the lowest dose necessary to control the symptoms they are meant to alleviate. Individuals taking these drugs should be examined periodically to detect the onset of tardive dyskinesia at the earliest possible time.

For more information, contact the Tardive Dyskinesia/Tardive Dystonia National Association, 4244 University Way NE, PO Box 45732, Seattle WA 98145; 1-206-522-3166.

Headaches

Headaches are so common that virtually everyone will experience them at one time or another. In fact nearly one-fourth of the disorders discussed in this book include headache as a possible symptom. However most headaches occur independently of other disorders, their onset is gradual, and they disappear after a few hours. Generally, headaches can be classified according to their cause: tension (or muscle-contraction) headaches, vascular headaches, and organic (associated with other symptoms) headaches.

HEADACHE WARNING SIGNS

Though most headaches are mild, short-lived, and benign, there are some warning signs that demand prompt medical attention:

- A severe headache accompanied by fever and a stiff neck that resists being bent forward may represent meningitis, an inflammation or infection of the membranes lining the brain that demands immediate medical treatment (*see* p. 97).
- A headache associated with impaired function, such as dizziness, paralysis, slurred speech, or double vision may be caused by bleeding, stroke, tumor, or abscess within the brain.
- Headaches that occur daily, require daily pain relievers, or that become progressively worse may represent high blood pressure or a brain mass, such as a tumor. Headaches that recur and are worse in the morning and get better during the day often signal high blood pressure.
- Sudden onset of excruciating headache, a so-called "thunderclap" headache, may represent brain hemorrhage.
- Pain at the temples in older people may represent *cranial arteritis*, a treatable condition that, untreated, may lead to blindness.
- Headaches occurring indoors or in a car that are accompanied by excessive drowsiness and/or nausea may represent carbon monoxide poisoning. Leave the room or car immediately.

Tension Headaches

Activity that places a strain on the muscles of the head and neck can lead to headaches, probably because the brain is not very good at localizing the precise area of tension when whole muscle groups are involved. Such factors as emotional distress (perhaps an argument, or a financial reversal) can lead to muscle tensing behavior and a headache. Activities that cause eyestrain or prolonged work in a hunched-over posture can also place strain on facial, eye, neck, or scalp muscles. Headaches are also associated with the temporomandibular joint (TMJ) syndrome, caused by tense jaw muscles and tooth grinding (*see* TMJ Syndrome, p. 278).

Vascular Headaches

The most common causes of headaches are those factors that cause constriction or dilation of blood vessels near the surface of the brain. These include the ordinary hangover, since alcohol dilates blood vessels. Certain foods rich in the amino acid, tyramine, also cause vascular headaches in susceptible individuals, as do nitrates and sulfites. Some foods that may cause problems include:

- Aged and processed cheeses
- Aged, canned, cured, or processed meats that contain nitrates
- Caffeine-containing foods or drinks, such as coffee, tea, colas, and chocolate
- Foods containing the flavor enhancer, monosodium glutamate (MSG)
- Foods made with soy sauce, yeast, or yeast extracts
- Wines, especially red wine, that contain sulfites

So-called "exertional" headaches are also vascular headaches. These occur after intense physical activities, including jogging, strenuous sports, or even sexual intercourse (post-orgasmic headache). Exertional headaches are usually mild and short-lived, but may be so excruciating as to prompt rushing to the emergency room. Numerous drugs and toxins (e.g., carbon monoxide) also cause vascular headaches.

Two special categories of vascular headaches are *migraine* and *cluster* headaches.

Migraines

Typically migraine headaches begin with a preliminary period, or *prodrome*, during which you feel unusually tired or out-of-sorts. This is followed by nausea, vomiting, visual disturbances, and often aversion to bright light (*photophobia*). This prodrome may last from several minutes to several hours and is followed by the headache itself. The headache may take many forms, and varies from one attack to another in the same individual, although with time, most sufferers of migraine can predict the kind of headache they will experience by the nature of the prodrome symptoms.

The name migraine derives from French and Greek and means "half a head" because the headache is often confined to one side of the head. The duration is variable, lasting at times up to 18 hours. The cause of migraine is unknown, although spasm of superficial brain arteries is known to be involved.

Cluster Headaches

These are a variant of the vascular headache, and typically strike the victim as a group of several headache episodes each day, often for days or weeks. Typically an attack begins at night, waking the unfortunate sufferer with an intense pain, often localized to one side of the head or around one eye. After one cluster headache, another may not occur for months or years. Like migraine, cluster headaches may be triggered by a particular food, by alcohol, or by stress.

Organic Headaches

Many headaches are associated with other symptoms, such as stiff neck (meningitis), fever (colds, flu, any severe infection), or intracranial disease (e.g., bleeding or brain tumor). Probably the most common organic headache is that associated with high blood pressure. If you have frequent headaches, you should certainly have your blood pressure checked.

Treatment. Simple tension and vascular headaches can usually be relieved by a pain reliever, such as aspirin or acetaminophen. Lie down and try to relax. Massage the muscles of your head and neck, or place a cool, damp compress over your forehead. Avoid alcohol and tobacco, and try to get a good night's sleep. If your headaches tend to recur, try to examine the stresses in your life to see whether, short of leaving your spouse or job, some simple adjustments can be made. For severe and recurrent headaches, you will need to see your doctor. Narcotics may be required for very severe headaches. Also ask your doctor about biofeedback techniques to control headaches.

For migraine and cluster headaches, several drugs are effective for some people, but none work for all. Such effective drugs include caffeine (black, undecaffeinated coffee), ergotamine (Cafergot, Migral), beta-blockers (propranolol, metoprolol, atenolol), calcium channel blockers (verapamil, nifedipine), and nonsteroidal anti-inflammatory drugs (ibuprofen, naproxen), steroids, and such tranquilizers as thorazine. In some patients, especially those who exhibit such symptoms of depression as lethargy, insomnia, and suicidal thoughts, antidepressants (Nardil, Tofranil, Elavil) may be useful.

Recent studies have shown that migraine headaches may be prevented in some people simply by taking one aspirin tablet every other day (just as is recommended for the prevention of heart attacks and stroke). Ask your doctor about the advisability of your taking aspirin regularly before doing so.

Information on the treatment of headaches can be obtained from the New England Headache Treatment Program, 1-800-245-0088.

Sleep Disorders

Sleep is a time-consuming activity; it takes up nearly one-third of our lives. It is as natural to us as eating. It is the last stop on every day's appointed rounds. Yet for a great many of us, nights are an agony of unwanted wakefulness, and days are interrupted by uncontrollable and often embarrassing fits of drowsiness. A study by the American Medical Association some years ago estimated that 20% of adults suffer from chronic sleeplessness. The Hamlets in our society appear to be legion; but unlike the days of the Gloomy Dane, we now know there is a lot that can be done for sleep problems.

The Normal Sleep Cycle

There are two phases of sleep that alternate through 5–6 cycles each night. These phases are called REM (Rapid Eye Movement) and non-REM sleep. Non-REM sleep accounts for 75–80% of total sleep time and varies in depth between level 1 (light sleep) and level 4 (very deep sleep from which arousal is seldom spontaneous).

During non-REM sleep, there is little muscular activity, brain activity is slow and regular, and sleep is dreamless. During REM sleep, there is rapid darting of the eyes, heartbeat and respiration speed up and become less regular, and brain activity increases. REM sleep characteristically begins about 90 minutes after the onset of sleep, lasts for about 10 minutes, and ends each sleep cycle. Most dreaming occurs during REM and stage 3 non-REM sleep. Most nightmares, sleep walking, and sleep talking occur in non-REM sleep stages 3 and 4.

Why do we sleep? No one knows for certain—perhaps it is a time for bodily repair, or for memory and other brain activities to sort themselves out. What we do know is that, when sleep patterns are interrupted, health and your sense of well-being quickly decline.

Insomnia

How much sleep do you need each night? Predictably, the number of hours required to make you feel rested varies greatly among individuals. The practical answer is: whatever number leaves you refreshed and ready for the new day. George Washington was said to have required no more than four hours of sleep each night. That, however, would soon lead to bleary eyes and daytime dozing for the average person, who needs from 7 to 8 hours sleep to function without complaint.

The amount of sleep needed also depends upon age. Infants sleep from 14 to 18 hours each day. After six months of age, sleep time declines and becomes increasingly nocturnal. By age 10–12, adult sleep patterns are established, and these change little until later in life, when sleep becomes more fragmented. After age 60 most people report an increase in the number and duration of nighttime awakenings, and sleep levels tend to be lighter. Perhaps because of this, complaints of insomnia are much more common among the elderly, who also account for the bulk of sedatives taken for sleeplessness.

There are basically three ways of getting a *bad* night's sleep:

- You toss and turn for hours before falling asleep.
- You awake after only a few hours of sleep (common when indigestion occurs or alcohol is drunk before bedtime).
- You awaken repeatedly during the night, attaining only light levels of sleep so that you feel unrested the next morning.

Everyone experiences insomnia from time to time. There are many causes. For example, jet lag may interfere with sleep when the body's biological clock is disrupted. Worry and depression frequently interfere with sleep patterns. Indigestion and gastric reflux (*see* Gastric Reflux, p. 279) almost invariably disturb sleep. Too, there are many people who simply have poor sleep habits: they spend too much time in bed, they nap during the day, depend overmuch on sleeping pills, or drink alcoholic beverages before bedtime. Sleep performance has been likened to sexual performance—the harder you have to try, the more anxious you become. This in turn makes success more difficult.

How To Get a Good Night's Sleep

Poor sleep habits account for most complaints of insomnia. Fortunately, there is quite a lot you can do if you recognize what you are doing to interfere with rest (*see* box on p. 115).

A side effect of the prolonged use of sleeping medications is an *inverted* sleep rhythm. With this condition, sleepless nights are accompanied by daytime drowsiness. At night, fitful, restless sleep prompts the wretched insomniac to take more sleeping pills, creating a vicious cycle. If sedation is increased, a confusional state may develop. This means it's time to see your doctor. But you can avoid this problem by *never* taking sleeping pills more than three nights in a row, and then only for reasons of temporary insomnia. For persistent insomnia, to which these suggestions fail to bring relief, ask your doctor for advice or referral to a sleep clinic to diagnose your problem.

If you do take sleeping pills, remember:

- Avoid alcoholic beverages.
- Don't take other sedatives or tranquilizers with the sleeping pills.
- *Don't take sleeping medications* if you have asthma, glaucoma, emphysema, chronic pulmonary disease, shortness of breath, difficulty in breathing, or difficulty in urinating because of enlargement of the prostate gland, unless directed by a doctor.

Snoring

Snoring is very common. Many people are awakened or kept awake by a partner's snoring, which is caused by vibrations of the air passages in the back of your throat that have relaxed during sleep. It is usually made worse by dry air, which dries your air passages, and by lying on your back (*see* box on p. 116).

For more information about sleep problems consult: *The Sleep Book: Understanding and Preventing Sleep Problems in People Over 50* by Ernest Hartman, MD, Scott, Foresman.

Sleep Apnea

The term *apnea* means "absence of breath" and in the condition known as sleep apnea, the victim actually stops breathing, often hundreds of times each night and for periods long enough to seriously lower blood oxygen, in some cases with fatal results. The usual cause of sleep apnea is airway obstruction, e.g., by swallowing the relaxed *uvula* (the little finger of tissue at the back of your throat that points downward toward your tongue). As a result, the sleep pattern may

How To Get a Good Night's Sleep

- Avoid caffeine-containing coffee, tea, and colas within 2–4 hours of bedtime. Understand, too, that decaffeinated coffee can cause gastric upset that may itself interfere with sleep.
- Dine early in the evening so that there's plenty of time for your stomach to empty before bedtime. But don't go to bed hungry.
- Avoid alcoholic beverages within 2–4 hours of bedtime. Even moderate amounts of alcohol can disturb sleep patterns, often producing light, unsettled sleep with episodes of wakefulness.
- Regular exercise is effective in promoting relaxation and easing psychologic tension. However, it is best to exercise in the afternoon or early evening. Avoid overexertion just before bedtime, since it may actually act as a stimulant to prevent sleep.
- I hate to sound like a nag, but *stop* smoking. Nicotine is a stimulant and interferes with deep and REM sleep.
- Relax before bedtime. Listen to music or read what you most enjoy. Warm baths are relaxing; avoid hot baths, which are stimulating. Good sex also relaxes.
- Avoid napping during the day.
- Do not go to bed unless you are sleepy. If you find yourself wide awake 20 minutes after retiring, get up, go to another room, and read or relax until you are sleepy.
- Try to make your bedroom quiet, dark, and not too warm. The best sleeping temperature is 65°F or less.
- Try a relaxation technique, such as relaxing muscle groups serially from fingertips to toes. Sheep counting, though much-caricatured and a boring remedy, promotes sleep for that very reason.
- Don't rely on sleeping pills. Most over-the-counter preparations contain antihistamines, which are ineffective as sleep promoters. And most prescription sleeping drugs interfere with natural sleep patterns. For example, barbiturates act like alcohol to reduce deep levels and REM sleep. Other drugs, e.g., Dalmane, are long-acting and may cause residual fatigue the next day. Virtually all sleeping drugs promote *tolerance*; that is, progressively more drug is needed to achieve the same level of sedation. Most sleeping medications also carry the risk of side effects, eventually producing daytime fatigue, jitteriness, depression. Older individuals are especially prone to such adverse effects as confusion, restlessness, slurred speech, and incoordination (sometimes mistaken for presenile dementia).

HOW TO ELIMINATE SNORING

Eliminating snoring is not easy, but here are things you can try:

- If bedroom humidity is low, consider getting a humidifier (*see* p. 233 for suggestions about humidifiers).
- Avoid dehydration. Take plenty of fluids before bedtime. Avoid alcohol several hours before bedtime, and eliminate tranquilizers and antihistamines, all of which tend to relax the throat muscles that cause snoring.
- Try attaching a rolled-up sock or tennis ball to the back of the snorer's pajamas to discourage lying on the back.
- Try elevating the head of the bed about six inches. Snoring is caused by partial airway obstruction, which may be relieved by assuming a more upright position.
- Snoring is three times more common among the obese, probably because fat tends to decrease the size of the air passages. Losing weight may reduce or eliminate snoring altogether.
- Consult an otolaryngologist to determine whether nasal obstruction from tonsils, adenoids, or a deviated septum may be the cause of snoring.
- Anyone who snores excessively and complains of daytime drowsiness may be suffering from sleep apnea.

---

be repeatedly interrupted with obstructive choking and startled awakening. Such interrupted sleep causes excessive daytime drowsiness, the most common initial complaint. People who suffer from sleep apnea often have a disastrous record of repeated automobile accidents, poor job performance, and other social and health disabilities.

Treatment. Those who suspect they suffer sleep apnea should be referred to a sleep clinic for diagnosis. In a sleep clinic, patients check in overnight to have their sleep patterns continuously monitored. This is done by recording breathing patterns, brain waves, heart rhythm, blood oxygen, penile tumescence, and other behavior during sleep in order to determine the levels of sleep achieved and the cause of interrupted breathing. Successful treatment may simply depend upon correcting the cause of snoring (*see above*). Some people may require a mask that forces air into the lungs during inspiration in order to keep the respiratory passages open. Others may be treated with drugs that stimulate respiration. In severe cases, a surgical procedure to enlarge the respiratory passages may be required. It should be recognized that sleep apnea is a serious, even potentially fatal, medical problem that demands treatment.

Nightmares

Nightmares are disturbing dreams that are usually associated with some emotional agitation, anxiety, or stress. If you suffer nightmares, try to examine the stressful situations in your everyday life and work out effective ways of dealing with them. Review the recommendations listed above on how to get a good night's sleep. If nightmares persist, see your doctor, who may advise psychologic consultation or referral to a sleep clinic.

Sleepwalking

Perhaps the strangest of all sleep phenomena—certainly to those who observe it—is sleepwalking. This unnerving habit is usually limited to children, among whom it is fairly common. Although sleepwalkers may go about with eyes wide open, they are actually at a fairly deep level of sleep and, if awakened, will be quite confused and unaware of what they are doing.

The best thing to do with sleepwalkers is to keep them out of harm's way and gently lead them back to bed. The old adage about not trying to wake someone who is sleepwalking has good foundation, because the response to being wakened may be violent. Take satisfaction that children usually grow out of their sleepwalking tendency. Sleepwalking in adults is thought to stem most often from stress or some disturbing psychological problem. Adults are also more apt than children to do harm to themselves. Professional help is advised.

Disorders of the Peripheral Nerves

The peripheral nervous system consists of the eight pairs of cranial and 31 pairs of spinal nerves that extend from the brain and spinal cord to supply all of the structures of the body. Most of these have both a sensory and a motor component. The sensory nerve fibers carry such sensory information as touch, pain, and position stimuli to the brain. The motor nerve fibers carry nerve impulses from the brain and spinal cord that control muscular activity. The principal disorders of the peripheral nervous system include trauma, degeneration, and tumors.

Neuralgia

Neuralgia is the pain that results from damage to or pressure on a nerve. The location of the pain depends entirely upon the particular nerve(s) affected. Usually, neuralgia is felt as a shooting pain along the affected nerve that is brief, but often repetitive. The condition may be temporary or chronic and may be quite debilitating in severe cases. Some examples include:

- *Trigeminal neuralgia*. Also called *tic douloureux*, this is a shooting pain felt in the face and jaw, which are supplied by the fifth (trigeminal) cranial nerve. The condition usually affects older people and is felt on only one side of the face. The pain lasts for a few seconds to a few minutes, is often excruciating, and may be triggered by such activities as chewing or brushing the teeth. It is now thought that the cause of trigeminal neuralgia is pressure on the fifth cranial nerve by an artery. Trigeminal neuralgia is treated by drugs (e.g., carbamazepine and phenytoin) that block or blunt the attacks. In severe cases the nerve is relieved surgically by separating it from the compressing artery.
- *Sciatica*. This pain, which shoots through the buttocks and down the back of your thigh, is most often caused by a prolapsed vertebral disc (*spondylosis*). Low back pain is discussed on p. 433.

Any neuralgia that persists for more than a few days should be seen by your doctor for diagnosis and treatment. Often a neurologist must be consulted.

Bell's Palsy

Bell's palsy is a paralysis of the muscles that control movement and expression on one side of your face. It is caused by damage to the facial nerve, which begins in the brain and exits the skull beneath the ear to innervate the facial muscles.

There are many causes of Bell's palsy. The most frequent is thought to be a swelling of the facial nerve, possibly by a viral infection such as herpes zoster (*see* p. 455). The facial nerve passes through a very small hole (foramen) in the skull. If the nerve swells, compression of the nerve may interrupt function of the nerve.

The symptoms of Bell's palsy are a drooping of one side of the face. When you move your facial muscles, as when smiling, only one side of your face moves, giving a distorted appearance. You may tend to drool on the affected side, since the muscles of the mouth are affected.

Occasionally, persons complain of pain behind the ear, in the jaw, or on the side of the face. If the muscles of the eyelid are affected, excessive tearing on that side occurs. If the affected eye does not close at night, the cornea may become dry, setting up the conditions for corneal ulcers.

Bell's palsy is relatively common, affecting one in 60 persons during a lifetime. Since tumors and strokes can also cause Bell's palsy, your doctor will probably suggest a CT scan and other brain examinations to rule out a central nervous system condition.

Treatment. Most causes of Bell's palsy are self-limited and recovery of function occurs with time. In some cases, your doctor may prescribe corticosteroids to reduce nerve swelling. If you develop dry eyes at night, your doctor can prescribe a temporary patch and ointment to be used while sleeping. Use of moisturizing eye drops, such as methylcellulose drops, can guard against excessive corneal dryness during the day.

Peripheral Neuropathy

This is a general term that indicates damage to any of the many peripheral nerves. Damage can result from a variety of causes, including trauma, nerve compression (e.g., carpal tunnel syndrome), infection (e.g., Herpes zoster, malaria, botulism), toxic agents (e.g., lead, mercury, arsenic, and the organophosphates found in many insecticides), and chronic diseases (e.g., diabetes mellitus, alcoholism, vitamin B_{12} deficiency).

The symptoms of peripheral neuropathy depend upon the nerve(s) involved. Often the onset is subtle with only numbness and tingling of the body part affected. Skin sensitivity may be present and the shooting pain of neuralgia *(see above)* may develop. In chronic cases, muscle wasting and paralysis may be features.

Treatment. The medical approach to peripheral neuropathy depends upon the underlying condition responsible. Your doctor will most likely refer you to a neurologist for diagnosis. Neuropathies caused by physical compression can usually be resolved by relieving the point of compression. If a toxic agent can be identified, its elimination will halt further progression of the disease. In chronic diseases such as alcoholism and diabetes mellitus, the nerve damage may be irreversible, but progression may be halted or slowed by control of the underlying disease.

Guillain-Barré Syndrome

Guillain-Barré syndrome is an acute form of peripheral neuropathy that often follows a few days after an otherwise innocuous viral infection or vaccination. The cause is not known; possibly it results from an allergic reaction to the virus.

The usual symptoms involve numbness, tingling, and weakness beginning in the legs and progressing to the arms and other parts of the body (polyneuropathy). In severe cases, cardiac irregularity and respiratory paralysis develop.

Treatment. Severe cases of Guillain-Barré syndrome require emergency care to maintain respiration and other vital functions. Plasmapheresis, a filtration treatment that removes certain antibodies from the blood plasma, may sometimes be effective. Improvement occurs gradually, though 30% of patients suffer a residual weakness that may require retraining, orthopedic appliances, or corrective surgery.

Neurofibromatosis (von Recklinghausen's Disease)

Neurofibromatosis is a rare hereditary disorder characterized by pigmented spots, skin tumors, and tumors of the peripheral nerves. The tumors may be few or exist by the thousands, and may also create grotesque deformities such as those that afflicted the main character in the play, *The Elephant Man*. Compression of peripheral nerves by nerve sheath tumors causes a variety of peripheral neuropathies. There is no effective treatment, save relief of neural compressions as they occur. Genetic counseling is advisable.

Pain and Pain Relievers

In this book, specific types of pain are discussed under the specific organ headings associated with the pain. Here I want to discuss the most common ways of relieving pain and provide some guidelines for selecting appropriate analgesic drugs.

The most common nonprescription pain medications are aspirin, acetaminophen (Tylenol, Panadol), and ibuprofen (Advil, Nuprin). All these drugs have one thing in common: they reduce the production of prostaglandins, the hormone-like substances produced by the body that trigger *inflammation, fever,* and *pain.* Aspirin and ibuprofen are effective in relieving all three effects of prostaglandins, whereas acetaminophen is effective in relieving fever and pain, but not inflammation. The following is a list of indications, as well as warnings and side effects, to help you decide which type of pain medication is most appropriate to use.

Aspirin

Aspirin has the widest range of applications, including simple head-aches, muscular aches and pains, arthritis, broken bones, rheumatism, toothache, and so on. Because aspirin inhibits clotting, it is often recommended in low doses (e.g., 300 mg/day) for older individuals to help reduce the risk of heart attack, stroke, and possibly colon cancer as well.

Aspirin also has the greatest number of side effects. About two percent of people, especially asthmatics, exhibit allergic reactions to aspirin, ranging from itching rashes to choking and labored breathing. Some individuals experience a ringing of the ears (*tinnitus*) that disappears when aspirin is stopped. In the high doses of aspirin used to treat arthritis, ulcers and bleeding occur quite frequently if measures are not taken to prevent them. Recently the prescription drugs, misoprostol and omeprazole (Prilosec), have been approved for use in patients at high risk of developing stomach ulcer complications while on aspirin or ibuprofen.

Aspirin should not be used by pregnant women during the last trimester, because it can cause bleeding in both mother and child. You should not use aspirin if you have an allergy to salicylates, or have ulcers, gout, or stomach bleeding. Aspirin (and other salicylates) are especially to be avoided by children under 18 years of age because of the risk of *Reye's Syndrome*. Reye's syndrome is an acute encephalopathy accompanied by liver dysfunction. It is usually associated with such viral diseases as flu and chicken pox, but may also be caused by salicylates, especially when given for a viral infection. The symptoms of Reye's Syndrome include severe tiredness, belligerence, and vomiting.

For adults who do not experience side effects, aspirin is usually the drug of choice for treating most minor aches and pains because of its long-proven safety, effectiveness, and low cost.

Acetaminophen

Acetaminophen produces fewer side effects and allergic reactions than aspirin. It is especially recommended for children under 18 because it is not associated with Reye's Syndrome. For adults it is probably less effective than aspirin and ibuprofen in reducing pain and fever, but it is useful for those who cannot take these drugs.

Acetaminophen should not be used in patients with liver and kidney diseases. Recent studies show that acetaminophen may cause liver or kidney failure in some who take it over long periods of time. Therefore, it is advisable to consult your doctor if you need to take this drug longer than 10 days.

Most "extra-strength" preparations of acetaminophen are just larger doses of the regular-strength drug, and offer little, if any, additional pain relief. They are, however, more expensive.

Ibuprofen

Ibuprofen is especially helpful for the relief of joint pain and inflammation caused by arthritis, as well as for fever, stiffness, toothaches, backaches, migraine, and the aches and fever of a cold. It is excellent for menstrual cramps and has an effect similar to aspirin in reducing blood clotting. Ibuprofen is less likely to cause ulcers than aspirin, though long-term use is known to result in ulcers and bleeding.

In general, it takes longer for ibuprofen to relieve pain than either aspirin or acetaminophen. Therefore, for rapid relief of such pains as headaches, the latter are probably more satisfactory.

Ibuprofen should not be taken by those with aspirin allergies because of possible cross-sensitivity, nor should it be taken for gout or ulcers, except under your doctor's advice. Ibuprofen should not be taken by pregnant women in the last trimester or by children under 12 years old without the advice of your doctor.

Recent studies have indicated that kidney failure may develop in some who use ibuprofen in large doses (more than 1600 milligrams per day) over prolonged periods of time. It is important to note that such instances of kidney failure were reversible after ibuprofen was stopped. Since such doses are taken by many with arthritis, make sure you discuss this possible complication with your doctor when taking more than 1000 mg per day of ibuprofen. Avoid dehydration by maintaining adequate fluid intake (8–10 glasses of nonalcoholic fluids daily).

Other Pain Relievers

Pain that is unusually severe or chronic, such as that associated with advanced cancers, shingles, kidney stones, and so on, must be treated by your doctor, who may prescribe tranquilizers, a narcotic, or other prescription drugs. All of these drugs have powerful side effects in addition to the potential for addiction, so they must be used cautiously.

Certain localized pain may be relieved by the application of weak electrical currents. This is done by means of a *transcutaneous electrical nerve stimulation* (TENS) device, a small battery-powered generator about the size of a deck of playing cards. The electrical pulses are thought to block the pain impulses flowing through the nerves below. Acupuncture may work in much the same way. Those who suffer from severe or chronic pain may obtain guidelines on choosing a pain clinic by contacting:

The American Chronic Pain Association, 257 Old Haymaker Road, Monroeville, PA 15146.

The National Chronic Pain Outreach Association Inc., 7979 Old Georgetown Road, Bethesda, MD 20814; 1-301-652-4948.

Cross-section of the eye

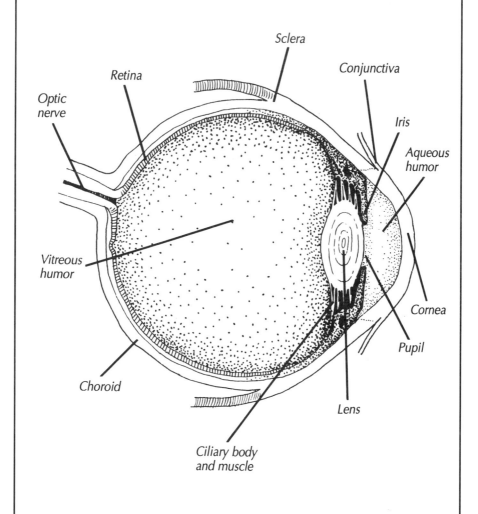

Your Eyes

How Your Eyes Work

Your eyes afford you an unceasing miracle—the power of sight, the most important of the five senses. The eye functions by detecting light rays emitted or reflected by objects around you. Light enters through the cornea, the transparent outer covering of the eye. The cornea bends (or refracts) the entering light—and serves as an important part of the focusing mechanism of the eye. Light passes through the fluid-filled front (anterior) chamber of the eye, and then through the pupil, which is merely the opening in the iris (the colored part of the eye). The iris is, in effect, a large circular muscle that adjusts the size of the pupil to admit more or less light, depending on its intensity. In dim light, the pupil dilates to admit more light, whereas in bright light, the pupil constricts.

Next the light passes though the lens, which changes shape to focus the image onto the retina lining the back of the eye. The closer the object is to the eye, the greater must be the curvature of the lens to keep the image in focus. Cells in the retina (the rods and cones) then convert the light rays into nerve impulses that are immediately transmitted by the optic nerve directly to the visual cortex at the back of the brain. There, the nerve impulses are reconstructed, interpreted, and integrated with memory so that not only do you see, but you understand what you see.

This is a complex process, and one that is incredibly sensitive. On a clear night, the eyes can detect a single candle burning 14 miles away. Your most sensitive vision is known as *central vision* in which the image of view is focused on the *fovea,* a portion of the retina especially dense in light-sensitive cells. This is the vision that allows you to read this page. You also have peripheral vision, which allows you to see objects and movement off to the side without moving your head or eyes. Unfortunately, many things can go wrong to alter or distort the visual process. However, there are also many steps you can take to help preserve good vision.

Color Blindness

Actually the term "color deficiency" is a more accurate description of the condition commonly known as *color blindness,* since very few people ever suffer a complete absence of color perception. Color is perceived by the specialized *cone cells* of the retina, whereas the retinal *rod cells* detect varying intensities of white light. Each cone cell contains a substance that is responsive to red, or green, or blue light. In those people afflicted with color deficiency, one of these substances is missing or deficient, making certain colors difficult to distinguish. Red–green deficiency, in which it becomes very difficult to distinguish certain shades of red and green, especially in dim light, is by far the most common of these.

People with color deficiency are often unaware of their condition; they assume that everyone sees things the way they do. Color deficiency can be detected by means of color testing, which is recommended for all children. Color-coded learning materials are used extensively in the primary grades, and teachers should be alert for pupils whose normal color perception is missing. In addition, color deficiency may affect career paths. Pilots and electricians, for example, do not do well with color deficiency. There is no cure for color deficiency, although color filters mounted on eyeglasses can enhance the ability to distinguish colors.

Errors of Refraction

Myopia (Nearsightedness)

Myopia, or nearsightedness, is a defect of vision in which near objects are seen clearly, but distant objects appear fuzzy or out of focus. This is a very common condition, affecting about 20% of the total United States population. Myopia is probably hereditary to some extent, but there is evidence that it can be brought on, or made worse, by too much close work. (The stereotype of the bookworm with glasses may therefore have some basis in reality.)

The arbitrary standard of "normal" vision is what is called 20/20 vision in both eyes. This means that your eye can read what a normal eye can read at a distance of 20 feet in daylight. You might have normal vision in one eye, but 20/50 vision in the other, which means that using that eye, you have to stand at 20 feet to read what a normal eye can read at 50 feet. The larger the second number is, the worse your vision.

Nearsightedness usually first occurs in school-age children, and almost always before the age of 20. In fact, nearsightedness is something to consider when children perform poorly in school. They also squint frequently in an attempt to focus distant objects. The actual cause of myopia is an eyeball that is too long to be able to focus light on the retina. The uncorrected image is blurred because the cornea and lens focus light rays from distant objects *in front of* the retina.

Treatment. Nearsightedness is easily corrected using concave lenses. Sometimes the condition worsens gradually with advancing age so that increasingly more correction must be applied. This is usually not a serious problem, however, because most myopics can be corrected fully with proper lenses.

Avoid working in bad light. Though it is a myth that reading in bad light will ruin your vision, you will be less prone to headaches in adequate glare-free lighting and your work and reading will certainly be more pleasureable.

The Russians have developed a surgical procedure called "radial keratotomy" to correct myopia. The operation changes the curvature of the cornea by means of a series of symmetrical incisions through the outer layers of the cornea that relax and flatten it. If the incisions are made precisely correctly, and if no other complication develops, the myopic individual's vision may be completely corrected. However, these are big IFs. Those who might consider this surgical procedure should be aware that a study by the National Eye Institute has shown that radial keratotomy reduces myopia in most cases, but not always enough to do away with glasses. In some cases it creates astigmatism, fluctuating visual acuity, or annoying glare after the operation. The results are sufficiently worrisome that the American Academy of Ophthalmology still classifies the operation as an investigative procedure. Simple nearsightedness is not a condition with which you should take risks. Keep in mind that eyeglasses are virtually risk-free and serve as a physical shield that actually protects the eye.

Hyperopia (Farsightedness)

In *hyperopia*, or farsightedness, the eyeball is too short for the focusing system, causing light rays to focus *behind* the retina. People who are farsighted often must hold objects at arms' length to bring them into focus. In expending extra effort to focus on objects, one may experience fatigue, tension, burning or aching eyes, and headaches. Farsightedness is easily corrected with convex lenses. However, with age the ciliary muscle, which controls the curvature of the lens, weakens, and it is common to require stronger lenses every few years.

Presbyopia

Though the eye as a whole reaches its full size by about the age of ten, the lens continues to grow. In the process it gradually loses some of its elasticity, with the result that focusing on near objects becomes difficult. This condition is known as *presbyopia* (meaning "old eyes"). Although it is often confused with farsightedness, in presbyopia the curve of the cornea and the length of the eye may be normal. Only the lens is faulty, being unable to increase its curvature sufficiently to focus near objects. Presbyopia is a normal aging phenomenon that usually becomes noticeable during the early or mid-forties.

If you have presbyopia, you may need to hold a book at arms' length to read it, and you probably also have difficulty with the fine print of telephone books. At times you may also experience eye fatigue and headache.

Treatment. If you have experienced no other problems with your vision, ordinary "reading glasses" purchased over the counter are usually sufficient to correct presbyopia. These are simply magnifying glasses. Since distance vision does not require correction, you can take the glasses off when close work is finished, or you can purchase half-lenses and merely look over the lower lenses to focus at distance.

When you select a pair of "reading glasses," try on several pairs. They are usually marked with a number from +1.00 (low magnification) to +4.00 (high magnification). Read the accompanying cards to make certain you are selecting the best pair for your personal vision needs. Start at a low number and work your way up the scale of magnifications, holding the card at a comfortable reading distance in a well-lighted room. As the power of your reading glasses increases, your usable range of vision (the distance you can move reading material and still keep it in focus) decreases.

Let me caution you, however, that buying readymade lenses does not substitute for an examination by your ophthalmologist (a medical doctor, or MD, who is trained not only in the measurement and correction of vision, but also in the diagnosis and management of medical and surgical problems of the eye) or your optometrist (a non-MD who is trained to examine the eyes and to correct visual disorders by dispensing glasses or contact lenses).

As you grow older it is especially important that your eyes be checked regularly for glaucoma and other diseases *(see below)*. For young people without vision problems, examinations every two years are usually sufficient. Because the incidence of glaucoma and other eye disorders increase substantially with age, yearly examinations by an ophthalmologist are highly recommended after age 40. Contact lens wearers should be examined at least yearly. If you experience blurring of vision, eye pain, changes in the appearance of your eyes or other eye symptoms, you should see your ophthalmologist at once.

People who suffer from nearsightedness, farsightedness, or astigmatism usually cannot get by with reading glasses alone as they become older. Rather, they often must have bifocal or trifocal lenses prescribed either as eyeglasses or contact lenses. The use of "monovision" lenses is becoming increasingly common. With the monovision technique, one contact lens is fitted for near vision and the other for far vision. The brain quickly learns which eye to use at any given distance, disregarding the image from the other eye. Marvelous how the brain works!

Astigmatism

With *astigmatism*, vision at all distances may be distorted. The usual cause is an irregularity in the shape of the cornea. Often the degree of astigmatism is different for each eye, and often, astigmatism may be a complicating factor in near- and farsightedness, adding to the lens correction requirements. Most problems of astigmatism can be corrected with properly fitted lenses.

Amblyopia (Lazy Eye)

Amblyopia, or lazy eye, is a condition of unknown cause in which the vision in one eye is markedly reduced. For some reason the brain is incapable or refuses to register the images from one eye. Only central vision is affected; peripheral vision remains intact. The condition probably stems from birth and first becomes detectable about the age of three. It affects from 2 to 4% of the population. The development of amblyopia after the age of six is rare. For these reasons it is important to have your child's eyes checked professionally, usually at age 3–4 and again at about age 13, when nearsightedness may develop.

Amblyopia is often accompanied by *strabismus* (crossed eyes). Usually children suffering amblyopia will favor one eye and occasionally they will bump into objects on the side of the amblyopic eye.

Treatment. Amblyopia should be treated early because the longer the condition goes untreated, the more resistant the eye becomes to recovering lost vision. Corrective lenses, prisms, contact lenses, and vision therapy are used. Vision therapy uses eye-exercise techniques to strengthen the amblyopic eye and coordinate vision with the unaffected eye. Occasionally, patching the good eye will stimulate the brain to register the central vision of the amblyopic eye.

Strabismus (Crossed Eyes)

In *strabismus*, better known as crossed eyes, the two eyes are not aligned with one another. In some cases, one eye looks directly forward, while the other is either turned away from the nose (wall-eyed) or toward the nose (cross-eyed). In other cases one eye may look up or down relative to the other (vertical misalignment). The cause is a weakness of one or more of the muscles that move the eyeball.

Parents often become aware of a misalignment in the position of a child's eyes by age 2 or 3. The most common sign is a tendency for one eye to wander, while the other eye is fixed on a target. In strabismus, the brain often disregards the image from the deviating eye, but sometimes it will use the eyes alternatively.

Crossed eyes that develop during adulthood usually stem from some other disorder, such as diabetes mellitus, high blood pressure, or muscular dystrophy. The result is double vision.

Treatment. In childhood, crossed eyes are treated by use of special lenses and eye exercises. In some cases an operation to shorten one of the eye muscles may be necessary. Therapy should commence early, because the condition only worsens with time. A new treatment for crossed eyes uses injections of botulin toxin into one of the eye muscles to relax it and thus overcome the eye deviation.

If you develop double vision as an adult, see your doctor, who will search for an underlying cause. Often, treatment of the underlying disorder will cure double vision. Until the problem is corrected, buy an eyepatch from your druggist to prevent double vision.

Contact Lenses

Thinking of getting contact lenses? They offer many advantages over eyeglasses, especially for those actively engaged in sports. Too, not everyone is as handsome as Gloria Steinem in aviator glasses. However, not everyone can wear contact lenses and there are some things you should know before rushing off to your eye doctor.

How They Work

Contact lenses are plastic or silicone discs that are curved to fit directly onto the cornea. The outer surface is ground so as to refract light directly onto the retina. When placed in the eyes, the lenses are held to the cornea by a thin layer of tears.

An important problem for contact lens manufacturers to overcome has been interference with the supply of fresh tears (and hence oxygen) to the cornea (since the transparent cornea has no blood vessels, the cells of the cornea must receive their supply of oxygen from tears). When the supply of oxygen is reduced, there is a danger of corneal swelling and infection. Hard lenses are made loose enough to permit tears to wash between the lens and the cornea. As the upper lid rises during blinking, it drags the lens upward, allowing old tears low in oxygen to drain away and be replaced by fresh tears. Although soft contact lens materials are permeable to gases, the oxygen needed by the cornea arrives mostly by the pumping action of the lids, as it does with hard lenses. All contact lenses require periodic care and close attention to hygiene to insure their comfort and safety.

Hard Lenses—Daily Wear

There are advantages to wearing hard, rather than soft, contact lenses. They are usually less expensive, they are more durable, and they frequently provide better vision. On the negative side, they may be uncomfortable to wear at first, and thus not all people can wear them. Because they are smaller and more loose-fitting than soft lenses, they may pop out of the eye, or wander off the cornea, more easily than soft lenses.

Hard lenses should be rinsed in plain water before and after wearing. They must be cleaned daily with a lens cleaner and placed in a disinfecting solution overnight, and this solution should be changed every night to avoid becoming contaminated. Some hard contact lenses are gas-permeable and these should be cleaned at least once weekly with an enzyme cleaner.

Soft Lenses—Daily Wear

These lenses have become very popular, because they are usually comfortable from the first day of wear. They also remain in place more effectively than hard lenses, and are thus favored by athletes. On the other hand, they are more expensive and they are easily damaged, seldom lasting longer than 18 months. They must be cleaned with a special solution and soaked overnight in a separate disinfecting solution. They must be treated with an enzyme once or twice weekly, and this may also require yet another special solution. Most soft lenses cannot be rinsed in tap water. Rather, they should be rinsed in saline to prevent (osmotic) distortion of the lens curvature. A soft lens that accidentally dries out can usually be returned to its normal condition in a few minutes by rehydrating it with saline.

Soft Lenses—Extended Wear

The requirement of a complicated daily cleansing ritual has provided ample stimulus to develop a lens demanding less fastidious care. To accomplish this, manufacturers have developed a very thin lens that is sufficiently permeable to oxygen that it can be worn during sleep. These lenses can be worn for up to 7 days between cleaning, although it is usually recommended that they be taken out more frequently to clean and give the eyes a rest. Because they are so thin, they are extremely fragile and tear easily. They also promote corneal swelling at night, which may then lead to corneal ulceration and infection. If this is not treated immediately, permanent damage or blindness can result. Consequently, you should carefully consider the need for this type of lens. Finally, extended-wear lenses are cleaned in the same manner as daily-wear soft lenses.

Soft Lens—Disposable

They sound great. Wear them for a week and throw them away. No tedious cleaning; no fumbling searches for your lens cases. But disposable lenses are not without problems. They still have many of the problems of regular extended or daily wear soft lenses.

Like other types of soft lenses, disposable lenses limit the amount of oxygen that gets to the cornea. They carry the same increased risk of infection and corneal swelling as other types of extended wear lenses. They are also very delicate and prone to tearing. And they are about twice as expensive as extended-wear lenses.

Good Contact Lens Practice

No matter what kind of contact lenses you have, there are certain precautions you must take:

- If your eyes become irritated or red for any reason, remove your contact lenses and place them in their disinfecting solution. Wear regular eyeglasses until the irritation or redness disappears.
- Avoid wearing contact lenses when using aerosol sprays, oil-base paints, or organic solvents to prevent eye irritation.

- Tobacco smoke, smog, and airborne irritants may preclude your wearing contact lens.
- Low humidity during dry weather, in airplane cabins, or on desert safari may cause excessive drying and eye irritation. Use your regular eyeglasses.
- Antihistamines and diuretics may decrease tear production and cause dry eyes.
- Pregnancy, menstruation, and birth control pills may be associated with water retention and unsatisfactory conditions for contact lenses. If this occurs, merely switch temporarily to regular glasses.
- No pain should be associated with wearing contact lenses. If pain or irritation develops, consult your eye doctor.
- Individuals who temporarily lose consciousness (e.g., epileptics) should carry a card indicating that they wear contact lenses.
- Don't wear your contact lenses while sleeping
- Out of doors you still need sunglasses to protect your corneas from ultraviolet light.
- Above all, follow the manufacturer's cleaning instructions exactly.

Selecting Sunglasses

Though most people are aware of the adverse effects that excessive sun exposure has on the skin, it is not so widely understood that sunlight also has adverse effects on the eye. Most eye damage comes from light in the ultraviolet spectrum of light, especially ultraviolet-B (UV-B). Acute exposure to intense ultraviolet light reflected from sand, water, or snow can actually burn the cornea, resulting in "snow-blindness" *(photokeratitis)*. The symptoms are pain, tearing, intense sensitivity to light, and a sense of having something in your eyes, usually developing 4–5 hours after exposure.

However, prolonged exposure to lower levels of ultraviolet light is believed also to be damaging to the eyes. For example, it is estimated that 10% of all cataracts in the United States are caused by excessive exposure to the sun, and are thus preventable. Macular degeneration *(see below)*, a common cause of reduced vision in the elderly, may also be largely caused by exposure to ultraviolet and blue light. It is especially important to wear sunglasses if:

- You are fair-skinned and blue-eyed.
- You spend much of your time outdoors, or live at a high altitude.
- You take tetracycline regularly (increases UV sensitivity).
- You have or have a family history of macular degeneration or have had cataracts (*see* p. 135).

HOW TO BUY SUNGLASSES

Here are some things to keep in mind:

- Buy sunglasses listing their ultraviolet (UV) absorption. "General-purpose" sunglasses should absorb at least 95% of UV-B, 60% of UV-A, and 60–92% of visible light. These sunglasses are recommended for most outdoor activities. If you are frequently exposed to bright sun combined with sand, snow, or water, you should buy "special-purpose" lenses that block at least 99% of UV-B and 60% of UV-A. If the transmission factor is not specified on the glasses, look at yourself in a mirror. You should not be able to see your eyes through the lenses.
- Select brown or amber lenses. They tend to block blue light, which is now thought to be injurious, along with UV light. They also reduce glare and increase contrast in haze and fog. Avoid red and purple-colored lenses because they distort real colors.
- Make sure the lenses are large enough to block most of the light coming around the outer rim of the glasses.
- Select lenses that are treated to block 100% of UV light. Remember that *photochromic* lenses (sunglasses that darken with increasing light) by themselves do not block UV light; they must be additionally treated.
- Reject lenses that distort vision. The way to tell whether glasses distort objects is to hold them at arms length and look at a straight line in the distance. The line should remain straight as you move the glasses across the line.
- Ask your optician about polarized lenses, mirrored lenses, and gradient lenses, all of which may offer particular advantages, depending on your personal outdoor activities.
- When buying regular eyeglasses, ask your optician to have them UVB-coated, which blocks most UV sunlight.

For more information about specific brands of sunglasses, their sources, special recommendations, and current prices, write to: Dr. Richard Young, Dept. of Anatomy, UCLA Medical School, Los Angeles, CA 90024-1763.

Spots and Floaters

From time to time, as you gaze into the distance or move your eyes suddenly, you may notice a dark spot, or a fine curly hair float across your field of vision. Most of these spots or floaters are quite harmless fragments of cellular debris from the retina, or drifting clumps of protein caused by changes in the composition of the vitreous humor, the transparent jelly-like fluid that fills the eye. Spots or floaters are common among older individuals and may change with time. They are harmless and usually of no concern.

Detached Retina

There are some danger signals that should warn you of the possibility of a detached retina, which is an acute eye emergency. These signs include sudden blurred vision with partial shading or veiling of the visual field, sudden increase in the number of floaters, or the sudden appearance of showers of flashing lights, especially when confined to one eye. Should you experience any of these phenomena, call your eye doctor or go to the emergency room at once.

When the retina detaches, it becomes separated from the *choroid*, the blood vessel-rich layer behind the retina that serves as its blood supply, and then bulges into the vitreous fluid of the eye. Ophthalmologists can repair the detachment by using laser therapy to "tack" the retina back onto the choroid, or by using cryosurgery to freeze the retina in place. Repair must be performed quickly, since the retina will soon degenerate without its blood supply.

Blood in the Eye

Streaks or blotches of bright red blood that occur spontaneously and without pain in the whites of the eyes are called "subconjunctival hemorrhages." They usually follow minor trauma, straining, sneezing, or coughing. They are caused by the rupture of small blood vessels within the conjunctiva. This kind of bleeding is quite harmless and disappears spontaneously within 2 weeks. Eye drops of any kind, especially decongestants, are of little help. If pain or fever accompanies bleeding in the eye, consult your ophthalmologist at once.

Cataracts

The term *cataract* refers to any cloudiness or opacity of the eye lens, which is normally perfectly clear. The name means "waterfall" and derives from the fact that the lens, when examined with an ophthalmoscope, somewhat resembles a miniature waterfall. Usually cataracts develop from a degeneration of protein in the lens, although secondary cataracts may form as a result of X-ray exposure, heat from infrared exposure, excess sun exposure, systemic diseases (e.g., diabetes), inflammations, and some medicines (e.g., steroids). Congenital cataracts occur in rare instances.

The early symptoms of cataracts include distortion and dimming of vision. Night driving, bright light, and back-lighting are also troublesome.

Treatment. Frequently, corrective lenses are adequate to maintain useful vision during cataract development. When reduced vision begins to affect daily life, cataract surgery is indicated. In most cases the opacified lens is removed under local anesthesia and replaced by a plastic implant. The past several years have seen many advances in implant design and technology. The complications of infection, bleeding, retinal detachment, implant dislocation, and glaucoma are now rare problems. After cataract extraction with lens implantation, correction of vision is usually possible with glasses or contact lenses.

Glaucoma

Glaucoma is a disease in which the internal pressure in the eye increases, caused most often by impaired drainage of the aqueous humor from the front (anterior) chamber of the eye. Increased pressure within the eye may eventually impair the circulation of blood supplying the retina, causing degeneration of the retina and optic nerve.

Glaucoma may be either acute or chronic. In the rare *acute glaucoma* (acute angle-closure or narrow-angle glaucoma), sudden obstruction of aqueous drainage from the eye develops. In such cases, rapid visual impairment, headaches, eye pain, haloes around lights, nausea, and vomiting should alert you that an eye emergency exists, one requiring immediate treatment to prevent irreversible optic nerve damage.

In chronic glaucoma, the buildup of pressure occurs much more gradually, and there may be no symptoms at all until degeneration of the retina and optic nerve gradually result in impaired vision. The diagnosis is made by "tonometry," which measures pressure inside the eye. This is why you should have periodic eye examinations, even if you experience no eye symptoms. In fact it is recommended that tonometry be a part of every complete physical examination. If your doctor does not do this examination, ask him to refer you to an ophthalmologist.

Chronic glaucoma is common, affecting about 2% of the population. In some cases it is a complication of inflammation, eye tumors, and certain types of cataracts. Prolonged treatment with steroids may also increase eye pressure.

People at greatest risk of developing glaucoma include:

- Those with a family history of glaucoma.
- Blacks.
- Anyone over age 65 (3% of this age group have glaucoma).
- Those with severe nearsightedness.
- Those taking certain blood-pressure medicines and long-term steroids.

Those over the age of 35 with any of the above risk factors should have an eye examination every year.

Treatment. At this time glaucoma cannot be prevented, but most cases can be treated with eyedrops that constrict the pupils *(meiotics)* and with oral diuretics. In cases of acute glaucoma, or in chronic glaucoma that does not respond to conservative treatment, a simple operation known as an *iridectomy* is performed (sometimes using a laser beam) to improve drainage of aqueous fluid.

If you have glaucoma, you should try to avoid emotional upset, the use of tobacco, and drinking large quantities of fluids in order to prevent raising your internal eye pressure. You should be aware that certain medications (for example, cold preparations containing atropine or scopolamine) may increase your internal eye pressure.

Diabetic Retinopathy

Diabetics especially need regular eye examinations to detect blood vessel changes in the retina that can lead to blindness. This problem is particularly severe in juvenile diabetes and insulin-dependent diabetes (*see* p. 168). The *retinopathy* (which means "disease of the retina") is caused by capillary leakage and hemorrhages into the retina, which result in gradually decreased vision.

The symptoms of diabetic retinopathy include blurred or cloudy vision, blind spots, and increased numbers of floaters (*see* p. 134). Ultimately blindness develops if the diabetes is not brought under control.

Treatment. Treatment consists of controlling the diabetes and lowering blood pressure if it is elevated. Although the retinal changes can often be stopped, they are usually not reversible. In some cases of severe disease, laser therapy and surgery may be effective. Low-vision aids include telescopic lenses for distance vision, microscopic lenses, magnifying lenses, and electronic magnifiers for close work. For more information, obtain *Low Vision* by Helen Neal (Simon & Schuster) from your library or bookstore.

NATIONAL EYE CARE PROJECT

This is a program of The Foundation of the American Academy of Ophthalmology designed to provide eye care to the elderly and to those who do not have access to an ophthalmologist. It is not a second-opinion program, and you are *not* eligible if:

- You are under 5 years of age.
- You are currently under the care of an ophthalmologist
- You have access to your regular ophthalmologist
- You have access to an ophthalmologist through a prepaid health plan (HMO) or through a government care facility, armed forces, or VA facility).

If you believe you may be eligible for assistance, contact: American Academy of Ophthalomology, PO Box 744, San Francisco, CA 94120-7424.

Macular Degeneration

The macula is the small area near the center of the retina that is responsible for seeing fine detail. In macular degeneration these central retinal cells are lost, usually in both eyes. The cause is unknown, but the disorder is thought to be hereditary, involving either a loss of eye pigmentation (visual purple) or a constriction of the blood vessels that supply the macula. It is one of the leading causes of vision impairment in the elderly. Macular degeneration affects vision in the following ways:

- Vision becomes blurred or fuzzy.
- Straight lines appear wavy, doubled, or tripled.
- Numbers and letters appear jumbled.
- Reading becomes difficult or impossible.

There is no specific treatment of macular degeneration. Smoking is thought to worsen the effects, and should be stopped. Your ophthalmologist can suggest a variety of low-vision aids. (*See* section above.)

Retinitis Pigmentosa

Retinitis Pigmentosa is a slowly progressive degeneration of the retina that often begins in childhood or adolescence. The cause is not known and currently there is no therapy available. The most common symptoms are night blindness and a gradual loss of peripheral vision. Children may stumble into objects that lie outside their central vision. Early detection can lead to career counseling that may direct affected individuals into areas not depending on night and peripheral vision.

Eye Infections

Sty

Technically, a *sty* is an infection of one or more of the eyelash follicles at the margin of the eyelid. It resembles a small boil, becoming red and painful, and gradually coming to a white, pus-filled head that bursts, draining off the pus. With proper care, a sty usually subsides after about a week.

Treatment. You can relieve the discomfort and cause a sty to burst earlier by applying hot compresses. Do not squeeze the sty, but instead pull out the lash, which will cause the pus to drain. If styes constantly recur, see your doctor, who may prescribe an antibiotic and possibly suggest changes in any eye makeup or cosmetics you may be using.

Conjunctivitis

Conjunctivitis is an inflammation of the conjunctiva, the transparent lining of the eyelids and outer margin of the eye up to the cornea. Bacterial or viral infections and allergies are the most common causes of conjunctivitis. Dilation of the blood vessels causes the white part of the eye to become reddened, with tearing and burning sensations. Your eyes may feel gritty, and frequently, crust forms around them in the morning.

Treatment. When you develop the symptoms of conjunctivitis, see your doctor, who will prescribe antibiotics and/or drops to soothe the tearing and burning. Wash your hands after you have touched your eyes and do not share washcloths or towels with others because many such infections are contagious. Use disposable tissues rather than handkerchiefs.

Be prudent in the use of eye makeup.

- When applying such makeup, wash your hands beforehand.
- Buy mascara in small amounts and don't share it with others.
- Don't use saliva to wet eye makeup or application devices.
- Don't try eye products from "testers" in department stores; these may have been contaminated by prior users.

Corneal Ulcers

Ulcers (small open sores) of the cornea most often result from a scratch or foreign body in the eye. The symptoms of corneal ulcers include irritation, tearing, and redness. The most common foreign bodies in the eyes today are contact lenses, which causes a localized infection that then forms an ulcer. Often, corneal ulcers are caused by the herpes simplex virus that also causes cold sores. If you have a cold sore, never put your hands to your eyes after touching your mouth.

Treatment. If you suspect you have a corneal ulcer, see your doctor at once. The usual treatments are antibiotics and eye drops to relieve the irritation. Untreated corneal ulcers may result in scarring of the cornea and reduced vision. Severe cases require a corneal transplant.

Iritis and Uveitis

Iritis is an inflammation of the iris (the colored part of the eye), usually of unknown cause. Symptoms include discomfort or pain in one or both eyes, redness, and sometimes, decreased vision. Cell debris may be visible through the pupil.

Uveitis is an inflammation of the *uveal tract*, which includes the iris and the choroid. Inflammations are usually caused by virus or are associated with some type of systemic disease, such as rheumatoid arthritis or sarcoidosis. The symptoms are similar to iritis.

Treatment. Your doctor will prescribe eye drops to reduce inflammation and to prevent the iris from becoming attached to the lens.

Watery Eyes

Excessive tearing, to the point that tears persistently overflow and run down your face, may be caused by a narrowing of the tear duct known as *dacryostenosis.* The narrowing may be either congenital or the result of a previous infection or trauma. The narrowing can usually be treated with simple dilation of the tear duct by your ophthalmologist.

Watery eye may also be caused by an inward growing eyelash, called an *entropion.* Such lashes rubbing against the conjunctiva set up a chronic irritation. Your doctor may be able to treat entropion by simply taping the eyelash outward with adhesive tape for a period of time. If this is not effective, a simple operation may be required.

Tears and Dry Eyes

Tears consist of water, protein, and oil in a combination that effectively lubricates and protects the eye. They also perform the vital function of delivering oxygen to the cornea, which has no direct blood supply of its own.

When tear production is inadequate to maintain moisture of your eyes (*keratoconjunctivitis sicca*), your eyes become reddened and irritated. This condition is most common in adult women. When the condition is associated with systemic diseases such as rheumatoid arthritis, it is termed Sjögren's Syndrome (*see* p. 270). If inadequately treated, corneal ulceration results.

Dry eye may also be caused by *ectropion*, a condition in which the lower lid hangs away from the eyeball, exposing the lower surface of the eye to drying.

Treatment. Frequent applications of artificial tears are effective in relieving dry eyes. Although many brands are available without prescription, those that are made without preservatives (for example, Refresh and Celluvisc) are least likely to cause irritation themselves. In mild cases of dry eye, humidifying your house and avoiding dry conditions and climates is all that is necessary to avoid symptoms. The use of contact lenses may also be helpful. In severe cases, surgical procedures to retard tear drainage may be indicated. Ectropion is treated by a simple operation on the tissues below the lower lid.

For further information, write to: Sjögren's Syndrome Foundation. For a brochure and sample issue of their newsletter, *The Moisture Seekers*, send a stamped, self-addressed envelope to: Sjögren's Syndrome Foundation Inc., 382 Main St., Port Washington, NY 11050.

Ptosis

Ptosis is a drooping of one, or rarely both, eyelids. It is most often caused by interruption of the seventh cranial (facial) nerve, which supplies the facial muscles of expression. It may result from a stroke, a brain tumor or injury to the nerve and lends to the face the appearance of a sleepy eye.

Treatment. The only consequence of ptosis is cosmetic. Often recovery is spontaneous if ptosis has been the result of a stroke. In the event of permanent ptosis, cosmetic surgery can greatly improve facial appearance.

Twitching Eyelids

Occasional twitching of the eyelids, though somewhat irritating, is usually benign and happens to most of us at one time or another. It most often disappears spontaneously. It is not known why the eyelids twitch; it may be caused by some irritation of the nerves that supply the eye muscles.

If twitching of the lids persists, it may result from eyestrain. If you work in an area of bright fluorescent lights, try reducing the level of illumination and add an incandescent light to your work area to "soften" the light. You may achieve relief by placing a hot, moist compress over your eyes twice daily to relax the eyelid muscles. If this is not effective, have your optician check the positioning of your glasses, or else consult your eye doctor.

There is a condition known as *blepharospasm* (*blepharo-* is the Greek combining form meaning "eyelid") that can be much more severe, involving exaggerated blinking and closing of the eye and even distortion of the entire face. This condition must be treated by an ophthalmologist. A recently developed treatment involves injecting tiny amounts of botulinum toxin (the bacterial toxin responsible for botulism) into the eyelid muscles.

Blepharitis

Blepharitis is an inflammation around the margins of the eyelids, often associated with dandruff. The eyelids become scaly, red, and itchy.

Treatment. Wash your eyelids twice daily with soap and warm water. Treat any dandruff condition with a medicated shampoo (*see* p. 446) and wash your face with the same preparation. If inflammation persists, see your doctor, who may prescribe an ointment.

Lumps on the Eyelid *(Chalazion)*

Chalazion is a painless swelling on the lid caused by blockage of one of the *meibomian* glands that lubricate the eye. You can usually treat small chalazions yourself using hot moist compresses and gently massaging the swelling with your finger to unblock the gland. If the swelling does not disappear after a few weeks, see your doctor. Larger chalazions may need to be incised.

Xanthelasma

Xanthelasma are small, hard yellowish nodules that form under the skin of the eyelids for poorly understood reasons. The nodules are harmless. You may wish to have them removed for cosmetic reasons, although they tend to recur.

Tumors of the Eye

Retinoblastoma

A *retinoblastoma* is a malignant tumor of the retina that occurs in children. Often the only symptom is crossed eyes, which is why this condition should always be examined by your doctor. If found early, the tumor can be treated by radiation or laser therapy. In advanced cases, the eye may have to be removed to prevent distant spread.

Malignant Melanoma

Malignant melanoma is the most common primary tumor of the eye. It usually arises in the choroid layer of the eye, and is generally discovered during routine eye examinations. If undetected, these tumors lead to gradual loss of vision in the affected eye.

Treatment. If the tumor is small, it may be treated with radiation or laser therapy and the eye saved. Larger tumors are treated by removal of the eye.

Eye Injuries

These are discussed under First Aid Procedures, p. 80.

Cross-section of the ear

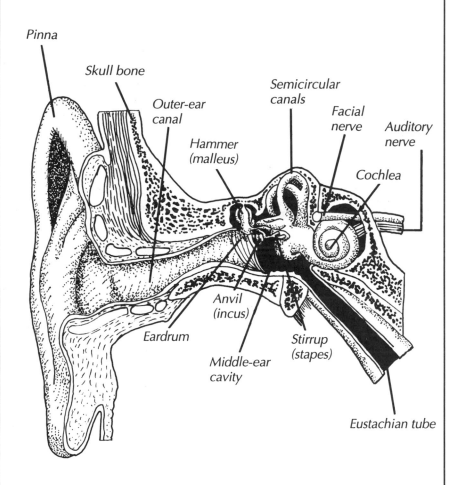

Pinna

Skull bone

Outer-ear canal

Hammer (malleus)

Semicircular canals

Facial nerve

Auditory nerve

Cochlea

Anvil (incus)

Eardrum

Stirrup (stapes)

Middle-ear cavity

Eustachian tube

Your Ears

How Your Ears Work

Your ear is conveniently divided into three parts:

1. The outer ear is the part you see and includes the ear canal leading down to the ear drum.
2. The middle ear contains the ear drum, the three tiny ear bones, and the surrounding air spaces (mastoid sinuses).
3. The inner ear contains the hearing organ, named the cochlea because it somewhat resembles a snail shell, and the auditory nerve.

Sound can be thought of as vibrating air that has two principal characteristics, intensity and frequency. These in turn are analogous to what we perceive as loudness and pitch, respectively. Sound waves travel down the ear canal and strike the eardrum, causing it to vibrate. These vibrations are transmitted to the cochlea by the ear bones. In the cochlea, the vibrations are transformed into nerve stimuli that are conducted to the brain by the auditory nerve.

The young ear can distinguish frequencies from about 20 cycles per second (Hertz), which is the sound produced by the largest and lowest-pitched pipe in an organ, up to about 20,000 cycles per second, which is close to the frequency produced by a shrill dog whistle. Neither of these two extremes is heard by most adults.

Hearing Loss

There are two general types of hearing loss: *conductive*, caused by abnormalities within the ear canal or middle ear; and *sensorineural* hearing loss caused by a lesion in the inner ear or the auditory nerve. Doctors can discriminate between these types of hearing loss by performing a series of auditory tests. If you suspect that you have impaired hearing, you should ask your doctor to recommend an auditory examination.

Conductive hearing loss occurs when the air passages are blocked, as occurs when earwax builds up, or when infection, such as a severe cold, causes fluid to collect in the middle ear, or when there is a blockage of the eustachean tube that connects the middle ear with the back of the mouth. Hearing losses that occur with middle ear infections, or during allergy season when your "ears become blocked," are usually temporary and subside when the infection, allergy, or other precipitating cause is treated.

Sensorineural hearing losses are more serious and are best prevented if it is possible in any specific case. It is estimated that one in ten Americans has a hearing loss that affects ability to understand normal speech. The incidence rises rapidly with age. Sensori–neural hearing loss or deafness can be caused by chronic ear infections, hereditary birth defects, certain drugs, head injury, aging, exposure to loud noise, and tumors. The most common cause of sensorineural hearing loss is deterioration of the inner ear structures as a result of the natural aging process. This is called *presbycusis*.

Sound intensity is measured in decibels (dB), units analogous to the Richter scale that measures seismic energy. Each 10-dB increase reflects a 10-fold increase in sound intensity. A quiet spot in the country may measure 20 dB; ordinary conversation takes place at about 60 dB, whereas a freight train runs up to 90 dB or more. Prolonged exposure to sound above 85 dB can result in measurable hearing loss. A common cause of such damage is playing loud music through headphones. Listening to headphones generating 90 dB for an hour or two can result in temporary hearing loss. Levels as high as 120 dB, which have been measured at rock concerts in front of the speakers, can result in immediate and permanent damage. Such noises do more than blow the mind!

How can you tell whether music or other sounds are too loud without having a decibel meter handy? Noise is probably too loud if:

- It hurts your ears.
- It causes ringing in your ears.
- You notice hearing impairment when the noise ceases.
- You must shout above the noise to make yourself heard.

What Can Be Done to Prevent Hearing Loss?

Sensorineural hearing loss is permanent in most cases. No treatment will recover it, but further loss can be prevented. If you must work in a noisy environment, you should wear hearing protectors. Such devices decrease the intensity of sound that reaches your eardrums. They come in two forms: earplugs and earmuffs.

Earplugs are small inserts that fit snugly into the ear canal. Earmuffs fit over the outer ears to reduce sound entering the ears. Properly fitting earplugs or muffs reduce noise by 15–30 dB. Using the two in combination may reduce sound by another 10–15 dB. If you have long hair or wear glasses, earplugs will be more effective than earmuffs. The American Academy of Otolaryngology offers a free booklet on *Noise, Ears and Hearing Protection.* The address is 1101 Vermont Ave. NW, Suite 302, Washington, DC 20005.

Hearing Loss with Aging *(Presbycusis)*

As noted earlier, the most common form of hearing loss occurs as a part of the normal aging process. It begins after the age of 20 and by age 65 affects almost 30% of Americans. Hearing loss affects the highest frequencies first, then gradually moves into the mid- and lower frequencies. Naturally there is great variability in individual losses. Men are affected more often and more severely than are women. Persons with mild hearing loss may have trouble hearing only certain sounds, such as *f, s,* and *th.* Or hearing may be difficult only when the sound source is far away or when there is loud background noise. Many of those with presbycusis describe the problem as being able to "hear" what others are saying, but being unable to understand what is being said. Another common complaint is that hearing seems normal when only one person is talking, but when several people are talking, an individual's speech gets lost in the "jumble." This condition can lead to withdrawal from personal interactions of all types. Family or friends may confuse this disorder with approaching senility, when in fact the mind is perfectly "sound."

Treatment. Most individuals with a handicapping sensorineural hearing loss can be helped dramatically with a hearing aid. If you have hearing impairment, you may be aware that you have difficulty hearing sounds that cause others no problem whatever. Some of the many signs of hearing impairment are listed below:

Hearing Impairment

Hearing impairment should be suspected in others if they:

- Respond inconsistently to sounds
- Turn their ears toward sounds
- Cup their ears with their hands
- Frequently ask those speaking to them to repeat, or
- Show other obvious signs of confusion or misunderstanding of speech.

SIGNS OF HEARING IMPAIRMENT

- You find yourself needing to raise the television or radio volume to a point that others complain of the loudness.
- You ever-more-frequently must strain to hear conversation at work or in a social setting.
- You frequently misunderstand or need to have things repeated.
- You find yourself watching people's faces intently when you are listening.
- You become irritated by people not speaking up. Remember, the problem may be with your ears and not that you live in a world of mumblers.

In such cases, ask your doctor for referral to an ear specialist, or contact the American Academy of Otolaryngology–Head and Neck Surgery at the address below. Detailed examination and testing must be done to determine the type of hearing loss you have and what, if any, treatment or hearing device you need. For information about ear specialists, audiologists, and speech and hearing clinics in your area, write to:

American Academy of Otolaryngology, Head and Neck Surgery, One Prince St., Alexandria, VA 22314.

The National Association for Hearing and Speech Action, 10801 Rockville Pike, Rockville, MD 20852, Phone: 1-800-638-8255. In Maryland: 1-301-897-5700.

Tinnitus (Ringing in the Ears)

Tinnitus is defined medically as the perception of sound in the absence of any acoustic stimulus. It may be a buzzing, ringing, roaring, whistling, or hissing sensation, and it may vary from time to time. It should be emphasized that tinnitus is a symptom of some underlying disorder within the ear. Contrary to what many people believe, tinnitus is not a disease itself.

There are many possible causes of tinnitus. The most common cause today is a deterioration of hearing as a result of the aging process, presbycusis, discussed above. Other causes include obstruction of the ear canal by earwax, ear infection, a hole in the eardrum, fluid in the middle ear, or stiffening (otosclerosis) of the middle ear bones. These problems are usually associated with hearing loss as well.

Tinnitus may also be caused by high blood pressure, allergies, tumor of the auditory nerve, diabetes, thyroid disease, excessive noise exposure, and head trauma.

Treatment. Most cases of tinnitus caused by external and middle ear disorders can be eliminated by treating the underlying disorder. However, treatment of tinnitus caused by sensorineural hearing loss often is not successful. There is a long list of medications and surgical proceedures that have been suggested to treat tinnitus, but none of them has proven effective. However, there are several things that can be done to help:

1. Avoid exposure to loud sounds and noises.
2. Have your blood pressure measured; if it is high, make certain your doctor gets it under control.
3. Decrease your salt intake.
4. Exercise regularly to improve your circulation.
5. Avoid stimulants such as coffee, soft drinks containing caffeine, tobacco, and marijuana. All adversely affect your hearing.
6. Avoid fatigue; it worsens tinnitus.
7. Attempt to reduce your stress level. Stress and anxiety have an adverse effect on tinnitus.
8. Your otolaryngologist will explain the possible benefits of biofeedback techniques and hearing aids. Some people with impaired hearing find that a hearing aid also reduces head noise. However, a thorough trial before purchase is advisable, because relief may be minimal.
9. Try one or more "masking" techniques. Tinnitus is usually more bothersome when it is quiet, especially when you are in bed. Devices that produce a low background (white) noise are often quite soothing. Electrical devices such as Sleep Mate, which emits a continuous low background noise, may please you. Try listening to FM music at low volume. Sometimes adjusting the dial slightly higher or lower than the broadcast frequency so as to "program" in background static creates the right effect. Electronic masking devices can be combined with hearing aids to relieve tinnitus and improve hearing at the same time.
10. "Self-help" groups have been formed in many communities for sharing information and coping strategies for living with tinnitus. For a list of such groups, contact: American Tinnitus Association, PO Box 5, Portland, OR 97207. For a free brochure on *Tinnitus*, write to: The Better Hearing Institute, 1430 K St. NW, Suite 600, Washington, DC 20005.

Dizziness and Motion Sickness

Dizziness has many causes and varies greatly in intensity, from "lightheadedness," or feeling "giddy," to true "vertigo," where the room seems to spin and the only position of relief is flat on your back. The term vertigo stems from the Latin verb "to turn" and the condition is frequently caused by a problem of the inner ear, which contains the organ of balance.

Motion sickness is related to vertigo in that the inner ear is probably affected. Many sufferers from motion sickness also experience dizziness, nausea, and even vomiting when riding in an airplane, boat (seasickness), or other vehicle. Motion sickness is usually temporary and seldom requires medical attention. However, some people are seriously affected, and even suffer symptoms for days after a trip.

The Complex Nature of Balance

Dizziness and motion sickness relate to the sense of balance and equilibrium. Researchers in space and aeronautical medicine call them disorders of "spatial orientation." Spatial orientation is the brain's notion of where the body is in space, both while moving and standing still. Spatial orientation is maintained by a complex interaction of several parts of the nervous system:

1. The inner ear (labyrinth), which monitors the directions of motion such as turning, up-down movement, etc.
2. The eyes, which monitor where the body is in space and also the direction of motion.
3. The skin pressure receptors in the feet and buttocks, which tell what part of the body is down.
4. The muscle and joint sensory receptors, which tell what parts of the body are moving.
5. The brain, which processes and coordinates all of the information coming from the above four systems.

The symptoms of dizziness and motion sickness develop when the *brain* receives conflicting messages from the other systems. For example, while riding in a car, reading a book, your inner ear detects all of the motion of travel, but the eyes see only the (apparently stationary) printed page. This conflicting information may lead to motion sickness. The same can occur on a boat or in an airplane.

Dizziness can also be caused by injury to, or a disorder of, the inner ear (for example, *Meniere's disease,* on the following page). Usually one ear is more affected than the other. In this case, the two ears may send conflicting signals to the brain, causing nausea or vertigo. Dizziness can be caused by inadequate blood supply to either the brain or inner ear. Hence those who suffer from arteriosclerosis, high blood pressure, diabetes, and heart disease may experience bouts of dizziness.

What You Can Do to Reduce Dizziness

1. Avoid rapid changes in position, especially from lying down to standing up or turning from one side to the other.
2. Avoid extremes of head motion, especially looking up. Avoid rapid twisting or turning of your head.
3. Avoid substances that impair circulation to your brain and ear, such as nicotine, caffeine, and salt.
4. Avoid hazardous activities when you are dizzy, such as driving, operating dangerous equipment, or climbing a stepladder.

What You Can Do to Reduce Motion Sickness

1. Try to ride where your eyes will see the same motion that your body and inner ears experience. For example, sit in the front seat of the car and look at distant scenery. In a boat, go up on deck and watch the motion of the horizon. In an airplane, sit by the window and look outside. Also select a seat over the wings where the motion is the least. In a boat, sit amidships.
2. Do not read while traveling if you are subject to motion sickness, and do not sit in a seat facing backward.
3. Avoid strong odors and spicy or greasy foods that do not agree with you just before or during travel. Folk wisdom has it that soda crackers and 7-Up are helpful. If they work for you, by all means use them!
4. There are several medicines that may reduce motion sickness. Dramamine, Bonine, and Marezine are over-the-counter preparations. If you have severe or debilitating symptoms, you should consult an otolaryngologist (an ENT specialist) for recommendations.

Recent air force studies have shown that the anti-seizure drug, dilantin, is effective in increasing tolerance to motion without the side effect of drowsiness that attends many antihistamines. Ask your doctor about it.

Meniere's Disease

A particularly disabling form of vertigo is known as *Meniere's disease*, named after the French physician who described it in the nineteenth century. It is characterized by recurrent, often prostrating vertigo, hearing loss, tinnitus, and frequently, a sensation of fullness in the affected ear. The cause is poorly understood, but the disease may arise from a failure of fluid drainage from the inner ear. The attacks of vertigo appear suddenly, last from several to 24 hours, and then gradually subside. These attacks are commonly accompanied by nausea and vomiting. Hearing in the affected ear tends to fluctuate, but progressively worsens over time.

Treatment. Meniere's disease must be treated by your doctor, usually with a combination of drugs and diet. In severe cases, surgery of the inner ear may be advised. The treatment is complex and highly uncertain. Because of this, it presents a ripe opportunity for charlatans recommending anything from vegetarian diets to megadoses of vitamins and homeopathic nostrums. My advice is to seek a board-certified otolaryngologist and avoid the numerous (and expensive) popular remedies that will relieve your purse before your symptoms.

Other Causes of Dizziness

If you get dizzy for a few seconds after standing up, you probably have a degree of "postural hypotension." This is caused by a temporary decrease in blood returning to your heart, so that the brain experiences a temporary lowering of blood pressure and its consequent oxygen deficit. This condition is accentuated by certain kinds of medicines, particularly those used to treat *high* blood pressure.

Another type of dizziness is caused by "hyperventilation," i.e., breathing too fast, usually a response to stress or anxiety. To test this, breathe more deeply and rapidly than usual through your mouth for half a minute. You should begin to feel somewhat lightheaded and your finger tips may tingle. If this is similar to your dizzy spells, hyperventilation may be the cause. Consult your doctor, who may recommend relaxation techniques (meditation is often effective), breathing into a paper bag, or possibly temporary use of tranquilizers.

One cause of severe dizziness and nausea is an inflammation of the labyrinth, known as *labyrinthitis*. The cause is usually a viral infection. If your doctor diagnoses labyrinthitis, the usual treatment is bed rest for several days, along with drugs to combat the nausea. Most cases clear up completely within a few weeks.

In rare instances, dizziness, particularly in adolescents, may be a manifestion of epilepsy. You should ask your doctor whether a neurologist should be consulted.

Ear Infections

Infections of the Middle Ear *(Otitis Media)*

Ear infections conjure for most parents sleepless nights, crying children, and expensive trips to the doctor. After the common cold, ear infections are the most frequent infection of childhood. About one third of all children have more than three ear infections during the first three years of life. By age 6, nearly 90% of children will have had at least one ear infection.

Causes of Otitis Media

The healthy middle ear is filled with air at the same atmospheric pressure as outside the ear. Air enters the middle ear through the narrow eustachian tube. When you swallow or yawn, a small amount of air enters the ear and you hear a small "pop" or click. This is repeated hundreds of times each day because the lining of the middle ear absorbs air continuously.

Bacteria entering the middle ear from the throat normally drain back out the eustachian tube. If the eustachian tube becomes blocked, as may happen during a throat infection or an attack of hay fever, bacteria cannot drain properly, and an infection known as *otitis media* ensues. Since air does not enter the middle ear, a vacuum is formed as the membrane lining the ear absorbs the air already trapped within. This causes the ear to fill with fluid, and as the infection develops, the pressure of the fluid increases, causing intense pain and ringing in the ears *(tinnitus)*. In some cases the eardrum will rupture and drain pus through the outer ear. For the child, misery is complete. Babies too young to verbalize the source of their agony will frequently tug at their ears, and they have difficulty sleeping because pressure in the ear is greater lying down.

Children under age 7 are especially prone to otitis media because their eustachian tubes are shorter and less rigid, and are thus more liable to collapse shut, preventing normal drainage. Too, they have more colds and sore throats that predispose them to ear infections. After age 7 or 8, growth changes occur that make otitis media relatively uncommon.

Treatment. The only thing to do is to get the child to the doctor as quickly as possible to begin antibiotic therapy. An antihistimine or decongestant to promote drainage of the ear is often prescribed, along with a painkiller such as ibuprofen (Advil, Nuprin) or acetaminophen

(Tylenol). Aspirin is not given to children because of the rare but dangerous complication of Reye's syndrome.

In some cases the eardrum must be lanced (a procedure called *myringotomy*) to promote healing. This dramatically reduces the pain.

In some instances, especially if the child has suffered repeated episodes of otitis media, your doctor may recommend indwelling drainage tubes (a procedure known as *tympanostomy*) to promote drainage while the infection is clearing. These tubes generally remain in place for about six months, when they spontaneously fall out of the ear and the eardrum heals itself. Removal of the tonsils and adenoids may also be recommended if they appear to be the focus of infection.

What Parents Can Do

Once specific medication has been prescribed, it is essential that your child take the antibiotic for the full duration it is prescribed, usually 10–14 days. This is important because the symptoms of infection will probably disappear before the infection is completely eliminated. Repeated infections are generally more severe than the first, and the chance of permanent hearing loss is increased

Parents can also be alert to the colds and throat infections that often precede ear infections. Your child should be taken to the doctor so that prompt treatment can be started. Although children with colds are often prescribed oral decongestants, these drugs do not prevent ear infections. They may also make your child either hyperactive or lethargic.

Children with a well-documented allergic history may benefit from antihistamines. These should be prescribed by your doctor.

Children should also enjoy a smoke-free environment. Recent studies show that exposure to smokers in the household can triple the risk of chronic ear infections. Remember not to bottlefeed a baby lying down because the milk can flow into the ear during swallowing and trigger a middle ear infection.

For parents with a child who has ear problems, a very comprehensive book has been written by a physician–parent team: *Ear Infection in Your Child—The Comprehensive Parental Guide to Causes and Treatments* by Kenneth Grundfast, MD, and Cynthia J. Carney, Compact Books, 283 pp., $14.95.

Air Travel and Your Ears

Air travel is associated with rapid changes in air pressure. If the eustachian tube is not functioning properly, an imbalance of pressure across the eardrum may cause sudden ear pain, particularly in infants and young children. This condition is known as *barotitis*.

What can *you* do to unblock your ears? Swallowing activates the muscle that opens the eustachian tube. Chewing gum or sucking hard candy is a good way to promote swallowing. Be sure to remain awake during descent, otherwise you will not swallow often enough to keep up with the pressure changes. The same is true for children. Awaken them when the flight attendant announces start of descent. Flight attendants often recommend yawning, which usually works well.

If swallowing or yawning is not effective you may try the following maneuver: Pinch you nostrils shut. Then take a mouthful of air. Using your cheek and throat muscles, force the air into your nose as if you were trying to blow your nose. When you hear your ears pop, you know your eustachian tubes have opened up. Do not force air from your lungs (i.e., with the glottis open) because the pressures you create are too high for the middle ear.

If you have a cold or are in a hay fever season, take an antihistamine or nasal decongestant an hour or so before boarding the aircraft. (Decongestants should be avoided by persons with heart disease, high blood pressure, irregular heart rhythms, and thyroid diseases, except by the advice of your doctor.)

Infection of the Outer Ear *(Otitis externa)*

Infections of the outer ear, called *otitis externa*, may be caused by either bacterial or fungal infections. Predisposing causes include water in the ear (hence "swimmer's ear") or such irritants as hair spray or hair dye, and of course the trauma caused by sticking things you shouldn't in your ears. The condition usually begins with itching and redness of your outer ear. If allowed to progress, acute otitis externa may develop. This is a serious infection characterized by pain, redness, and swelling, with drainage of a milky, and sometimes foul-smelling, fluid. Pain produced by pulling on the earlobe tends to distinguish otitis externa from otitis media.

Treatment. Early-stage infections can often be treated with dilute acetic acid drops (vinegar solution) for a week, which discourages bacterial growth. Once swelling and pus have developed, your doctor will probably prescribe topical antibiotics and cortisone.

Infected pimples (furuncles) in the outer ear are treated effectively by gentle cleansing with an alcohol sponge twice daily. Dry heat is helpful in relieving pain and speeding healing.

EARWAX

The amber-colored wax found in your ears is produced by special glands near the outer ear canal. This wax keeps water, dust and dirt away from the eardrum. Usually the wax accumulates a bit, and then dries and falls out of the ear, carrying trapped dust and debris with it. Sometimes earwax accumulates sufficiently to block the ear canal, causing impaired hearing and/or tinnitus. Paradoxically, this can happen as a result of sticking things in your ear to clean it of wax. You should not probe your ears with cotton-tipped applicators, bobby pins, or twisted napkins; such objects just serve as ramrods to push the wax in deeper.

Your doctor can clean your ears. However, you may wish to try such over-the-counter wax softeners as Debrox, which contains carbamide peroxide. Currently this is the only safe and effective medication for use in softening earwax. It is instilled twice daily for two or three days.

After a few minutes, flush your ear gently with warm water, either in the shower or using the rubber syringe supplied with the drops. Do not use preparations that fizz in your ear, because pressure can build up and perforate your eardrum. *Do not use any preparation if you know you have a hole in your eardrum*, because this may result in a middle ear infection. If you are uncertain whether you have a perforated eardrum, consult your doctor. No product should be used in children under 12 except on your doctor's advice.

Swimmer's Ear

Swimmer's ear is an inflammation or infection of the outer ear caused by bacteria in water trapped in the ear. It can be prevented by instilling antiseptic drops in your ears after swimming. Some over-the-counter preparations are Aqua Ear, Ear Magic, and Swim Ear. If you get water in your ears after swimming or showering, bend your head to the side with your ear up, pull your earlobe upward and backward, and instill the eardrops. Wiggle your ears to get the drops down into the canal. Then turn your head down to let them drain out.

You can make up your own eardrops using plain rubbing alcohol. It absorbs the water, helps dry out the ear, and may kill the organisms that cause swimmer's ear. You can also mix vinegar half and half with alcohol. The vinegar also kills bacteria and fungus and leaves the ear with a low pH, an environment unfavorable for growth of these organisms.

Your druggist will supply you with a dropper bottle. If you have a tendency to develop swimmer's itch, use antiseptic drops regularly after swimming or showering. Properly fitting ear plugs also prevent water from entering your ear canals.

Dry Ears

If you develop itchy ears only during winter, it may be that you produce insufficient wax to lubricate your ears during dry periods.

Treatment. Keep your ears dry when bathing and swimming. Use earplugs if necessary. Protect them from shampoos, hair coloring, and hair sprays. Use a cortisone cream (e.g., Cortaid) applied daily to the affected area.

Foreign Bodies in the Ear

Gnats may fly into the ear and become trapped in the earwax. Larger insects such as flies and roaches generally become trapped because they cannot crawl backwards or turn around in the ear canal. Needless to say the result is not pleasant. Gnats are usually washed out with warm water gently instilled from a rubber bulb syringe. The latter is a handy device that used to be a common item in the home medicine cabinet, but is curiously uncommon nowadays.

If larger insects chance into your ear, fill the ear with mineral oil or olive oil. This suffocates the insect by plugging its breathing pores. It takes five to ten minutes to do the culprit in, but be patient. In the meanwhile you can be calling the doctor to stand by to extract it.

Children have an astonishing tendency to fill the void they sense in their ears with whatever is at hand—from beads and beans to rice and dice. Do not attempt removal. This is one for the doctor who can also tell whether the eardrum has been perforated.

Trauma

A blow to the ear may result in the external ear becoming a shapeless, reddish-purple mass, called a *hematoma*. Because the swelling may cut off the blood supply to the ear, the hematoma must be surgically removed. Failure to do so may result in "cauliflower ear"— common to boxers—not a pleasing consequence.

Perforation of the eardrum can result from objects thrust into the ear canal, a slap to the side of the head, swimming and diving accidents, or even by kissing (a big smooch can create a lot of negative pressure!). The result is sudden pain, followed by bleeding from the ear, loss of hearing, and tinnitus. Closure will usually occur spontaneously if the perforation is small, but you should see your doctor, who will probably prescribe prophylactic antibiotics to prevent infection.

If you have loss of hearing and/or dizziness following injury to your ears, consult your doctor immediately.

The Endocrine System

Hypothalamus

Pituitary gland

Thyroid gland

Parathyroid glands

Adrenal glands

Pancreas

Your Endocrine Glands and Their Disorders

Your endocrine glands are the small, but essential organs that secrete all the important hormones regulating body functions. They include the pituitary, thyroid, parathyroid, adrenal, and pancreas glands. The interrelationships between these glands and the alterations that occur to cause endocrine diseases are extremely complex. We will discuss only the more common problems.

Disorders of the Pituitary Gland

The pituitary gland is a thimble-sized organ that lies just beneath the brain. It has been called the "master gland" because its secretions control the activity of the other endocrine glands and it is itself responsible for growth and development. The pituitary in turn is controlled by a part of the brain called the hypothalamus. Most disorders of the pituitary occur because the gland produces either too much of or too little of one of its six hormones. Some examples include:

Dwarfism

Dwarfism occurs when the pituitary fails to produce enough *growth hormone* during childhood, resulting in retarded development, or dwarfism. Sexual development is also usually retarded. This is a relatively rare disorder; nutritional deficiencies and congenital heart disease are more common causes of stunted growth. If your child fails to achieve expected growth guidelines, your doctor will measure growth hormone levels in your child's blood as well as investigate more common causes. Pituitary dwarfism can be treated with injections of bioengineered human growth hormone when discovered early.

Gigantism

Gigantism occurs when the pituitary produces too much growth hormone during childhood, and all parts of the body are stimulated to excessive growth. The usual cause of such excessive growth hormone production is a pituitary tumor, which results in overly rapid growth and development of the child or adolescent. Here too, sexual development may be retarded. Pituitary tumors are ordinarily treated by irradiation to control the output of hormone.

Acromegaly

Acromegaly occurs when excess growth hormone production arises during adulthood; height is not affected, because vertical growth stops at the end of adolescence. Rather, the most common signs are enlargement of the hands and feet, excess body hair, and overgrowth of the jaw and other facial features. Also common are fatigue, profuse sweating, arthritis, and generalized stiffness. Again, the usual cause of this excess of growth hormone is a pituitary tumor, which is treated by surgical removal or irradiation.

Diabetes Insipidus

Diabetes insipidus develops when the pituitary produces too little *antidiuretic hormone*, often as a result of brain injury. This hormone acts on the kidneys to conserve body water. When too little is produced, the kidneys fail to reabsorb water, resulting in excess urine production. This in turn gives rise to unquenchable thirst. The treatment consists of oral and nasally inhaled drugs that control urine formation.

When diabetes insipidus is caused by a pituitary tumor, surgical removal of the tumor is often effective.

Thyroid Disorders

The thyroid gland is the small organ that lies in the lower neck, just in front of your trachea (windpipe) and just below your larynx (voice box). The thyroid gland produces the hormone, *thyroxine*, sometimes called T4, as well as a similar hormone, T3, which regulate the rate of metabolism in your body. The principal disorders of the thyroid are *hyperthyroidism*, caused by overproduction of thyroxine, *hypothyroidism*, caused by underproduction of thyroxine, and various types of lumps and tumors.

Hyperthyroidism
(Grave's Disease, Toxic Goiter, Thyrotoxicosis)

In *hyperthyroidism*, the thyroid gland, or a tumor of the thyroid produces excess T3 and T4, thus speeding body metabolism. Hyperthyroidism is much more common in women than men. In some cases the gland may become visibly enlarged, in which event, a *goiter* is said to be present. The most common symptoms are nervousness and a shaking tremor of your hands; increased sweating; oversensitivity to heat; a rapid, pounding heart (palpitations); weight loss despite an increased appetite; inability to sleep; muscle weakness; and diarrhea. In some cases, the eyes may become widened and bulge prominently, a feature called *exophthalmia*. Interestingly, most of these symptoms can also be found in those patients with hypothyroidism who overdose themselves with thyroid medication, a condition called *thyrotoxicosis factitia*.

In very severe cases of hyperthyroidism, known as *thyroid storm*, rapid heart rate, cardiac irregularities, and high temperature can lead quickly to prostration and death. Thyroid storm is a true medical emergency.

Treatment. There are three general methods of treating hyperthyroidism. The first is to take antithyroid drugs that interfere with the production of T3 and T4. These drugs may cure some people, but all too often the symptoms return when the drugs are stopped. Surgical removal of a portion of the gland cures about 90% of patients, but involves such complications as voice changes should the laryngeal nerve be severed and calcium disturbances when the parathyroid glands *(see below)* are inadvertently removed.

The treatment chosen by most patients is radioactive iodine, which can be taken orally and involves no surgery. The thyroid concentrates iodine to manufacture thyroxine. The gland cannot distinguish radioactive from natural iodine. In concentrating the radioactive iodine, the gland is selectively irradiated, with very little radiation to the rest of the body. If just enough radioactive iodine is given, a normally active gland may result.

In a large number of individuals, the gland is rendered permanently hypothyroid (by either surgery or radioactive iodine), in which case thyroid pills must be taken for life. This, however, is a simple and relatively complication-free treatment. *(Please read the next section.)*

Hypothyroidism (Myxedema)

In *hypothyroidism*, the thyroid does not produce enough thyroxine and consequently body metabolism slows down. The symptoms, which are often subtle and gradual in onset, are in striking contrast to hyperthyroidism. You are apt to feel tired, have minor aches and pains, move more slowly than usual, become intolerant of cold, and exhibit an increased tendency to gain weight. Your face may take on a dull, puffy appearance and your tongue may become thickened. Your hair may become sparse and your skin is apt to become dry and scaly. Hypothyroidism is much more common in older individuals and many of the symptoms may be mistaken for natural changes associated with aging. In advanced cases, the mental slowing that occurs with hypothyroidism may be misinterpreted as early senility (*see* Dementias, p. 104). In some severe cases, drowsiness, markedly reduced activity, and even coma (called myxedema coma) can develop. The diagnosis is made easily through appropriate blood tests that measure thyroid hormones and the pituitary hormone, TSH.

Treatment. The treatment is quite simple: a daily oral dose of a synthetic thyroid hormone preparation. The dose must be adjusted to your particular requirements and must be taken for life.

Recently it has been recognized that *overreplacement* of thyroid hormone can cause osteoporosis, particularly in postmenopausal women. Osteoporosis is a metabolic bone disease that causes bone loss and fractures (discussed in detail on p. 405) The usual symptoms associated with excess thyroid hormone replacement, called *thyrotoxicosis factitia*, are nervousness, jitteriness, weight loss, and difficulty sleeping. However, the slight overdoses that can lead to osteoporosis cause no symptoms, and such overdoses have been difficult to diagnose. Although newer, more sensitive blood tests for the pituitary hormone, *thyroid stimulating hormone* (TSH), promise to make this diagnosis easier.

TSH is produced by the pituitary in response to reduced levels of circulating thyroid hormones, T3 and T4, stimulating the normal thyroid to increase production. Correspondingly, when there is excess circulating thyroid hormone, TSH production is turned off. If you are taking thyroid replacement pills, your doctor will most likely monitor your progress by TSH measurement. Your thyroid hormone replacement dose must be selected so that not only are the symptoms of hypothyroidism prevented, but also that the same thyroid hormones do not have an adverse effect on your bones. The blood levels of TSH are the best indication that the thyroid hormone replacement dose is correct. Ask your doctor about the newer measures for TSH.

Subacute Thyroiditis

Subacute thyroiditis is an inflammation of the thyroid, probably caused by a virus. The symptoms are neck pain—often mistaken for a sore throat—and low-grade fever. Your thyroid may become swollen and tender to the touch. Rarely, the symptoms of hyperthyroidism *(see above)* develop when the inflammation causes a rapid release of stored thyroid hormone.

Treatment. Your doctor will probably prescribe aspirin to reduce inflammation and relieve soreness. In severe cases steroids may be prescribed. The inflammation seldom lasts longer that a few months.

Hashimoto's Thyroiditis

Hashimoto's thyroiditis is a chronic inflammation of the thyroid and is thought to be an autoimmune disorder, i.e., your body manufactures antibodies against your own thyroid as if it were a foreign tissue. There is painless enlargement (*goiter*) of the gland and gradually the symptoms of hypothyroidism develop.

Treatment. The treatment is the same as for hypothyroidism.

Thyroid Nodules

Thyroid nodules are localized enlargements or swellings in an otherwise normal gland. They may be single or multiple. There are four common types of thyroid nodules:

1. Soft fluid-filled cysts.
2. Localized swelling caused by bleeding. These may be temporarily painful.
3. Benign tumors (adenomas). These may or may not produce thyroxine and the symptoms of hyperthyroidism *(see above)*.
4. Thyroid cancer. These also may or may not produce thyroxine.

If you should feel—or see—a nodule in your neck, consult your doctor for a diagnosis. The type of nodule can usually be determined through a combination of blood tests, radioisotope scans, ultrasound scanning, and biopsy.

Treatment. Fluid- and blood-filled cysts usually require no treatment. The fluid may be aspirated with a needle if the cyst is large. Benign tumors may often be suppressed by giving thyroid hormone, during which many shrink or disappear completely. Thyroid cancers are treated by surgical removal, followed by treatment with radioactive iodine. The long-term prognosis of most thyroid cancers is excellent if treated early and correctly.

For more information about thyroid cancer, call the National Cancer Institute Information Center, 1-800-4-CANCER.

Parathyroid Disorders

The parathyroid glands are four pea-sized organs located behind the thyroid gland. They secrete *parathyroid hormone*, which, along with vitamin D and the thyroid-produced hormone, *calcitonin*, helps build strong bones and teeth. Disorders of the parathyroid involve either over- or underproduction of parathyroid hormone.

Hyperparathyroidism

Overproduction of parathyroid hormone is usually caused by a benign tumor (*parathyroid adenoma*) or else by uniform enlargement (*hypertrophy*) of one or all of the glands. The excess parathyroid hormone causes calcium to be drawn out of the bones, which eventually become weakened and prone to fracture. The increased blood calcium must be excreted by the kidneys, which become prone to develop kidney stones (*see* p. 330). It is often the onset of such stones that gives the first indication of parathyroid disease.

Treatment. Surgical removal of the enlarged parathyroid(s) usually cures the disease.

Hypoparathyroidism

In the rare condition known as *hypoparathyroidism*, the parathyroid glands do not produce enough parathyroid hormone, causing the blood level of calcium to fall. The result is often painful cramp-like spasms in the hand and feet, known as *tetany*.

Treatment. Oral doses of calcium and vitamin D usually prevent tetany and restore blood levels of calcium to normal. Treatment must be continued for life.

Disorders of the Adrenal Glands

The *adrenal glands* are two pyramid-shaped organs that lie one on top of each kidney. They contain an outer cortex and an inner medulla. The medulla is responsible for producing *epinephrine* (adrenalin) and *norepinephrine* (noradrenalin), which help regulate blood pressure, heart rate, and vascular tone.

The cortex produces three different types of steroid hormones. The first group, the *mineralocorticoids*, helps regulate mineral balance. The most important of these is *aldosterone*. The second group helps regulate carbohydrate metabolism, as well as inflammatory responses. The most important of these is *hydrocortisone*. The third group includes the sex hormones, especially *androgen*, *estrogen,* and *progesterone,* all of which are also produced in the testicles and ovaries and are responsible for sexual development. Both sexes produce all three types of hormones in the adrenal cortex, although androgens predominate in males and estrogen and progesterone predominate in females. Disorders of the adrenal glands primarily involve either excess or insufficient production of these various hormones. Only the most common disorders will be discussed here.

Cushing's Syndrome

Cushing's syndrome is a disorder that actually encompasses several abnormalities, all of which cause an excess of adrenal hormones circulating in the blood. The most common cause is the intentional administration of steroid medications by your doctor for some other condition, such as arthritis, asthma, and many chronic inflammatory conditions. In rare cases the excess may be caused by a tumor or enlargement of either the adrenal gland itself, or else of the pituitary gland, which regulates the adrenal glands.

The symptoms of Cushing's syndrome develop only after several weeks or months of elevated blood steroids. The face becomes fat, rounded, and red, sometimes called a "moon" face. A fat pad often develops about the shoulders, which produces a rather humped back. Muscle mass is lost from the arms and legs. Patients become weak and tire easily. The skin may be blotchy and bruise easily. In prolonged cases, osteoporosis also develops (*see* p. 405).

Treatment. If the cause of Cushing's syndrome is excess steroid medication, your doctor will most likely attempt to reduce the dosage, depending upon the nature and severity of the disease being treated. Never stop taking these medicines yourself without your doctor's advice, because sudden withdrawal can have catastrophic consequences. In cases in which a pituitary tumor is responsible, surgical removal or radiation therapy is often curative. In rare instances, the adrenal glands themselves must be removed.

Addison's Disease

In *Addison's disease,* the opposite of Cushing's syndrome exists, namely an insufficient secretion of adrenal hormones from the cortex. The most common cause is an atrophy of the gland for unknown reasons. In some cases infection may destroy the glands.

The most common symptoms include weakness, tiredness, and weight loss. The skin may become strikingly dark. In some cases vomiting and diarrhea occur. The disease is diagnosed by discovering low levels of steroid hormones circulating in the blood. The treatment consists of daily oral steroid hormone replacement for life. Usually this consists of oral hydrocortisone twice daily. Increased doses will most likely be administered by your doctor should you develop an infection or other condition that places greater stress on your body.

Adrenal Tumors

Adrenal tumors and enlargement (hypertrophy) usually produce an excess of a specific hormone. In most cases treatment is by surgical removal of the tumor. The most common conditions include:

1. *Pheochromocytoma.* This is a benign tumor of the adrenal medulla (core of the gland) that produces excess epinephrine and norepinephrine. The symptoms include attacks of rapid heart beat, pallor, sweating, weakness, and headache. During these attacks, the blood pressure is usually very high.
2. *Aldosteronism.* Excess production of aldosterone may be caused by a tumor or by enlargement of the adrenal cortex. The chief symptom is high blood pressure, which is relieved only by removal of the tumor or enlarged gland.
3. *Virilizing syndrome.* Here a tumor or enlargement of the adrenal cortex produces excess sex hormones. The signs and symptoms are more marked in women than in men, and include excess hair, acne, deepening of the voice, enlargement of the clitoris, menstrual irregularity or cessation, and decreased breast size.

Endocrine Disorders of the Pancreas

The pancreas has two special functions. The first of these is to produce enzymes that help digest food (*see* p. 299 for a discussion of malabsorption syndromes). The second is to produce the hormones, *insulin* and *glucagon*, which are responsible for regulating the glucose level in the blood. Glucose is the principle energy source for all the body's cells.

Diabetes Mellitus

Diabetes mellitus occurs when the pancreas fails to produce enough insulin to maintain normal levels of blood glucose (sugar). There are two types of diabetes mellitus: Type I (also called juvenile-onset or insulin-dependent diabetes) and Type II (also called adult-onset or insulin-independent diabetes).

Type I Diabetes

Type I, or *insulin-dependent diabetes,* is usually diagnosed during childhood or adolescence. Children with this type of diabetes most likely have an autoimmune disease in which the body's immune system produces antibodies that destroy the insulin-producing cells within the pancreas. Without insulin, the blood glucose level soars, but the body is unable to make use of the excess glucose, which is excreted in vast quantities in the urine. Such diabetics must take insulin injections for life to maintain normal blood glucose.

Type II Diabetes

Type II diabetes, also known as *adult-onset or insulin-independent diabetes,* begins later in life, the incidence increasing steadily with age. In Type II diabetes, the pancreas continues to produce insulin, but not in sufficient quantities to maintain normal blood glucose. This type of diabetes is often controlled by weight reduction, diet, and in severe cases, oral diabetic medications or injectable insulin. Type II diabetes is much more common than Type I. There are several known risk factors that increase the likelihood of developing diabetes:

- Blacks, Hispanics, and North American Indians all have higher than average rates of diabetes. For example, black women have twice the incidence of diabetes as white women.
- Having at least one family member with diabetes increases your chance of developing diabetes, suggesting a definite hereditary disposition to developing both types of diabetes.
- People who are overweight and inactive have a higher incidence of diabetes. Nearly 80% of blacks with diabetes are obese.
- Women who have experienced temporary diabetes while pregnant are more apt to develop diabetes later in life.

What Are the Symptoms of Diabetes?

Since glucose cannot be metabolized without insulin, your body's glucose is excreted in the urine, carrying with it large quantities of water. This makes you urinate often, sometimes every hour or two both day and night. Naturally this water requirement makes you constantly thirsty. Because glucose provides food for

---

MANAGING YOUR DIABETES

Regardless of the type of diabetes you have, certain habits are important to maintaining good health:

- Do not smoke. Smoking promotes development of atherosclerosis and constricts blood vessels, thus compounding the adverse effects of peripheral neuropathy.
- Take special care of your feet to prevent ulcers and gangrene. *See* p. 202 for a discussion of proper foot care.
- Pregnancy greatly alters the need for insulin. See your doctor at once if you believe you are pregnant.
- If you require insulin, try to take the same quantities of foods at the same times each day. If you are unable to eat according to your usual schedule, take additional glucose drinks rather than reducing your insulin dose.
- Ask your doctor for a card or bracelet (MedicAlert bracelet) that identifies you as a diabetic so that appropriate treatment can be given quickly in case you become incapacitated.
- Always tell your doctor and dentist that you are diabetic so that they can take appropriate precautions.

---

bacteria, urinary tract and vaginal infections are common. Infections of many types are common in uncontrolled diabetes.

Since your dietary glucose cannot be utilized, fats are burned and weight loss is common. You are also likely to tire easily. Women are apt to experience menstrual irregularities and some men develop impotence.

Diabetics, especially those whose blood glucose has been poorly controlled by diet or insulin injections, are at risk for developing several serious diseases, including diabetic retinopathy (*see* p. 137), peripheral neuropathy (*see* p. 117), atherosclerosis (*see* p. 175), and kidney failure (*see* p. 332).

Diagnosis and treatment. The diagnosis of diabetes is made by demonstrating glucose and ketones in the urine. Ketones are a product of fat metabolism. In some cases of Type II diabetes, ketones are not present. In this event your doctor may order a glucose tolerance test in which your blood glucose is measured before and after your consumption of a test glucose drink.

Type I Diabetes. This form of diabetes is treated with a combination of diet and daily insulin injections. There are different types of insulin and your doctor must decide which is best for you. Insulin lowers the blood glucose, but too much insulin can lead to dangerously low levels of glucose, a condition known as *hypoglycemia* (*see* next section). Consequently, the blood glucose must be carefully monitored by frequent measurements of urine and blood glucose. Currently there are several electronic devices that can determine the amount of glucose in the blood from a test strip to which a drop of blood from the side of your finger has been added. Blood glucose measurements are more reliable than urine glucose measurements in determining the correct dose of insulin or the need for additional food. To obtain an accurate reading of blood glucose, you must follow the manufacturer's instructions carefully and be trained by your doctor in the instrument's use. Urine glucose can easily be measured by adding a drop of urine to a test tablet (Clinitest) or a paper test strip (Tes-Tape, Diastix, or Clinistix).

Currently too, there are devices, both internally and externally worn or implanted, that can automatically administer insulin to provide a more uniform dose and thus even out the inevitable wide swings of blood glucose that result from subcutaneously injected insulin. In juvenile-onset diabetes, parents must usually administer their child's insulin until about age ten, at which time they can usually take responsibility for their own injections.

Equally important to administering the prescribed dosages of insulin is to adhere to the diet your doctor recommends in order to avoid hypoglycemia. Since additional exercise and such stresses as infections and trauma consume more glucose, your doctor may prescribe extra food during these occasions.

Type II Diabetes. In many cases diet alone can control this form of diabetes, especially if you are overweight. It is usually recommended that you maintain an ideal weight for your sex and height (*see* p. 314) and eat small portions of carbohydrates at regular intervals to avoid wide swings in blood glucose.

If diet alone does not control blood glucose, your doctor may recommend one of several oral antidiabetic drugs. The most frequently prescribed is glyburide (marketed as Micronase and DiaBeta). The techniques for measuring blood and urine glucose are the same as described above.

For more information about diabetes and for resources available in your area, contact the American Diabetes Association Inc., 1660 Duke St., Alexandria, VA 22314, 1-800-232-3472.

Hypoglycemia

Hypoglycemia is the condition in which the blood glucose level is reduced and the body's cells become starved for food. One of the most common causes is an overdose of insulin in patients with "brittle" diabetes, i.e., those who experience wide swings of blood glucose from very high to very low. Another common cause is *reactive hypoglycemia*, in which a meal stimulates an excessive outpouring of insulin that lowers blood glucose to symptomatic levels. Other causes include alcohol in sensitive individuals, an abnormal reaction to certain types of foods and drugs, liver disease, pregnancy, high fever, and in rare instances, an insulin-producing tumor of the pancreas known as an *insulinoma*.

The symptoms include faintness, dizziness, weakness, jitteriness, rapid heart beat, sweating, hunger, and nervousness. Some people also experience confusion, disorientation, unsteadiness, and even aggressive behavior. In the latter cases, hypoglycemia may be mistaken for drunkenness. When caused by eating, the onset of symptoms is characteristically within 2–4 hours after the meal.

The diagnosis of hypoglycemia is made by measuring a low blood glucose level during an attack. You should carefully consider the circumstances that occurred prior to an attack to give your doctor an idea of the precipitating cause. If the attacks occur after insulin injections, the cause is obvious.

Treatment. The symptoms of hypoglycemia can be relieved within a few minutes of ingesting sugar, candy, or anything with sugar. One convenient method is to stir three tablespoons of granulated sugar into a glass of fruit juice or water. Another common treatment is to self-administer *glucagon* subcutaneously. Glucagon is a pancreatic hormone that releases glucose into the bloodstream from the liver.

If you are subject to attacks of hypoglycemia, you should carry sugar tablets or candy with you at all times and take these as soon as you become aware of the first symptoms in order to prevent a full-blown attack. If attacks occur after meals, a diet high in proteins and low in carbohydrates is often recommended. If you become dizzy or tend to pass out, your doctor may advise that you carry injectable glucagon with you at all times. Parents, spouses, and close associates should be taught how to inject glucagon in case you lose consciousness. The usual dose is 0.5 to 1.0 milligram. Finally, if you tend to have severe reactions, you should not drive, swim alone, or operate machinery.

Cross-section of the heart

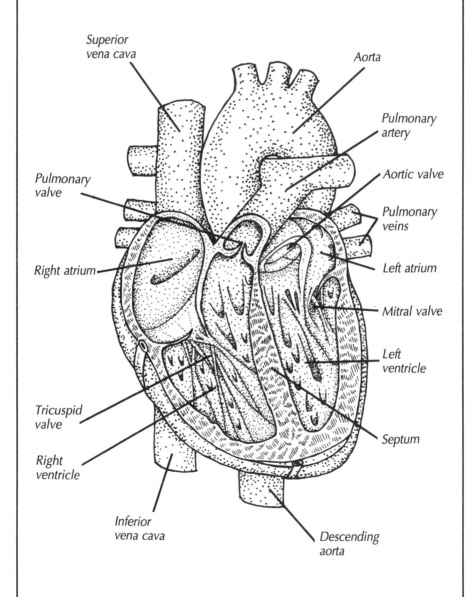

Superior vena cava

Aorta

Pulmonary artery

Pulmonary valve

Aortic valve

Pulmonary veins

Right atrium

Left atrium

Mitral valve

Left ventricle

Tricuspid valve

Septum

Right ventricle

Inferior vena cava

Descending aorta

Your Heart and Circulation

How Your Heart Works

Every minute your heart pumps about five quarts of blood through-out your body, carrying oxygen and nutrients that sustain all your body functions. The heart is essentially a four-chambered pump as shown on opposite page. Venous blood from the body enters the upper chamber on the right (right atrium) and flows from there into the right ventricle, which pumps the blood out through the pulmonary artery to your lungs. There carbon dioxide is released and oxygen is taken up. The freshly oxygenated blood returns to the left atrium by way of the pulmonary veins and flows into the left ventricle.

The left ventricle pumps oxygenated blood into the aorta, the main artery of your body. From the aorta, blood is delivered throughout your body through progressively smaller arteries and ultimately to the capillaries, where oxygen diffuses into the tissues and excess carbon dioxide is picked up. From the capillaries, blood flows into increasingly larger veins, thence into the vena cava, and back into the right atrium.

The heart itself is supplied with blood through three coronary arteries. It is disease in these arteries that causes most heart attacks, and many other heart diseases as well. Let us first look at blood vessel diseases in general.

Arteriosclerosis and Atherosclerosis

Arteriosclerosis has also been called "hardening of the arteries" because part of the muscle in the arterial wall is replaced by fibrous tissue that makes the vessel less elastic. This is a widespread process that affects all arteries of the body and hence gives rise to diseases in many organs: the heart (heart attacks), brain (strokes), kidneys (kidney failure), and others. Arteriosclerosis may be part of the normal aging process, since it occurs in all people and begins at an early age. Fortunately in most people it progresses very slowly.

Atherosclerosis is the most common feature of arteriosclerosis and involves chiefly the medium and large arteries. In this condition the linings of the arteries become thickened and irregular with plaque-like deposits of fats and cholesterol called *atheromas*. These atheromas protrude into the central channel *(lumen)*, obstructing the flow of blood. Atheromas may also become eroded, encouraging the formation of blood clots *(thrombi)* that further narrow the vessel channels. If a blood clot breaks off, it becomes an *embolus* or *thromboembolus* that travels downstream until it finally becomes lodged in a smaller artery, cutting off the blood supply to whatever organ that artery supplies. If the involved artery is in the brain, for example, a stroke results; if in the heart, a heart attack occurs.

Angina Pectoris

Angina means pain and *angina pectoris* means chest pain and refers to the pain caused by too little oxygen to the heart muscle. It is usually brought on by exertion, or other factors (high blood pressure or rapid heartbeat) that stress the heart. Angina most often results from atherosclerosis of the coronary arteries, which reduces blood flow to the heart muscle *(ischemia)* without actually resulting in muscle damage *(infarction)*.

The pain of angina is highly variable. It is most commonly felt beneath the sternum (breastbone) and often radiates to the back or to the left shoulder and arm. It is seldom located directly over the heart. It may be mistaken for indigestion. The pain is usually triggered by exercise and lasts only a few minutes, subsiding with rest. Angina is worsened by exertion after a meal when more of the total blood volume is drawn to the gastrointestinal region. It is frequently worse during cold weather, so that the exercise that is pain-free in summer may in winter cause angina. It may occur at night, when it is called *nocturnal angina*. Any change in the character or pattern of anginal pain is called *unstable angina*, and this is a danger sign that your heart requires immediate medical attention.

Diagnosis and Prognosis

Chest pain has many causes other than angina, such as that caused by gastrointestinal and lung disorders, and your doctor will undertake appropriate tests to rule out causes other than your heart. Such tests may include an electrocardiogram (ECG) both at rest and during exercise to detect the changes that occur when the heart is not receiving enough oxygen. In doubtful cases ultrasound or radioisotope tests may be performed to determine how efficiently your heart is working. In other cases, you may be referred to a cardiologist for cardiac catheterization and coronary angiography (the injection of dye into the coronary arteries and taking of X-rays) to determine the extent of coronary artery narrowing by atherosclerosis.

The major risk factors that determine whether you will go on to have a heart attack *(myocardial infarction)* are your age, the extent of coronary disease (determined by cardiac catheterization), the severity of your symptoms, and your heart's response to exercise. Approximately 1.5% of patients with angina die each year. With high blood pressure and an abnormal ECG, more than 10% die each year.

Treatment. There are three principal drugs used to control angina:

1. *Nitrates.* Nitroglycerin, taken as tablets placed under the tongue, is especially effective in relieving acute attacks of angina and preventing pain during exercise. Dramatic relief is usually obtained within a minute or two. Nitroglycerin relaxes arterial muscle, causing the arteries to dilate. This in turn lowers blood pressure, placing less stress upon the heart. If nitroglycerin is prescribed, you should carry the tablets at all times. Nitroglycerin is also available as a spray, and as an ointment or as a patch to provide slow, sustained absorption through the skin. Nitroglycerin deteriorates rather quickly, losing its potency. Buy tablets frequently in small quantities. Keep the bottle tightly closed. Do not take more of any cardiac medicine than your doctor directs.

   Amyl nitrite is an especially potent blood vessel dilator that should be used only for severe angina. It comes in a crushable ampule to be carefully inhaled. Inhalation is practically the equivalent of an intravenous injection. Only two or three inhalations are required to relieve pain.
2. *Beta-blocking drugs,* such as propranolol and atenolol, block nervous stimulation of the heart, reducing blood pressure, heart rate, and the force of heartbeat, thus reducing oxygen consumption.
3. *Calcium blockers* (e.g., verapamil, nifedipine, diltiazem) may be effective in a special type of angina caused by muscular spasm of the coronary arteries. These drugs act to relax arterial muscle, allowing more blood to flow to the heart muscle.

Coronary artery bypass operations and angioplasty are also used to treat severe angina, just as they are used following heart attacks (*see* p. 179).

AVOIDING ANGINA

There are several things you can do to prevent or reduce the severity of your angina attacks:

- *Avoid overeating.* Large meals place extra stress on your heart. Rest after eating. Reducing your weight will also reduce the workload on your heart and permit you more exercise before angina begins.
- *Reduce dietary fats and cholesterol.* Some evidence suggests that lowering blood cholesterol may reduce atherosclerotic narrowing of the coronary arteries.
- *Avoid persons, topics of conversation, and other situations that make you angry.* Tension makes the heart work harder.
- *Stop smoking.* Nicotine constricts blood vessels, the exact opposite of what is desired for angina.
- *Reduce alcohol consumption* to no more than an ounce or two of hard liquor a day (4–8 ounces of wine; 12–24 ounces of beer).
- *Exercise.* Ask your doctor to prescribe an exercise program designed to gradually increase your exercise tolerance. Walking is especially good. Avoid either very hot or very cold weather. If you become short of breath or develop pain, sit down and rest immediately and take nitroglycerin, if this has been prescribed for you. Do not continue until you feel rested.
- *Avoid sex if you are tired or have just had a heavy meal.* If you experience chest pain during sex, stop at once. Consult with your doctor about how best to renew your sexual activity.
- *Avoid activities that rapidly tire you or cause you shortness of breath,* such as heavy lifting, strenuous cleaning, or gardening. If you get tired for any reason, stop what you are doing and rest.
- *Humor yourself and others.* Laughter is good for the heart as well as the soul.

Heart Attacks *(Myocardial Infarction)*

A heart attack occurs when one or more of the coronary arteries or their branches become blocked so that blood cannot reach the heart muscle. Without oxygen and nutrients, the affected heart muscle dies *(myocardial infarction)*. The usual cause of a heart attack is the gradual formation of a blood clot *(thrombus)* on an atherosclerotic plaque *(atheroma)* that already partially blocks the vessel. As the vessel clogs more completely, there is a rapid loss of blood flow to the heart.

The dead and injured muscle left in the wake of a heart attack causes your heart to lose some of its efficiency, since the amount of blood the heart can pump depends on muscle contraction. When more than about 50% of the *myocardium* (heart muscle) is lost—as a result of either previous scarring or new infarction—shock and death result because the heart simply cannot supply enough blood to sustain life.

The symptoms of a heart attack depend upon how much heart muscle is injured. Nearly 20% of victims experience no symptoms at all and are unaware they have suffered a heart attack (the so-called "silent" attack). Thus, you may learn about your heart attack only when your doctor discovers evidence of an "old infarct" on your electrocardiogram.

Most heart attack victims, however, suffer chest pain or discomfort. This may range from a persistent feeling of "indigestion" to a crushing chest pain or pressure under the breastbone that radiates to the back, jaw, or left arm. Other symptoms include weakness, shortness of breath, sweating, and nausea. A person who has just had a heart attack is often pale, cold, and sweaty. Sudden death results from the first heart attack in almost one-fourth of heart attack victims. Few diseases entail this degree of mortality.

Treatment

Emergency Measures

Since about half of all people who succumb to heart attacks die within the first few hours, emergency management is critical. If you experience chest pain, you should seek medical help as soon as possible. A major reason for treatment delay is the victims' denial that their symptoms represent a life-threatening condition. If you are the victim, play it safe and have someone get you to a hospital emergency room immediately. Otherwise, dial 911 and say "chest pain" and give your name, address, and telephone number. Try to remain calm, any exertion will increase the pain, as well as your danger. Don't try to drive yourself to the hospital if anyone can take you. Don't delay seeking help while trying to convince yourself you are not having a heart attack. Denial is not a river in Egypt!

If the victim's heart stops, cardiopulmonary resuscitation (CPR) can often maintain life until an ambulance and medical treatment are available. If you desire training in CPR, call your local chapter of the American Heart Association or the American Red Cross for informa-

tion about classes. Do not attempt CPR yourself unless you are trained
in the technique.

Hospital Measures

In recent years medical advances have greatly reduced the hospital mortality of heart attack victims. Here are the most important measures taken:

- Pain and anxiety are relieved with such analgesics as morphine.
- Drugs such as nitroglycerin are given to dilate the coronary blood vessels, which often constrict during a heart attack.
- Oxygen is administered to make up for reduced pumping efficiency by the heart.
- The patient is placed on continuous heart monitoring to record the heart rhythm. Irregular heart beat *(arrhythmia)* is the usual forerunner of fatal ventricular fibrillation. Arrhythmias are treated with a variety of intravenous drugs or by electrical defibrillators that apply an external shock that often restores the heart to an effective rhythm or starts the heart beating again if it has stopped *(cardiac arrest)*.
- Potent enzymes, such as *streptokinase* or *tissue plasminogen activator*, can be administered. These dissolve the coronary artery blood clot that initiated the heart attack and thus prevent further muscle damage. Such measures must be started soon after the heart attack to be effective.
- Anticoagulants, usually heparin, are frequently administered to prevent formation of more blood clots.
- According to recent studies, aspirin given in conjunction with clot-dissolving enzymes can reduce the mortality from heart attacks by about 50%.

After a Heart Attack

Aside from general supportive measures, the mainstay of treatment is to prevent blood clots from recurring. Currently, low-dose aspirin appears to be the most safe and effective drug for this.

At some time during recuperation from a heart attack, most individuals suffer from depression and a feeling of helplessness. Hence, they need strong reassurance that they are likely to get well. A gradual program of increasing exercise will be prescribed. If the patient has been a smoker, a stay in a coronary care unit is a potent stimulus to give up the habit, and this notion is one that should be reinforced by everyone who cares for and about the patient.

Recurrent chest pain (angina) is not uncommon following a heart attack. In most instances this pain can be relieved by appropriate drugs (*see* p. 177). In a few patients, particularly those with continued cardiac failure and atherosclerotic involvement of all three coronary arteries, coronary bypass surgery may be recommended. This surgery involves grafting a piece of leg vein between the aorta and a point below the coronary artery obstruction.

Coronary bypass surgery is a major operation. Some patients may be candidates for a simpler procedure that can be performed under local anesthesia, called *percutaneous transluminal coronary angioplasty*. In this procedure, a balloon-tipped catheter is advanced into the coronary artery to the point of obstruction. It is then inflated to open up the narrowed vessel. Unfortunately, relief by this means is usually temporary. Currently under investigation are an astonishing variety of cutting, scraping, and laser-melting procedures to unclog arteries. Be sure to ask your doctor the pros and cons of each procedure.

Prevention of Coronary Artery Disease

Who Is at Risk?

Heart disease is the leading cause of death in most industrialized countries. Coronary heart disease (atherosclerosis) accounts for about 70% of all deaths from heart disease and about a quarter of deaths from all causes. These figures should convince everyone of the importance of thinking about their own risks for heart disease and what they may do about them.

There are seven major risk factors that promote the development of atherosclerosis and consequently of the coronary artery disease that causes heart attacks:

- High blood pressure
- High blood cholesterol
- Cigaret smoking
- Obesity
- Male sex
- A family history of heart attacks, especially in the father, mother, grandparents, and siblings
- Diabetes mellitus

Other "presumed" risk factors include physical inactivity, increasing age, stress, and the hardness of your drinking water.

Cigaret smoking is the most important risk factor for coronary heart disease that you can easily modify. Smokers are at more than twice the risk of heart attack as nonsmokers. Also, a smoker who suffers a heart attack is more likely to die from it, and is more likely to die suddenly than a nonsmoker.

Encouragingly, when you stop smoking, regardless of how long you've smoked, your risk of heart disease rapidly decreases. In fact, ten years after quitting, your risk of death from heart disease is almost the same as if you had never smoked. By stopping smoking you also reduce your exposure to several types of cancer, and to peripheral vascular disease. *See* p. 492 for tips on how to quit smoking.

Smoking seems to be an especially serious risk factor for women. One study estimates that 55% of heart attacks in women under 50 can be attributed to smoking. And the combination of smoking and the use of birth control pills entails the most serious risks of all.

Diabetes mellitus greatly increases the risk of heart disease, particularly if it goes untreated. Your doctor can easily determine whether you have diabetes and prescribe changes in your eating habits, exercise, and body weight to bring the disease under control.

The Use of Aspirin to Prevent Heart Attacks

For a long time it has been known that aspirin reduces the tendency of platelets to form clots within blood vessels. The platelets are said to become less "sticky." It has been the fond hope of many scientists that small amounts of aspirin will reduce heart attacks. These hopes were given a big boost by a Harvard University study in which male doctors were followed for several years, half taking one aspirin tablet every other day and the other half taking a placebo (sugar pill). The group taking aspirin were found to have about half the number of heart attacks as the placebo group.

Before you begin taking aspirin to prevent a heart attack—and you may well be someone who can benefit from this simple prophylaxis— you should consult your doctor, who will determine whether you really need aspirin. Your doctor will also decide whether you have some condition that aspirin might worsen, e.g., aspirin allergy, liver disease, peptic ulcer, gastrointestinal bleeding, or uncontrolled high blood pressure. Remember, too, that it is probably unwise to combine aspirin prophylaxis with any other anticlotting regimen, such as fish oil or anti-inflammatory drugs. The danger of serious bleeding, especially of a hemorrhagic stroke, may exist.

High Blood Pressure *(Hypertension)*

Blood pressure is a measure of the force of the blood against the walls of the arteries generated by the pumping action of the heart. It is measured in terms of the higher *systolic* pressure, i.e., the pressure following complete contraction of the left ventricle, and the lower *diastolic* pressure, i.e., the pressure during filling of the left ventricle. Most healthy young people have a blood pressure around 120/80 millimeters of mercury (read "120 over 80"). Since blood pressure often goes up as adults age, a reading up to 140/85 is considered normal between ages 18 and 50. When blood pressure exceeds 140/90, it is time to see your doctor, regardless of age.

High blood pressure is usually classified as *primary* (also known as *essential hypertension*) or *secondary*. Secondary hypertension is associated with kidney disease, thyroid disease, and certain endocrine tumors and usually disappears when these diseases are treated. Also, many drugs can cause temporary high blood pressure. However, only a small percentage of people with high blood pressure have secondary hypertension. The cause of primary high blood pressure, which accounts for 90% of cases, is not known. What is known is that high blood pressure tends to run in families, is more common in men than women, is more likely to occur after the age of 35, is more common among blacks, and is associated with obesity, excess alcohol consumption, diabetes, and the use of oral contraceptives. It used to be thought that high blood pressure in the elderly was a normal process of aging. However, it is now known that high blood pressure in older people must be treated just as vigorously as in younger persons to reduce the risk of their suffering heart attacks, stroke, and kidney failure.

It is not known why blacks more often suffer high blood pressure than whites. In fact, American blacks have one of the highest rates of high blood pressure in the world. As a result, strokes are 1.5 times more frequent and kidney failure is 15 times more common among blacks. Though the reasons for these differences are not fully understood, they may in part result from a greater sensitivity to salt. Nevertheless, it is of special importance that blacks have their blood pressures checked regularly.

The effect of high blood pressure, which itself is often symptomless, is to accelerate the development of arteriosclerosis and atherosclerosis (both described earlier). On average, individuals with

Assessing Your Own Coronary Risk

The following questionnaire was prepared by the American Heart Association to help adults who have no evidence of heart disease assess their risk of developing symptomatic coronary heart disease. Read each question and circle the number that best describes you. Total the numbers you circled for all ten questions and compare them to the risk groups at the end of the questionnaire.

1. *What is your family history of heart disease?*
     Count parents, grandparents, brothers, and sisters only.

No heart disease	0
1 Relative with heart disease over age 60	2
2 Relatives with heart disease over age 60	3
1 Relative with heart disease under age 60	4
2 Relatives with heart disease under age 60	6
3 Relatives with heart disease under age 60	7

2. *What is your family history of diabetes?*
     Count parents, grandparents, brothers, and sisters only.

No diabetes	0
1 Relative with diabetes	2
2 Relatives with diabetes	3
I have diabetes beginning after age 60	4
I have diabetes beginning between ages 20–60	6
I have diabetes beginning before age 20	7

3. *What is your stress level at work and home?*

No stress	0
Occasional mild stress	2
Frequent mild stress	3
Frequent moderate stress	4
Frequent high stress	5
Constant high stress	6

4. *What are your smoking habits?*

Never smoked	0
Quit cigarets more than 1 year ago	0
Quit cigarets less than 1 year ago	1
I smoke 10 cigarets per day maximum	2
I smoke 20 cigarets per day	4
I smoke 30 cigarets per day	6
I smoke 40 or more cigarets per day	8

5. *What is your current level of exercise?*

Regular aerobic exercise program	−1
Intensive occupational and recreational exercise	0

Moderate occupational and recreational exercise	2
Sedentary work and intense recreational exercise	3
Sedentary work and light recreational exercise	5
Sedentary work with no exercise	6

6. *What is your saturated fat and cholesterol intake?*

Total vegetarian	0
Almost total vegetarian; rare egg yolk, no butterfat, and lean meat only; two meatless days per week; no whole milk products	2
Meat (mostly lean), eggs, cheese 12 times per week, nonfat milk only	3
Meat, cheese, eggs, whole milk 23 times per week	6
Meat, cheese, eggs, whole milk over 24 times per week	8

7. *What is your upper blood pressure reading?*
Use 140 if you do not know your blood pressure.

Less than 120	0
130 maximum	2
140 maximum	3
160 maximum	4
180 maximum	6
Over 200	8

8. *Compared to the healthy weight for your age and height (see p. 314), what is your body weight?*

Underweight	0
Healthy weight; up to 9 lbs excess	2
10 to 19 lbs excess	3
20 to 29 lbs excess	5
30 lbs or more excess	7

9. *What is your sex and age group?*

Female under 40 years	0
Female between 40 and 50 years	1
Female over 50 years	2
Male under 40 years	3
Male between 40 and 50 years	4
Male over 50 years	5

10. *What is your age?*

10–20 years	0
21–30 years	1
31–40 years	2
41–50 years	3
51–60 years	4
Over 60 years	5

EVALUATING YOUR RISK OF HEART ATTACK		
Total score	*Your risk*	*Suggested course of action*
6–15	Well below average	Continue the good work. You are within acceptable limits
16–21	Average	Take note of risk factors in the highest point categories and try to modify the the controllable ones. Ask your doctor for help.
22–29	Borderline	Contact your doctor for a cardiovascular program to lower those risks that fall in the highest categories.
30–39	Moderate	Contact your doctor for a complete physical examination including an ECG test.
40–50	High	
50+	Dangerous	Your risk factors must be lowered. *Act Now!*

uncontrolled high blood pressure are three times as likely to develop coronary artery disease, six times as likely to develop congestive heart failure, and seven times as likely to have a stroke as individuals with controlled blood pressure. Therefore, if you have high blood pressure, it is important to have it treated.

Diagnosis

The diagnosis of primary high blood pressure is made by (1) demonstrating that either the systolic or diastolic pressure is higher than normal, and (2) excluding causes of secondary high blood pressure. Always remember that a single elevated blood pressure reading does not mean that you have hypertension, but it is a sign that further measurements are required. If your blood pressure is found to be elevated during the course of a routine medical examination, it may be merely because of the anxiety of being in the doctor's office. Never accept a diagnosis of hypertension from a single measurement.

Treatment. There is no cure for primary high blood pressure, but diet and specific therapy can modify its course and prevent such complications as heart attack, kidney disease, and stroke. In fact, the life expectancy of hypertensive individuals with controlled blood pressure is the same as for normals. The most important control measures are:

Diet

More than half of all overweight Americans have high blood pressure. For many of these, weight loss alone will bring the blood pressure down to normal. If you are overweight, every effort should be made to bring your weight into the healthy range for your height and age. Your doctor can prescribe a diet, or you may find it helpful to consult a registered dietitian; they are often very clever in overcoming the strong resistance to losing weight that most of us have. Combined with a modest dietary restriction of sodium, drug therapy may be unnecessary for those with only moderate high blood pressure.

The Question of Salt?

Doctors talk about "sodium sensitivity" as a probable cause of high blood pressure (salt as sodium chloride is the largest source of sodium in our diet). The nature of sodium sensitivity is not well understood, but about half of all Americans with high blood pressure are thought to be sodium sensitive, i.e., their blood pressure will fall with a diet of salt restriction. Much of the evidence for salt sensitivity comes from studies of societies where salt intake is low. For example, African tribesmen, who eat very little salt, have a low incidence of high blood pressure. When these tribesmen enter military service and begin eating a high-sodium institutional diet, their rate of high blood pressure approaches the very high rate among American blacks. When they leave service and return to their villages, the rate returns to the low tribal rate.

Does this mean that restricting salt will prevent high blood pressure? No one knows. But both the American Heart Association and the National Heart Lung and Blood Institute recommend that everyone, regardless of blood pressure, reduce their salt intake by about half or to no more than about 5 grams per day. This is the amount of salt in about 1 teaspoon and is equivalent to about 2 grams of sodium, since salt is 40% sodium by weight. Your body actually only needs about one-tenth this amount of sodium, and the average American eats 2–4 times this amount. To know how much two grams of sodium is, you need to begin to learn how much sodium is contained in several varieties of foods. Ask your doctor for dietary salt guidelines. Learn to read labels. Processed foods contain much more salt than you are likely to suspect. And fast foods are notorious.

You will probably find that food tastes bland and unappetizing when you first try to cut down on salt. This is because your palate has adjusted to a higher salt concentration in food, not because your body needs more salt. There are several things you can do to reduce your dependence on salt and "re-educate" your palate to a lower salt level:

1. *Add small amounts of lemon juice to food.* The sharp acid taste enhances flavors and accentuates the taste of salt already in the food. Be careful in using flavor enhancers that you do not add products such as soy sauce or Worcestershire sauce, which contain large amounts of salt.
2. *Leave salt out of cooked foods* and use a salt shaker to add salt at the table. Studies have shown that salt consumption is much lower when adjusting salt taste with a salt shaker. Later you can remove the salt shaker, or use a salt substitute.
3. *Use spices and herbs* to add flavor and zest to foods.
4. *Reduce your salt usage gradually* and avoid overly salted foods such as chips, crackers, canned meats and vegetables, and preserved meats and vegetables.
5. *Switch to a salt substitute* that contains potassium instead of sodium salts if your doctor advises.
6. *Avoid fast food chains.* Most of the foods they prepare contain huge amounts of salt.

For more information, consult: *Cooking Without Your Salt Shaker* from the American Heart Association, or: *Sodium Content of Your Food,* USDA Home and Garden Bulletin No. 233, Superintendent of Documents, US Government Printing Office, Washington, DC 20402 (Send $4.25).

Alcohol

People who have high blood pressure also need to limit the amount of alcohol they drink. Not only does alcohol contribute nonnutritious "empty" calories, thus promoting obesity, alcohol also seems to elevate blood pressure biochemically. You should consume no more than 2 oz of hard liquor daily, or no more than 8 oz of wine or 24 oz of beer.

Calcium

Recent studies show that low dietary calcium may contribute to high blood pressure. The American diet is moderately low in calcium, especially with increasing reluctance to consume meats and dairy products, because of their cholesterol content. In some studies, calcium supplements have caused elevated blood pressure to return to normal. The mechanism of calcium's action is thought to be in relaxing smooth muscles in the arterial walls. Though calcium supplements are not recommended, except on a doctor's advice, you should consider increasing such calcium-rich foods in your diet as low-fat dairy products, fish, green vegetables, and nuts. The daily intake of calcium should be 800 mg and 1200 mg, respectively, during pregnancy and breastfeeding.

Potassium

A diet rich in potassium appears to lower high blood pressure somewhat. Eat more servings of grain products, fresh fruits, and vegetables each day to increase potassium intake. Potassium supplements are probably not worthwhile unless you are also taking diuretic drugs (*see below*). Also ask your doctor about magnesium supplements.

Caffeine

Numerous writers have tried to pin a rap on caffeine, especially in coffee, perhaps because so many Americans (8 of 10 adults drink coffee) consume so much of it (half the world's brewed coffee). Indeed one can find scientific studies that show caffeine raises, lowers, or does not change blood pressure; increases, decreases, or does not alter heart rate; raises or does not raise metabolic rate; raises or does not raise blood cholesterol. Why all of this contradictory evidence? Part of the reason is that these studies have been performed on different groups of people. If caffeine is give to someone who never drinks coffee or tea, it will raise all of these factors. However if the caffeine equivalent of 2–3 cups of coffee is given to an habitual coffee drinker, none of these parameters is affected at all. Thus if you feel you need coffee or tea to pep you up, moderate amounts (3–4 cups) probably won't hurt you. There is no evidence that caffeine is associated with increased risk of cancer, including cancers of the breast, bladder, and pancreas. The most recent studies also show no correlation between caffeine consumption and fibrocystic disease of the breast (despite much early brouhaha about this relationship). Apparently drip or filtered coffee is better than boiled coffee. Some studies have shown that boiled, but not filtered, coffee raises blood cholesterol levels.

Caffeine does have some harmful effects, however, definitely causing irregular heartbeat (*arrhythmia*) in some people, especially those with known heart disease. Such individuals should avoid caffeine altogether, including caffeine-containing soft drinks. Caffeine also increases stomach acid (both regular and decaffeinated coffee do this).

How can you quit drinking coffee or tea? Caffeine is a weakly habit-forming drug and may give rise to mild withdrawal symptoms: drowsiness, lethargy, headaches, irritability, depression, etc. when heavy users try to give it up. To avoid these symptoms, give up coffee or tea gradually, cutting back a cup a day until the habit is gone.

Exercise

A regular exercise program helps you strengthen your heart, lose weight, and reduce stress, all of which may help lower your blood pressure. Most experts recommend aerobic exercises for 20–30 minutes three times a week to lower mildly elevated blood pressure.

Medication

If the above measures fail to bring blood pressure below 140/90, you will need to take medication. There are numerous drugs available to reduce high blood pressure. Broadly, these include:

- *Diuretics* to promote excretion of salt and water (e.g., hydrochlorothiazide, furosemide, chlorthalidone).
- *Beta blockers* to reduce sympathetic nerve stimulation of the heart, slow the heart, and reduce systolic blood pressure (e.g., propranolol, metoprolol, atenolol, pindolol, etc.).
- *Nerve blockers* to relax smooth muscles and dilate the arteries (e.g., guanethidine, methyldopa, clonidine, prazosin).
- *Calcium blockers* to dilate arteries and decrease vascular resistance (e.g., diltiazem, nifedipine, verapamil).
- *Blood vessel dilators* such as hydralazine and minoxidil.
- *Enzyme inhibitors* to prevent natural blood vessel constrictors from becoming active (e.g., captopril, enalapril).

Not everyone responds alike to these drugs. For example, beta blockers, widely used to treat high blood pressure in whites, don't work well for blacks. Everyone reacts somewhat differently to these drugs and they all have unwanted side effects for some people (especially lassitude, mental slowness, and occasionally, impotence). Therefore, you can expect a trial period before your doctor finds the drug or combination of drugs that works best for you. The starting doses of these drugs should be relatively low to minimize early side effects.

Another factor to bear in mind is that antihypertensive drugs are more effective and can usually be used in smaller doses with fewer side effects when you maintain a healthy weight, exercise regularly, and reduce your salt intake.

Many people quit taking their high blood pressure medications because they do not feel as well after they begin taking the medications as they had felt before doing so, usually as a result of one of the side effects mentioned above. If this happens, ask your doctor to recommend a substitute drug or combination of drugs.

Monitoring Your Own Blood Pressure

Taking your blood pressure at home is a useful way to monitor your progress with diet, exercise, and drugs. Before you buy your own blood pressure cuff *(sphygmomanometer)* you should do some comparative shopping, since there are different types, and quality and prices vary widely. The easiest type to use employs a digital readout and does not require a stethoscope to hear the blood sounds. If you buy one, take it to your doctor to learn how to use it and to calibrate it against the more accurate mercury column set. I suggest you consult a *Consumer Reports* comparison before buying or ask for the pamphlet, *Buying and Caring for Home Blood Pressure Equipment* from your local American Heart Association.

Low Blood Pressure

Although high blood pressure is a serious problem, blood pressure that is moderately lower than average is of no special concern. Many people have pressures of 100/60 or lower with no ill effects. There is only one kind of low blood pressure that may cause a problem, the so-called *postural hypotension*. This condition occurs when you stand up after sitting or lying down for some time. In standing up, gravity tends to drain blood downward, away from the heart. Dizziness or even fainting may occur if the blood returning to the heart is insufficient to maintain adequate blood flow to the brain.

Normally, postural hypotension is avoided by automatic constriction of the blood vessels upon standing to prevent blood from flowing downward. In some people, however, this reflex may be defective. The most common cause is medication prescribed to control high blood pressure. In this case, it is usually sufficient to lower the dose of the medication to avoid postural hypotension; or you may ask your doctor to consider a change of medication. Postural hypotension may also be a temporary complication of pregnancy, or the result of diabetes and certain blood vessel diseases. Usually the temporary dizziness can be avoided by making a habit of first sitting up, and then standing up slowly. If the condition is chronic and symptoms severe, consult your doctor.

High Blood Cholesterol

Like high blood pressure, high blood cholesterol is a silent *(asymptomatic)* condition that you first learn about from blood tests. The major fats *(lipids)* found in the blood are of two kinds: cholesterols and triglycerides. Of these, cholesterol is by far the more important as a risk factor in coronary artery disease and stroke.

Cholesterol does not circulate freely in the blood, but rather is bound to large protein molecules called *lipoproteins* that transport it to and from the liver and the fatty tissues of the body. Most of the cholesterol is bound to *low-density* lipoproteins (LDL). Normally, LDL is removed from the blood by the liver. However, when the amount of LDL circulating in the blood is high, or when liver function is compromised, a portion of LDL is removed by special cells in the arterial walls, thus contributing to the formation of atherosclerotic plaque in them. For this reason, LDL has been termed the "bad cholesterol."

Cholesterol is also bound to *high-density lipoproteins* (HDL), which have been dubbed "good cholesterol" because they help remove cholesterol from the blood. The blood concentration of HDL is inversely related to the risk of coronary artery disease. Thus if your total cholesterol is high, your doctor will probably want to measure both your LDL and HDL to determine your risk for coronary heart disease.

What is normal blood cholesterol? Since blood cholesterol tends to rise with increasing age, it used to be stated that values greater than 180 mg/dL plus your age should be considered abnormal (dL stands for deciliter, which equals one-tenth of a liter, or 100 milliliters). Recently it has been determined that the increased cholesterol associated with advancing age is itself a risk factor and the upper limit is now considered to be 240 mg/dL for all persons who have no other risk factors for heart disease. The National Institutes of Health recommends a maximum cholesterol level of 200 mg/dL if you have other risk factors for heart disease, such as high blood pressure, heart disease that runs in your family, or obesity, if you smoke cigarets.

Furthermore, any HDL level lower than 40 mg/dL is also considered to contribute to coronary heart disease risk.

How to Lower Your High Blood Cholesterol

There are three ways of lowering your blood cholesterol: diet, weight reduction, and medication. Most people can lower their cholesterol 30–50 mg/dL by dieting and exercise alone, without resorting to medications. The key to dieting is to reduce the amount of cholesterol and saturated fats in the foods you eat. There is no need to have any cholesterol in your diet since your body can easily make all it needs from other foods.

Cholesterol is found only in foods of animal origin, especially such foods as meats, eggs, dairy products, and organ meats (liver, kidneys, sweetbreads). Often merely limiting yourself to two or three eggs per week and reducing your intake of cheese and whole milk products is sufficient to lower your cholesterol. You should learn which foods contain cholesterol and how much, and then plan a daily dietary intake of 300 mg or less (one egg yolk contains about 200 mg of cholesterol).

Saturated fats (those containing high amounts of hydrogen) also tend to raise blood cholesterol levels. These are found primarily in animal products, particularly fatty meats and dairy products. They are also contained in coconut oil (use it for moisturizing, not cooking), palm kernel oil and palm oil, and such hydrogenated oils as margarine. You can help lower your cholesterol by substituting polyunsaturated fats (especially from vegetable oils) for saturated fats in your diet. Ask your doctor to prescribe a cholesterol-lowering regimen for you. You may also write for: *Eating to Lower Your High Blood Cholesterol*, NIH Publication No. 87-2920, Sept., 1987, from your local American Heart Association, or from the National Heart, Lung, and Blood Institute, National Institutes of Health, Bethesda, MD 20892. Remember, you must maintain a low-cholesterol, low-fat diet for life to keep your blood cholesterol level normal.

Diets high in fiber can lower blood cholesterol by 10–15%. The theory behind this effect is that soluble fiber, like such drugs as cholestyramine resin and colestipol, act by binding bile salts in the small intestine and preventing their reabsorption. Bile salts are largely made of cholesterol and are usually reabsorbed from the colon for reuse. If they are bound to soluble fiber and eliminated, the liver must manufacture more bile salts from the pool of circulating cholesterol, thus lowering blood cholesterol.

Fish oil. One of the most recent dietary fads is the consumption of fish oil to reduce blood cholesterol and protect against heart attacks. Actually there may be good reason to do so. Certain fish, particularly those that live in deep, cold water, e.g., salmon, mackerel, bluefish, herring, and cod (only cod livers, however, contain substantial quantities of a fatty acid known as *eicosapentanoic acid,* or EPA). This marvelous substance appears to have a number of nifty properties: It interferes with the production of LDL-cholesterol (the bad kind), thus lowering blood cholesterol. It also interferes with the production of another substance, *thromboxane,* which causes blood platelets to become sticky and clot more easily. Because of this anticlotting property, fish oil is thought to help protect against heart attacks and strokes.

All of this is somewhat speculative. Few carefully controlled studies have been published to substantiate any of these claims. Nevertheless, substitution of fish for red meat twice a week is probably a good idea. You should be careful about taking cod liver oil for its cholesterol-lowering properties. Cod liver oil is high in vitamins A and D; it can be toxic if you take more than 1–2 tablespoons per day.

If your blood cholesterol is greater than 200 mg/dL or your LDL-cholesterol is greater than 130 mg/dL, your doctor will prescribe a diet and exercise program. If after 4–6 months your cholesterol is not within normal limits, he may prescribe a cholesterol-lowering medication, of which there are several.

Niacin. I should insert a word of caution about taking the vitamin niacin to lower blood cholesterol. Niacin has indeed been found to lower cholesterol and to reduce the rate of nonfatal heart attacks. However, it appears to do so only when taken in such large doses as 3000 milligrams per day, which is 150 times the Recommended Daily Allowance of 20 milligrams. At such levels, niacin is no longer considered a vitamin, even though you can buy it at drug and health food stores. Rather it is a drug that can cause such serious side effects as irregular heartbeat, impaired regulation of blood sugar, and liver abnormalities. Niacin is not a drug that you should take on your own, but only under the supervision of your doctor.

Abnormal Heart Rhythm

The normal heartbeat arises from electrical impulses that begin in pacemaker cells found in the small *sinoatrial node* in the right atrium of the heart. From there, the impulse spreads throughout the right and then the left atrium, and finally to the right and left ventricles, resulting in a coordinated muscular contraction that pumps blood throughout the body. The normal heart rate is between 60 and 100 beats per minute, with an average of 72–78 per hour. In athletes and very fit individuals, the resting heart rate may be as low as 40 or 45, and the normal heart rate in infants may be as high as 150. In most people, the heart rate increases slightly with inspiration and decreases slightly with expiration. This is called *sinus arrhythmia* and is normal.

Slow Heart Rate

A heart rate less than 60 per minute is called *bradycardia*, from the Greek "brady," meaning slow. Such slow heart rates are associated with hypothyroidism, jaundice, some gastrointestinal disturbances, heart disease, and certain drugs, especially excess digitalis. As noted earlier, a slow resting heart rate is common in athletes.

Heart rates between 40 and 60 per minute generally do not cause symptoms. A slow heart rate that does not increase with exercise or emotion is usually a sign of *heart block,* and you should consult your doctor. Sudden onset of a heart rate of less than 40 beats per minute, especially if accompanied by chest pain, fatigue, or shortness of breath, suggests a recent heart attack and is a medical emergency.

Rapid Heart Rate

In adults a heart rate greater than 100 per minute at rest is called *tachycardia,* from the Greek "tachy," meaning "rapid." There are many causes, including hyperthyroidism, heart failure *(see above),* anemia, bleeding, infections, and drugs (e.g., nicotine, caffeine, alcohol, marijuana). If you are aware of a persistent rapid pulse, or pounding in your neck or chest, see your doctor.

Occasionally, you may experience the sudden onset of a rapid heart rate, known as *paroxysmal atrial tachycardia.* This condition usually starts during youth, and attacks may recur throughout life. Frequently, there is no identifiable heart abnormality and the condition is essentially benign, though you may feel weak and faint during the attack. These paroxysms may be brought on by emotional upset, fatigue, indigestion, alcohol, or drugs. The heart rate may range from 140 to 250 per minute. Several cardiac drugs are available to prevent these attacks. When an episode begins, lie down and remain calm. Standing only accentuates an attack's severity. Once you are familiar with these attacks, certain physical maneuvers may be used to interrupt them. These, however, should be demonstrated by your doctor once the diagnosis has been firmly established.

Other causes of tachycardia include atrial flutter, atrial fibrillation, ventricular tachycardia, and Wolff-Parkinson-White syndrome. All of these are serious and require an ECG and other tests to identify.

Irregular Heart Rhythms

There are numerous causes of irregular heart beats, or arrhythmias. Most, if not all cases of irregular heart rhythm that last longer than a few minutes, should be investigated by your doctor.

One cause of irregular heart beat that most people experience now and then is quite benign: it is caused by *atrial premature beats* (APBs). These beats are usually recognized by a fluttering sensation in your neck or chest, caused by periodic heartbeats that are extra forceful. The cause of APBs is a periodic electrical stimulus that begins in the muscles of the atrium instead of the sinoatrial node. Usually APBs are benign and most people ignore them unless their frequency becomes alarming. They are commonly caused by drugs that stimulate the heart, e.g. nicotine, caffeine, marijuana, and alcohol. Avoidance of these usually prevents APBs, unless there is underlying heart disease. If they become frequent, or if you become alarmed, you should see your doctor. There are several drugs that can reduce or prevent them. In exceptional cases, a *pacemaker,* an electronic device that initiates the heartbeat, may have to be implanted beneath the skin to sustain a normal heart rhythm.

Alcohol and Your Heart

Long-standing alcohol abuse can have several effects upon the cardiovascular system. Social drinking is often associated with mild increases of blood pressure. In heavy drinkers, elevated blood pressure can be substantial and may contribute to the higher incidence of strokes, heart enlargement, and heart failure among alcoholics. Whether high blood pressure is permanently reversed with abstinence is not known.

Alcohol can cause a variety of arrhythmias. These usually occur during and after heavy alcohol intake and then subside with sustained abstinence. The exact cause of these arrhythmias is not known, but it is thought that alcohol has a toxic effect on the heart. The great danger from arrhythmias, of course, is the danger of sudden death from *ventricular fibrillation,* a condition in which the heartbeat becomes so rapid and irregular that the cardiac output cannot sustain life.

Heart Failure

The heart is said to "fail" whenever it cannot pump enough blood to meet the body's demand for oxygen. There are numerous causes of heart failure and the condition may be temporary, as during a severe infection, or chronic, as in alcohol-induced heart disease *(alcoholic cardiomyopathy)*. The most common causes of heart failure are diseases that affect the heart muscle's ability to contract. These include previous heart attacks, diseases of the heart muscle itself *(cardiomyopathies)*, and diseases of the lining of the heart. Diseases of the heart valves *(valvular heart disease)* and abnormalities of heart rhythm *(cardiac arrhythmias)* also cause the heart to pump inefficiently. Congenital heart defects can affect heart muscle, the heart valves, or the flow of blood, all of which can cause heart failure. Finally, certain diseases of the lungs and thyroid, and several anemias, can cause heart failure.

When the heart fails to meet the body's demand for blood, a complex sequence of adjustments takes place. One of the most important of these is retention of salt and water in order to increase the total blood volume and maintain cardiac output (the amount of blood pumped per minute). The first signs and symptoms of heart failure are swelling of the legs and ankles *(edema)*, fatigue with exertion, and shortness of breath *(dyspnea)* with mild exercise. If heart failure worsens, fluid may accumulate inside the lungs *(pulmonary edema)*, causing wheezing, coughing, and shortness of breath at rest. Pulmonary edema also causes *orthopnea*, in which you require more than one pillow to rest comfortably. By this time urgent medical help is needed.

Treatment. The treatment of heart failure includes reduced activity and rest, preferably in a chair, if symptoms are severe. Try to avoid becoming bedridden. Leg exercises and elastic stockings may be useful to prevent blood clots *(thrombosis)* in your legs. Elastic stockings should always be prescribed by your doctor and you should be instructed in their proper wear.

Your doctor may prescribe a mild sedative if anxiety prevents adequate rest. Anticoagulants may be given to help prevent blood clots. For long-term management, diuretic drugs and salt restriction are essential to prevent reaccumulation of excess fluid. Dietary salt should be restricted to 5 grams per day (this equals about 2 grams of sodium). Your doctor may prescribe digitalis to strengthen your heart muscle. In addition to these measures, every effort will be made to identify the exact cause of heart failure and address such specific treatable causes as anemia, hyperthyroidism, and high blood pressure. In cases of progressive heart damage that cannot be arrested, heart transplantation may be the only life-saving measure available.

Diseases of the Heart Valves

The heart has four chambers and each has a one-way check valve that keeps blood flowing in the proper direction. The tricuspid valve separates the right atrium from the right ventricle. The pulmonic valve prevents backward flow from the pulmonary artery into the right ventricle. The mitral valve separates the left atrium and left ventricle. The aortic valve prevents back flow from the aorta into the left ventricle.

The two principal problems that affect the heart valves are excessive narrowing *(stenosis)* and insufficiency, which permits back flow *(regurgitation)*. These are precisely the kinds of problems that occur with any plumbing valve.

Tricuspid Valve

Tricuspid stenosis occurs when the valve between the right atrium and right ventricle becomes narrowed, usually as a complication of rheumatic fever. If the stenosis is severe, blood backs up in the great vein *(vena cava)* and causes enlargement of the liver and a fluttering sensation in the neck because of distention of the neck veins. At the same time, not enough blood is pumped through the lungs, causing fatigue and shortness of breath. Only rarely is the stenosis so severe that surgical correction is required.

Tricuspid regurgitation is usually caused by some congenital abnormality that enlarges the right ventricle to the point of insufficiency of the valve with leakage of blood into the right atrium during ventricular contraction. The symptoms are usually the same as in stenosis of the valve. Surgery is not often required.

Pulmonary Valve

Pulmonary stenosis, which restricts outflow of blood to the lungs, causes severe cyanosis (poorly oxygenated blood) in infants ("blue baby") and may be a surgical emergency soon after birth. An operation to reroute blood around the narrowed valve is life saving. In less severe cases, cyanosis does not occur until later in childhood, when growth outstrips the ability of the heart to supply sufficient blood to the lungs. Again, surgical correction is required. Pulmonary stenosis occurring in adulthood is usually a result of rheumatic fever, which damages the valve leaflets.

Mitral Valve

Mitral stenosis in adults is often a complication of rheumatic fever. The chief symptoms are fatigue and shortness of breath, especially with exertion, owing to reduced cardiac output. Some cases can be treated medically with drugs that slow heart rate and prevent coagulation. If these fail, either surgical opening of the valve, or its replacement by an artificial valve, is then indicated.

Mitral regurgitation also results from valve damage caused by rheumatic fever, or in some cases, by rupture of the muscular cords that attach to the valve (a complication of heart attack). The symptoms are palpitations and heart failure. Patients who cannot be managed medically are treated by artificial valve replacement.

The mitral valve may undergo bulging or buckling on closure, a condition known as *mitral valve prolapse*. There are several causes, most of which are benign. Most often there are no symptoms; the diagnosis is suspected on routine physical examination when your doctor hears a "systolic click" when listening to your heart. If prolapse is associated with mitral regurgitation, then chest pain, palpitations, irregular heart beat, and fatigue may be experienced. Usually heart surgery is not required.

Aortic Valve

Aortic stenosis often results from a congenital narrowing, or may be caused by calcification of the valve following rheumatic fever. The classic symptoms are fainting, chest pain, and shortness of breath, all caused by failure of the heart to supply the body with enough blood. The usual treatment is surgical replacement of the valve.

Aortic regurgitation may also be congenital or result from the damage caused by rheumatic fever. Symptoms usually only appear with advanced disease. These are shortness of breath, and occasionally palpitations and chest pain. Treatment is by surgical replacement of the valve when symptoms become disabling.

Rheumatic Fever

Rheumatic fever begins as a throat infection caused by the Streptococcus bacterium. In rare individuals, when the throat infection is not treated, or is inadequately treated, a subsequent inflammation develops, most commonly in the heart and the joints. These inflammations are not caused by the bacteria, but by the body's immune defenses against the bacteria. The most common heart valves affected are the mitral and aortic valves. Inflammation of the valves may result in either stenosis from scarring, or regurgitation that results from physical alteration of the valves so that they do not close completely *(see above)*. These complications may not become evident until years later. The most common joints affected are the knees and ankles.

Treatment. Drugs that reduce inflammation include salicylates (aspirin) and corticosteroids. Often lifelong antibiotic prophylaxis is recommended to prevent a recurrent attack that will result in further heart and joint damage.

Endocarditis

The endocardium is the internal lining of the heart chambers and valves. In rare instances these structures may serve as the sites of growth for colonies of bacteria and fungi. Not only do these colonies damage the endocardium directly, but small clumps of bacteria may break off to form infective emboli that travel through the arterial system until they become lodged, there to grow and form distant abscesses. The direct damage to the heart caused by such growing organisms may lead to heart failure and low grade fever.

Treatment. Once the diagnosis has been made, prolonged treatment with antibiotics is required to quell the infection. If you have had endocarditis, it is wise to have prophylactic antibiotics before subsequent surgery and dental procedures to prevent recurrence.

Myocarditis

Myocarditis is an inflammation of the heart muscles and is usually a rare complication of infection elsewhere. The symptoms are mild chest pain, shortness of breath, and low-grade fever. The diagnosis is made from changes in the patient's ECG, and by biopsy of the heart muscle. The treatment is aimed at identifying and eliminating the underlying infection.

Pericarditis

The *pericardium* is the membranous bag that surrounds the heart. In pericarditis, the pericardium becomes inflamed, usually as the result of a viral infection, or one of the connective tissue diseases, e.g., *systemic lupus erythematosus*. The symptoms include chest pain that is made worse by coughing or deep breathing. You also may experience fatigue and shortness of breath. In chronic cases, scarring of the pericardium may result in a condition known as *constrictive pericarditis,* which leads to heart failure (*see* p. 197).

Treatment. Viral pericarditis usually resolves by itself in 1–2 weeks. In some cases your doctor will prescribe corticosteroids to reduce inflammation. In rare cases, fluid accumulates between the heart and pericardium (*pericardial effusion*). If this effusion interferes with the pumping action of the heart, the effusion must be drained through a needle inserted into the pericardium. With constrictive pericarditis, a heart surgeon must remove the pericardium to relieve heart failure.

Disorders of Blood Vessels

The vascular system is divided into the pulmonary circulation and the systemic circulation. The pulmonary circulation carries blood from the heart and through the lungs, where it is oxygenated. At the same time, the heart pumps blood through the systemic circulation that serves the rest of the body. The most common disorders of the systemic blood vessels are described below.

Arteriosclerosis *(Hardening of the Arteries)*

As people grow older their arteries tend to become less elastic, a process known as *arteriosclerosis.* They may also develop fatty deposits within the arteries, called *atheromas,* in a process known as *atherosclerosis,* discussed on p. 175. If atherosclerosis is extensive, blood flow to the limbs, especially the legs, may become so impaired as to produce symptoms, known as *intermittent claudication,* caused by lack of oxygen to the muscles. This is characterized by aching and cramping of the leg muscles, or a tired feeling that occurs when walking or running. The onset is gradual and becomes worse with time. The muscles most often involved are those in the calf, but muscles in the feet, thighs, hips, and buttocks may also be affected. The pain is quickly relieved by resting.

Since arteriosclerosis is a progressive obliterating disease, it may advance to the point where pain occurs even at rest. Such pain is aggravated by elevating the legs and is relieved by hanging them over the bed, or sitting in a chair. The feet may appear pale and feel cold and numb. The skin of the feet and lower legs often becomes dry and scaly, and the nails and hair grow slowly (*see* Stasis Dermatitis, p. 446). Ulcers may develop on the toes, heels, and ankles. Ultimately gangrene may develop (*see* p. 205). The affects of arteriosclerosis are made worse if you also have diabetes, anemia, or heart failure.

TAKING CARE OF YOUR FEET

Proper care of your feet is essential whenever you have impaired circulation to your legs:

1. Inspect your feet every day or have someone do this for you. If you notice any redness, new swelling, cracks in your skin, calluses, corns, or sores, consult your doctor or podiatrist.
2. Bathe your feet daily in lukewarm (not hot) water, using a mild soap. Afterward, dry them gently and thoroughly. You may use a nonmedicated powder, such as talcum, if your feet become moist. Change your socks daily.
3. Apply a lubricant such as lanolin if your skin is dry.
4. Trim toenails straight across, not too close to the skin. Do not use sharp instruments to dig into the corners of your toenails. If your eyesight is poor, have a podiatrist trim your toenails.
5. Corns and calluses should be treated by your podiatrist. Never cut them with a razor or sharp knife.
6. Avoid over-the-counter corn plasters. They often contain an acid that destroys tissue and increases the possibility of infection.
7. Wear properly fitted shoes with firm soles and soft uppers, and without either open toes or open heels. There should be about three-fourths of an inch of space between your big toe and the shoe. Change your shoes daily to avoid moisture buildup. Wear new shoes for only short periods until they become broken in. Never walk barefoot; even slight trauma will heal slowly and complicate your daily foot care. Foot deformities such as bunions and hammer toes (*see* p. 431) require special orthotic shoes.
8. Avoid restricting circulation to your feet, such as sitting with your legs crossed or wearing garters. Do not smoke; nicotine constricts peripheral arteries and may hasten gangrene.
9. Avoid burns to your feet, including sunburn. Do not put your feet into hot water or add hot water to a bath without testing the water temperature with your hands or a thermometer. Do not use hot water bottles or heating pads. People with poor circulation usually have decreased perception of heat and pain.

Treatment. If you have leg pain only while walking, rest until the pain is relieved and then walk again. It is important to walk at least an hour each day to maintain circulation to your legs. Gradually you will increase the distance you are able to walk without pain, both as a result of physical training and by development of collateral blood vessels that bypass the disease-blocked arteries. At night elevate the head of your bed 4–6 inches for greater leg comfort.

Several drugs relieve intermittent claudication. One of these, pentoxifylline (Trental) improves blood flow and increases the oxygen delivered to tissues. Your doctor may also prescribe aspirin to prevent blood clots. Beta-blocking drugs (e.g., propranolol, atenolol), often used to treat atherosclerotic heart disease, may worsen intermittent claudication. Tobacco in all forms must be avoided because it dramatically constricts peripheral arteries, reducing blood flow.

In some cases, your doctor may suggest a surgical bypass. This is a procedure in which a vein in the leg is removed and grafted onto the artery above the region of constriction in order to channel blood around the clogged artery. Another procedure is balloon angioplasty, which entails inserting a balloon-tipped catheter that is then blown up to dilate the plaque-narrowed artery. A new technique just now being developed uses a laser-tipped catheter inserted into the diseased artery that literally vaporizes the atherosclerotic obstruction to open up the channel.

Acrocyanosis

This is a relatively common condition, especially among women, in which the hands and feet sometimes look bluish *(cyanosis)* and feel cold and sweaty. It is caused by spasms of the small arteries that supply the hands and feet. This condition is not associated with arteriosclerosis. The cyanosis is usually made worse by exposure to cold.

Treatment. No treatment is necessary. Avoiding exposure to the cold weather helps prevent the spasms.

Raynaud's Phenomenon

This is a distressing condition in which the blood vessel response to a cold stimulus is grossly exaggerated, so that when exposed to cold weather, touching an ice cube, or even walking into an air-conditioned room can result in a vasoconstricting reaction. Fingers or toes suddenly turn white, then blue, and become cool to the touch. Numbness and tingling often occur. As the attack subsides, the digits flush and may tingle or ache. In some cases, nervousness or an embarrassing situation may trigger the reaction.

Raynaud's attacks are much more frequent in women, typically occurring between the ages of 15 and 40. In men, the phenomenon usually has a later onset. The cause is not known, but it is thought to be a local reaction within the peripheral arteries, rather than an abnormal sympathetic nervous reaction. Raynaud's phenomenon may also be more common in people who suffer migraine headaches.

A particularly severe type of Raynaud's phenomenon is known as *secondary* Raynaud's, in which such underlying diseases as systemic lupus erythematosus, scleroderma (which causes fibrous tissue to build up in the skin and internal organs), thyroid disease, and rheumatoid arthritis may be responsible for the abnormal vascular response. In sensitive individuals, such drugs as nicotine, ergot alkaloids and beta-blocker drugs (e.g., propranolol) may trigger secondary Raynaud's.

Treatment. The diagnosis of Raynaud's phenomenon is usually made from the patient's history. The phenomenon can often be induced by asking patients to immerse their hands in cold water and observing the characteristic white, blue, red color sequence in their skin. The therapeutic approach to Raynaud's is primarily preventative: proper dress in cold weather to avoid chilling, the use of gloves when handling cold objects, avoidance of excessive air conditioning, wearing mittens and socks to bed, using insulated cups for cold drinks, and the like. Obviously the avoidance of nicotine and any drug known to bring on an attack is necessary.

There are some other therapeutic approaches that you may ask your doctor about. Biofeedback techniques have had some success in training patients to bring the temperature of their fingers and toes under voluntary control. Some patients are able to stop a Raynaud's attack by using a maneuver described by a doctor in Vermont: swing the arms rapidly in 360-degree circles for a few minutes to move blood by centrifugal force to the fingers. In severe cases, calcium-channel blockers such as nifedipine may be prescribed to dilate blood vessels. Others have found relief through the use of prazosin, a drug that counteracts natural vasoconstricting hormones.

Acute Artery Occlusions

The sudden occlusion of an artery in the arm or leg produces abrupt onset of pain, coldness of the hand or foot, numbness, and pallor. The cause of such an acute occlusion may be a blood clot that breaks loose from the left ventricle and lodges in a distant artery (*see* embolization p. 209), an aneurysm, or an acute thrombosis (blood clot). These represent acute medical emergencies. For treatment of pulmonary embolism (*see* p. 209).

Gangrene

Gangrene is simply dead flesh. It can occur anywhere, but is most common in the extremities, where it results from reduced or absent blood flow. It is characterized by blackening and sloughing of the skin, and can be either dry or wet. Wet gangrene is caused by infection, whereas in dry gangrene there is no infection. There are numerous causes of gangrene. The most common include diabetes and arteriosclerosis, both of which result in progressive narrowing of small arteries to the point that they cannot sustain healthy living tissue. Frostbite is the most common accidental cause of gangrene (*see* p. 82). Other causes include Buerger's disease, which is caused by an inflammation of small arteries that results in thrombosis (blood clot) and gangrene; and Raynaud's disease (*see* p. 203).

Wet gangrene is a consequence of infection, usually by the bacterium *Clostridium*, which grows in the absence of air and releases toxins that destroy tissue. They also produce gas to form *gas gangrene.*

Symptoms. When dry gangrene forms in the foot of someone with poor circulation, the foot may at first feel cold or numb. Later a dull aching pain develops that increases with walking. Clear warning signs are pallor, cold, and pain in one or both feet. If wet gangrene develops, the infected area will quickly become discolored and have an unpleasant smell.

Treatment. Frank gangrene of either type is usually treated by amputation at a level high enough that adequate circulation remains to ensure wound healing. Wet gangrene is also treated with a combination of antibiotics and antisera to combat the bacteria's toxins. In some cases the victim must be placed in a *hyperbaric chamber,* a large chamber filled with oxygen under pressure that forces oxygen into the dead tissues. Clostridia cannot live in the presence of oxygen.

The prevention of gangrene of the foot is outlined above in the box on *foot care.*

Bed Sores

Patients who are confined to bed for prolonged periods of time can develop ulcerations as a result of decreased blood flow to pressure points on the pelvis and heels. Older patients with vascular insufficiency are particularly prone to such bed sores. They can largely be prevented by frequently moving patients who are confined to bed, through the use of pillows, sheep skin, and other cushioning to distribute the body weight over a greater surface area, and by keeping the patient clean and dry. If a bed sore should develop, call the patient's doctor at once so that intensive treatment and antibiotics can be commenced and routine bed care be reviewed.

Varicose Veins

Varicose veins are superficial veins that have become twisted and dilated, causing bulging discolorations, most often noticeable on the legs. The cause is absent or damaged valves inside the veins. These valves are thin folds of tissue lining the veins that close to prevent backflow and engorgement. Varicose veins in the legs tend to run in families and they are four times more common in women. Age also plays a part, since they usually develop after age 40.

There are three types of veins in the legs: the *superficial veins* that lie close to the skin, the *deep veins* that lie deep within the leg muscles, and the *perforator veins* that connect the two. The heart cannot pump venous blood against gravity from the legs to the heart. Rather, peripheral blood is pumped by muscular activity that forces the blood higher and higher until it reaches the heart. Backflow is prevented by the venous valves. However, if the valves are incompetent, either from congenital absence or from damage by previous blood clots, or are distended from prolonged standing, this pumping action is interfered with and the superficial veins, which have thin, fragile walls, become stretched and distorted in their typical ropy varicosities. When varicose veins develop in the anus for similar reasons, they are known as hemorrhoids. Varicose veins can also develop inside the vagina during pregnancy.

Symptoms. The earliest signs of varicose veins are the appearance of enlarged, twisting, purplish veins that pop out in the lower legs upon standing. Small groups of tiny blue or red veins under the skin called *spider bursts* accompany varicose veins. Sometimes varicose veins occur in only one leg. Often there are no symptoms. Otherwise you may have a sense of fullness or pain after prolonged walking or standing. Your legs and feet may swell, itching is common, and nighttime leg cramps may interfere with sleep. Many women have more discomfort during their menstrual periods. If the condition is severe, the skin may become discolored and skin ulcers may develop (*see* Stasis Dermatitis, p. 446). Inflammation of the veins (*see* Thrombophlebitis *below*) is also fairly common.

Treatment. Mild cases of varicose veins require no treatment. You can reduce symptoms by sitting down and elevating your feet to promote drainage. Try to avoid long periods of standing and do not sit with your legs crossed or hanging down. Get plenty of exercise to keep your leg muscles pumping and the blood from pooling. Avoid tight clothing, garters, girdles, and pantyhose. Losing excess weight also helps retard the development of varicose veins.

Ask your doctor about graduated compression stockings. These are elastic stockings that fit most tightly at the ankles and gradually decrease pressure as they go up. *Do not* try to fit yourself with elastic stockings, nor try to use elastic bandages without proper instruction.

In more symptomatic cases of pain, swelling, and limitation of activity, or where the varicose veins are cosmetically objectionable, your doctor will most likely recommend surgery wherein the large leg veins are stripped out and the smaller, perforating veins tied. Another treatment is the injection of sclerosing agents that cause the veins to close by scarring. After both types of treatment, normal circulation is taken over by surrounding veins. If varicose veins recur after surgery, they can usually be treated by injections.

Thrombophlebitis

Phlebitis is an inflammation of veins, usually caused by injury or infection. Blood clots (thrombi) then form on the inflamed blood vessel walls. *Thrombophlebitis* is most common in the superficial veins of the legs, and frequently occurs in those who have varicose veins (*see above*). The area around the inflamed vein becomes tender, warm, and red. The vein can usually be felt as a hard cord running the length of the vessel.

Treatment. You should see your doctor, who will be able to distinguish superficial thrombophlebitis from the much more serious deep venous thrombosis (*see below*). If superficial thrombophlebitis is confirmed, aspirin or ibuprofen may be prescribed for discomfort. Warm compresses over the involved vein may also bring relief. If itching develops, use one of the zinc oxide preparations. If you develop a fever, it may indicate the presence of an infection, in which case you should see your doctor to determine whether an antibiotic is appropriate. Most cases of superficial thrombophlebitis clear within about a week.

Deep Venous Thrombosis

When a blood clot forms in one of the deep veins of the leg or arm, the condition is much more serious than is the case with superficial thrombophlebitis (*see* p. 207), because of the possibility of the clot breaking off to form an *embolus* that may then travel to the blood vessels of the lungs (*pulmonary embolism; see* next article).

Two conditions increase the risk of developing deep venous thrombosis: slowed venous circulation and an increased tendency to clot. Slowed circulation is common in those on bed rest, particularly after an injury or surgery. Heart failure slows the circulation. So does pregnancy by compressing the veins in the pelvis that receive blood from the legs. Obesity—that old bugaboo—also predisposes to deep venous thrombosis.

Increased clotting tendency is found in those who take high doses of estrogens in contraceptives (*see* p. 368), as well as in victims of cancer, kidney diseases, and certain blood diseases such as polycythemia vera (*see* p. 223).

Symptoms. There may be no symptoms of deep venous thrombosis at all until the sudden onset of chest pain caused by pulmonary embolism (*see* next article). However, more commonly, redness, pain, and swelling of the involved leg or arm will indicate the presence of thrombosis. Prominence of the superficial veins and a bluish skin discoloration may also be present. Pain usually occurs on standing or walking and is relieved by lying down. It is often difficult to distinguish the pain of thrombophlebitis from muscle pain.

If you suspect you have deep venous thrombosis, see your doctor at once. The diagnosis is usually confirmed by duplex ultrasound in which high frequency sound waves are passed into the legs to detect the presence of a clot and the reduced blood flow that it causes. In some instances venography, in which dye is injected into the veins and X-rays taken to outline the clot within the venous channels, will be performed.

Treatment. The primary treatment goal for cases of deep venous thrombosis is to prevent pulmonary embolism. Your doctor will most likely place you in the hospital on bed rest and administer such anticoagulants as heparin to prevent further clot formation. Analgesics are given for pain. After release from the hospital, you will most likely be given an oral anticoagulant such as coumadin and advised to wear elastic stockings. Most venous clots resolve themselves.

Prevention. If you are bedridden, your doctor may prescribe elastic stockings. You will be encouraged to move your toes and ankles and bend your knees frequently to keep the blood in your legs flow-ing. Practice periodic deep breathing, because the negative pressure in your chest also helps propel blood upward toward your heart. In some cases your doctor may order plastic sleeves placed around your legs that inflate and deflate mechanically, thus pumping blood up from your legs. Your doctor will also get you up and walking to improve circulation as soon as your condition permits.

Pulmonary Embolism

Pulmonary embolism occurs when a blood clot from one of the deep veins in the legs or pelvis breaks off, travels to and through the heart and out into the pulmonary artery, where it soon lodges in an artery of the lungs too small to pass further. Here the clot obstructs the lung blood flow, preventing oxygenation of the blood. If the clot is very large, the result can be disastrous. In fact about 30% of people who have a pulmonary embolus will die as a result. Those at risk for pulmonary embolism are the same as those at risk for deep venous thrombosis discussed above.

Symptoms. Small pulmonary emboli do not cause any symptoms at all. Larger emboli may impair oxygenation of blood in the lungs sufficiently to cause shortness of breath, dizziness, faintness, chest pain, and occasionally blueness around the mouth or coughing bloody sputum. Massive pulmonary emboli can cause collapse and death within minutes.

Diagnosis. The diagnosis of pulmonary embolism is made by radio-active lung scans, which demonstrate absent blood flow to a region of the lungs, and by pulmonary angiography, in which dye is injected into the heart and X-rays are taken to outline the clot within the lung's blood vessels.

Treatment. If the diagnosis of pulmonary embolism is made early enough, the embolus can sometimes be dissolved by enzymes, includ-ing *streptokinase, urokinase,* and *tissue plasminogen activator.* Your doc-tor will also most likely order anticoagulation drugs to prevent the formation of new blood clots. In serious cases a mechanical filter can be inserted by means of a catheter into the great vein, the vena cava, to trap emboli before they can reach the heart and lungs.

The prevention of pulmonary emboli is achieved by the same measures as those taken to prevent deep venous thrombosis, as described above.

Disorders of the Blood, Bone Marrow, and Lymphatic System

Blood Disorders

Blood is considered a body tissue because it consists of groups of cells, each with their own special function, all suspended within a liquid medium, the plasma. Most blood disorders arise from alterations of the blood cells.

There are two main types of blood cells: red and white. The great majority of blood cells are red cells that carry oxygen from the lungs and deliver it through the circulatory system to all of the tissues of the body. Red cells also carry waste carbon dioxide from the tissues back to the lungs, where it is released and expired. The ratio of the volume of red cells to the volume of whole blood (the cells plus plasma) is known as the *hematocrit*. This percentage is normally about 40–45 percent. In anemias the hematocrit is less.

The white cells account for only a small fraction of the total blood cells, but they are vital. They have two principal functions: destroying bacteria and producing antibodies. Most white cells are *neutrophils* (also called *granulocytes*) that attack and ingest bacteria and other foreign substances that find their way into the body. The other main white cell, the lymphocyte, is responsible for producing antibodies and performing other essential immune functions.

There is a third general type of blood cell, the platelet. Platelets are responsible for initiating the clotting of blood whenever the integrity of a blood vessel is broken. Once initiated, other chemicals from the plasma join with platelets to form a blood clot that seals the wound.

There are four general types of blood disorders: infection, decreased hemoglobin, which causes anemias; inadequate clotting, which causes bleeding and bruising; and cancer, namely the leukemias.

Septicemia

Infections of the blood known as *septicemia* are those in which bacteria and their toxins enter the bloodstream, usually from a localized site of infection, such as an abscess, and thus spread throughout the body. The symptoms can range from mild sweating, to cyclical chills and fever, to shock and prostration, depending on the type of bacterium responsible and the number of organisms entering the bloodstream. The diagnosis of septicemia is made by demonstrating the presence of bacteria isolated from blood cultures.

Treatment. Septicemia is a serious infection that usually requires hospitalization and intensive antibiotic therapy. In addition, every effort is made to localize the site of the primary infection, the treatment of which usually eliminates the septicemia.

Infectious Mononucleosis

Infectious mononucleosis, often referred to as "mono," is an infection of the leukocytes by the Epstein-Barr virus (EBV). The infection occurs primarily in young people, especially teenagers. It is characterized by fever, sore throat, fatigue and weakness, loss of appetite, swollen lymph nodes, and often stiffness of the muscles. This infectious disease is believed to be spread by infectious saliva, with an incubation period of 7–14 days. Generally, infectious mononucleosis is not a serious disease. However, in some severe cases, hepatitis and jaundice can develop and the spleen may become so enlarged as to cause pain and abdominal fullness.

Your doctor can make the diagnosis of infectious mononucleosis by the *monospot* test, which detects antibodies to the EBV. The major symptoms usually disappear in 1–14 days, although it is often 1–3 months before easy fatigability disappears.

Treatment. As with most viral infections, there is no effective treatment that is specific for mononucleosis. Treatment is supportive and includes bed rest, plenty of fluids, and a nourishing diet (despite a lack of appetite). Gargling with warm salt water may be soothing to the throat and acetaminophen may be taken as needed. Antibiotics are not recommended unless a secondary bacterial infection develops. A sudden sharp pain in the left upper part of the abdomen (which may result from the rare rupture of an enlarged spleen) should alert you to call your doctor at once.

Chronic Fatigue Syndrome

A syndrome is a collection of symptoms that appear together and define an illness, but whose cause is usually unknown. This is certainly the case with chronic fatigue syndrome, which is discussed here because it resembles chronic infectious mononucleosis in many respects. However, in most cases the Epstein-Barr virus is not demonstrable.

Fatigue is a feeling of tiredness severe enough to interfere with your everyday activities. Chronic fatigue occurs when the tiredness lasts more than a few days or weeks, so that it can't be attributed to a lack of sleep or a flu.

Diagnosis. Because chronic fatigue syndrome is such a vague illness, doctors have defined certain criteria that must exist before this diagnosis is considered appropriate:

1. You must suffer from recent severe fatigue and weakness that has impaired your ability to work productively for 6 months.
2. All other known diseases, infections, or psychiatric illness that might cause these symptoms must be ruled out.
3. You must have experienced four of the following:
   • Low-grade fever (99.5–100.5°F) or chills
   • Sore throat
   • Painful lymph nodes in the neck or armpits
   • Generalized headaches
   • Unexplained muscle soreness
   • Migratory joint pain without redness or swelling
   • Forgetfulness, irritability, or confusion
   • Sleep disturbance

Fatigue is also a frequent manifestation of depression. Though most people do not like to admit that they have psychological problems, such conditions as depression are usually relatively short-lived and are treatable. However, your doctor will want to rule out other conditions before concluding that your fatigue is the result of depression.

Treatment. Since there is no known cause of chronic fatigue syndrome, it follows that there is no specific treatment. The symptoms are treated with appropriate amounts of rest and exercise, according to individual tolerance. Mild analgesics are appropriate for pain and soreness. The syndrome will eventually disappear.

For more information about this difficult-to-diagnose condition, the following sources may be helpful.

Chronic Fatigue and Immune Dysfunction Syndrome Society, PO Box 230108, Portland, OR 97223.

Chronic Fatigue and Immune Dysfunction Syndrome Association, PO Box 220398, Charlotte, NC 28222, 1-800-442-3437.

For a packet of information, send a self-addressed stamped business-sized envelope to Box CFS, National Institute of Allergy and Infectious Diseases, Bldg. 31, Rm 7A32, NIH, Bethesda, MD 20892.

Anemias

All anemias have one thing in common: decreased hemoglobin in the blood. Hemoglobin, you may recall, is the protein in red blood

Common Types of Anemia

Cause	Comments
Blood loss	May be caused by acute hemorrhage or chronic loss, as from slow intestinal bleeding
Iron deficiency	Caused by chronic blood loss or lack of iron absorbed from the intestine
Vitamin B$_{12}$ deficiency	Vitamin B$_{12}$ is needed in red cell production
Folic acid deficiency	Folic acid is needed in red cell production
Hemolysis	Red cells destroyed prematurely
Sickle cell disease	Congenital deformity of red cells that causes hemolysis
Thalassemia	Congenital lack of red cell hemoglobin
Chronic disease	Often seen in rheumatoid arthritis, hepatitis, cancer, and chronic infection. Disappears when the underlying disease is treated
Marrow replacement	Occurs when cancer or fibrous tissue displaces normal bone marrow cells

cells that carries oxygen. The deficiency of hemoglobin may be caused by either too few red cells (such as after you suffer a hemorrhage), or too little hemoglobin per red cell (which occurs when you have an iron deficiency). The table above lists the most important types of anemias.

Regardless of cause, all anemias have certain symptoms in common: pallor, weakness, and fatigue. If severe, anemias also cause headaches, faintness, breathlessness, drowsiness, and sometimes jaundice, loss of libido, missed menstruation, and bizarre behavior.

Iron Deficiency Anemia

Iron is an essential component of hemoglobin. When you have insufficient iron stores in your body, the bone marrow responds by making smaller red cells that carry too little hemoglobin. This is the most common cause of anemia and is more common in women because of menstruation. Normally what little iron is lost from your body is easily made up by iron in your diet. There are three main causes of iron loss.

The most common cause of iron deficiency is chronic blood loss. Frequent causes of bleeding include heavy menstruation, bleeding from gastritis, stomach ulcers, stomach cancer, or inflammatory bowel disease. Even severe hemorrhoids may cause enough blood loss to make you anemic. Your bone marrow responds to blood loss by making more red cells. This draws upon the stores of iron in the bone marrow and liver. When these stores are inadequate to keep up with the increased demand, anemia results. A much rarer cause of iron loss is from excessive red cell destruction (hemolysis) and excretion of hemoglobin in the urine.

The second reason for inadequate iron is diminished absorption from the intestines, which occurs in the malabsorption syndrome (*see* p. 299). The most common cause is removal of part of the stomach for such conditions as stomach ulcer or cancer, since stomach acid is necessary for iron absorption.

The third cause of iron deficiency anemia is a lack of iron in the diet. This is occasionally seen in children during the first two years of life if iron in the diet is inadequate for the demands of rapid growth. Adolescent girls may become anemic when the demands of growth are compounded by the onset of menstruation. People who have very restricted diets or bizarre eating habits may also have inadequate iron intake.

Symptoms. The symptoms of all anemias are similar: pallor, weakness, fatigue, and breathlessness. In severe deficiency, the tongue may take on a glossy appearance and a condition known as *pica*, in which very anemic persons crave to eat dirt or paint, may develop.

Treatment. If you suspect you are anemic, see your doctor. Do not attempt to treat yourself, because there are many different types of anemia, all of which are treated differently. You cannot tell what type you have without laboratory tests. If iron deficiency is diagnosed, your doctor will probably recommend iron injections or oral iron supplements. If dietary restriction is the likely cause, you may have to adopt new eating habits. Foods rich in iron include meat, eggs, cereals, and beans

Vitamin B$_{12}$ Deficiency Anemia *(Pernicious Anemia)*

Vitamin B$_{12}$ is necessary for the production of red blood cells. Usually the liver stores enough vitamin B$_{12}$ to maintain normal red cell production for 3–5 years. Most diets contain adequate amounts of vitamin B$_{12}$, which is absorbed in the small intestine. However, absorption of this vitamin depends on a substance known as *intrinsic factor*, which is produced by cells lining the stomach. In some people intrinsic factor secretion is diminished, a condition that will ultimately lead to anemia when stores of the vitamin in the liver become depleted. Less common causes of vitamin B_{12} deficiency include intestinal malabsorption (*see* p. 299) and insufficient dietary intake among strict vegetarians.

Symptoms. The symptoms of vitamin B_{12} deficiency are similar to those of other anemias, described above. Because of the large liver storage capacity and the fact that malabsorption is seldom total, the onset of symptoms is usually very slow. Ultimately, weakness, pallor, fatigue, and shortness of breath develop. The tongue may become inflamed (glossitis) and produce a burning sensation. In very severe disease, the nervous system also is involved, causing difficulty walking and maintaining proper balance.

Treatment. Once lost, the ability to absorb vitamin B_{12} is not regained. This necessitates life-long injections of the vitamin or high doses of oral vitamin supplements. Once the liver stores have been replenished, you can expect to receive injections once monthly or daily vitamin pills. You may be able to give injections to yourself if your doctor agrees. The anemia is corrected in about six weeks. If neurologic symptoms have developed, these may take as long as 18 months to correct.

Folic Acid Deficiency Anemia

Folic acid is another vitamin essential to the production of red cells, although in this case, the most common cause of the anemia is inadequate amounts in the diet. The body can only store a few months' supply of folic acid. Since folic acid is found primarily in green vegetables and is destroyed by overcooking, a diet deficient in fresh vegetables may lead to anemia. It is especially common in chronic alcoholics and that group of individuals known as "tea and toasters," who through apathy or simply bad habit, adopt a very bland and restricted diet. This is common among the elderly who live by themselves. Intestinal malabsorption and prolonged treatment with certain antibiotics can also lead to folic acid deficiency. The symptoms are similar to those of vitamin B_{12} deficiency anemia without the neurological symptoms.

Treatment. Your doctor will likely prescribe folic acid tablets at first, and will also instruct you on a well-rounded diet, which should provide all the folic acid you need. Foods rich in folic acid include leafy green vegetables, beans, peas, and liver.

Hemolytic Anemias

Hemolysis is defined as premature destruction of red blood cells. Red cells are normally destroyed in the spleen, liver, and bone marrow at the end of their life span of about 120 days. When for some reason this life span is shortened, the bone marrow must increase production to maintain a normal number of circulating red cells. When the bone marrow cannot keep up with the rate of destruction, anemia results.

There are numerous causes of hemolysis. The body may produce antibodies that attach themselves to the red cell, thus marking the cell for early destruction. Certain drugs and bacteria can cause hemolysis. In other cases, the spleen may become overactive (*hypersplenism*) and destroy too many red cells before they complete their normal life span. Hereditary defects in the red cell membrane can also cause hemolysis, e.g., *hereditary spherocytosis.*

Symptoms. The symptoms of hemolytic anemia are the same as those of other anemias: pallor, weakness, fatigue, and breathlessness. If the destruction of red blood cells is severe, jaundice, and dark-colored urine may develop. Sometimes chills, fever, and pain in the back occur.

Treatment. Treatment varies with the cause of the hemolysis. Hemolysis caused by drugs or antibiotics will be cured by changing the drug therapy. In some cases, surgical removal of the spleen, the site of most red cell destruction, considerably improves the disorder.

Sickle-Cell Anemia

Sickle-cell anemia is a hereditary disorder that affects mostly blacks and is caused by the presence of an abnormal hemoglobin molecule, hemoglobin-S, in the red cell. To develop sickle-cell anemia, the abnormal gene must be inherited from both parents. If only one gene is inherited, "sickle-cell trait" is said to exist and half of the hemoglobin in the red cells is normal. Only a few symptoms are associated with sickle-cell trait.

When red cells containing all hemoglobin-S enter a tissue containing decreased levels of oxygen, the cell becomes deformed, or "sickled." These cells are unable to flow smoothly through capillaries and small blood vessels. Rather they tend to clog the capillaries, causing the surrounding tissues to become starved for oxygen. This is known as a sickle-cell "crisis" and can be very painful.

Symptoms. The symptoms of sickle-cell anemia are quite variable. In severe cases, all of the symptoms of anemia are present, including weakness, fatigue, and breathlessness. In addition there may be episodes of jaundice and *sickle-cell crises*. Crises are characterized by bone and joint pain caused by localized destruction *(necrosis)* of bone. There may also be nausea, vomiting, and abdominal pain that is difficult to distinguish from an acute abdominal emergency. Infections are common, as are kidney failure (*see* p. 332) and pulmonary embolism (*see* p. 209), and the disease is generally associated with a reduced life expectancy.

Treatment. There is little that can be done to treat the basic disease; however, pain can be alleviated with painkillers and antibiotics can be administered when infections occur. Those with sickle-cell anemia should avoid flying in unpressurized planes or going to altitudes above 6000 feet in order to avoid suffering a severe sickle-cell crisis caused by the reduced level of environmental oxygen.

Thalassemia

This is a group of inherited anemias particularly common in persons of Mediterranean, African, and Southeast Asian ancestry. These disorders are all characterized by production of abnormal hemoglobin molecules that cause premature red cell destruction.

Symptoms. The symptoms of thalassemia vary in severity. In the form known as *thalassemia major* (abnormal genes inherited from both parents), all of the symptoms of full-blown anemia occur, including weakness, fatigue, pallor, and breathlessness. The spleen may become huge and cause abdominal tenderness. This anemia may also impair normal growth, resulting in a short, slight stature. Persons with "thalassemia trait" (inheritance of the abnormal gene from only one parent) usually have few or no symptoms.

Treatment. Thalassemia major usually requires regular blood transfusions throughout life. Since most of the iron from these transfusions is retained, it must be removed by iron-chelation therapy (drugs that remove iron) to avoid liver, heart, and kidney damage. Persons with thalassemia minor require no treatment.

Bleeding and Bruising

Bleeding, both internal and external, is halted by a complex set of physical and chemical reactions to produce a blood clot. First, the local blood vessels constrict in order to reduce flow to the damaged vessel. Second, platelets in the blood become "sticky" and clump together. Finally, fibrin and other substances in the plasma combine with the platelets to form a clot that seals off the broken blood vessel. Serious bleeding can occur if any of these processes fails.

Easy Bruising *(Purpura simplex)*

This is probably the most common of all bleeding disorders and develops more often in women. You may notice bruises, especially on your thighs, buttocks, and upper arms without having injured them. Usually there is no other symptom, and all laboratory tests of bleeding function prove normal.

Treatment. If you bruise easily, see your doctor, who will test your blood for a serious bleeding disorder. If none is found, you will probably be advised to avoid aspirin and aspirin-containing drugs, which prolong bleeding time. Otherwise the condition is not serious.

Some older people may develop deep purple bruises that persist for a long time on their arms and backs of their hands. This is known as *senile purpura* and is thought to be caused by previous sun exposure. There is no treatment, and the condition is benign, although the bruises, which later turn a permanent brownish color, may be cosmetically objectionable. Long sleeves are the best solution.

Thrombocytopenia

In *thrombocytopenia* you have too few platelets in your blood, which in turn makes you bleed easily. There are several reasons why your platelet count may become low: failure of platelet production in the bone marrow, increased utilization from clotting, increased platelet destruction caused by either the formation of platelet antibodies or a drug reaction.

The symptoms of thrombocytopenia are easy bruising, prolonged bleeding from minor cuts, or nosebleeds. You may also develop a characteristic rash consisting of tiny, bright red dots on the skin, especially your legs. These are actually tiny areas of bleeding into the skin. If fever, malaise, muscle aches, and joint pains accompany a rash, an underlying infection is usually responsible.

Treatment. Your doctor will probably stop any drugs you are taking, because many drugs can cause platelet destruction. Corticosteroids may be prescribed if platelet antibodies are found to be responsible. In serious cases, removal of the spleen *(splenectomy)* is required, because this is the site of platelet destruction. Transfusions of platelets may also be required to stop bleeding.

Hemophilia

As noted earlier, the clotting of blood is a result of a complex series of physical and chemical interactions that requires the presence of several *clotting factors* normally present in the blood. In hemophilia there is a hereditary absence of one or more of these clotting factors, so that bruising and bleeding become a frequent occurrence. The most common type of hemophilia is known as hemophilia A, in which a substance known as factor VIII is missing or markedly reduced. Because of the way hemophilia is inherited, only males have the disease, but it is passed from generation to generation by mothers who carry the defective gene.

Symptoms. The symptoms of hemophilia are easy bleeding and bruising, usually starting as soon as the child becomes active and crawling. In some cases the condition is mild and may not become apparent until adulthood. Bleeding into joints can cause joint stiffness. A major injury can be fatal because of uncontrolled bleeding.

Treatment. Acute bleeding can usually be stopped by intravenous transfusions of factor VIII. Naturally hemophiliacs must be careful to avoid injury and such anticoagulant drugs as aspirin. Even minor surgery requires careful preparation to limit bleeding, and should only be done at a medical center experienced in treating hemophilia. Those with known hemophilia in their family should seek genetic counseling before beginning a family.

Hemophiliacs remain at increased risk of contracting hepatitis and AIDS because they require periodic transfusions of blood products. However, with current universal testing procedures, this risk has been greatly diminished.

More information about hemophilia and recognized treatment centers can be obtained from: National Hemophilia Foundation, 19 West 34th Street, New York, NY 10001.

Leukemia

Leukemia is a cancer of white blood cells in which groups of white cells grow without control and without performing their natural functions. Instead of dying after a useful lifespan, these leukemic cells continue to live and multiply, often infiltrating other organs and crowding out normal cells from the bone marrow, usually with disastrous consequences. The cause of human leukemias is not known. In animals, leukemias are known to be caused by viruses, but this has not been proven for most human leukemias.

There are two kinds of leukemias involving the two types of white blood cells, the lymphocytes and the neutrophils (also called granulocytes). Leukemias are also either acute or chronic, depending on how mature the leukemic cells are. Thus, acute leukemias are those in which the leukemic blood cells are relatively immature, whereas in chronic leukemia, the leukemic cells are more mature. In general acute leukemias tend to have a more rapid, malignant course than chronic leukemias when untreated. Treatment, however, may reverse this trend.

Acute Leukemia

There are two kinds of acute leukemias: acute lymphocytic leukemia and acute nonlymphocytic leukemia (also called acute granulocytic leukemia), depending on the cell type that becomes cancerous and grows out of control. Acute lymphocytic leukemia is mostly a childhood disease, with a peak incidence between ages 3 and 5, although it may occur in adolescents and young adults. This is the most common childhood cancer.

Acute nonlymphocytic leukemia occurs at all ages and is the most common acute leukemia in adults. This leukemia is thought to be caused by prior irradiation or as a result of prior use of anticancer drugs for another type of cancer.

In both types of acute leukemia, the leukemic cells crowd out normal bone marrow cells, disrupting the production of white cells, red cells, and platelets. As the leukemic cells enter the bloodstream they invade several organs of the body, including skin, liver, spleen, and brain, causing these organs to become enlarged and interfering with their functions.

Symptoms. Because bone marrow is replaced by masses of leukemic cells, an anemia results from the loss of red cell production, infections and fevers result from the loss of granulocyte production, and bleeding results from loss of platelet production. Progressive weakness, tiredness, and pallor are common. The liver and spleen enlarge and invasion of the brain can result in neurologic symptoms and eventually coma.

Untreated, acute leukemia is almost always fatal. The diagnosis is made by discovery of leukemic cells in the blood and bone marrow.

Treatment. The aim of treatment is to wipe out the entire line of leukemic cells so that normal bone marrow function can take place. This is usually accomplished with a wide variety of anticancer drugs, the type and combinations of which are constantly changing as new information is gained and as new drugs are developed. Bone marrow irradiation is also used to destroy the leukemic cells. In some cases restoration of normal function requires a bone marrow transplantation, usually from a close relative or sibling. During the prolonged and often arduous treatment, supportive care consists of periodic transfusions of blood cells and antibiotics to fight infection. This treatment is only undertaken in specialized treatment centers with a highly trained staff fully familiar with the treatment of leukemias.

Prognosis. Before modern treatment was available, the average victim of acute leukemia survived only about four months. With modern treatment, 50% of patients survive five years or longer. With bone marrow transplants, the chances of long-term survival are even greater. Still the prognosis depends on the exact type of leukemia cell present and how successfully doctors can prevent infection and bleeding until a normal bone marrow can be reestablished.

For more information contact:

Office of Cancer Communication, National Cancer Institute, Bethesda, MD 20892, 1-800-4-CANCER.

Leukemia Society of America, 800 Second Avenue, New York, NY 10017, 1-212-573-8484.

Bone Marrow Transplant Registry maintains a list of potential bone marrow donors; its hotline is: 1-800-745-2452. Call 1-800-726-2824 for information concerning costs and resource centers.

Chronic Granulocytic Leukemia
(Chronic Myelocytic Leukemia)

In this leukemia there is an overproduction of granulocytes (neutrophils), the white blood cells responsible for fighting infections. It is more common in adults and is rare before the age of 10 years.

Symptoms. The symptoms include fatigue, weakness, loss of appetite, weight loss, fever, and night sweats. In some cases bleeding and easy bruising occur if the platelets fall to low levels (*see* Thrombocytopenia *above*). Often the spleen swells and a "dragging" sensation is felt in the left abdomen. The diagnosis is made by the discovery of leukemic cells in the blood and bone marrow.

Treatment. The treatment of chronic granulocytic leukemia is generally the same as in acute leukemia: anticancer drugs and irradiation followed by bone marrow transplantation if a suitable donor can be found. In some cases the spleen will also be irradiated or removed surgically.

Prognosis. The average patient with chronic granulocytic leukemia survives 3–4 years after the onset of symptoms. Anticancer drugs are usually successful in relieving symptoms temporarily, but in time the leukemic cells become more malignant and the clinical course is then usually rapidly downhill. In cases where bone marrow transplantation is successful, complete cure is possible.

For more information, contact the resources listed above.

Chronic Lymphocytic Leukemia

In this type of leukemia, the lymphocytes undergo malignant transformation and grow out of control. This is generally a disease of older people, usually over the age of 60, and is 2–3 times more common in males. The cause is unknown.

Symptoms. The onset of symptoms is gradual. In some the first signs of illness are enlarged lymph nodes in the neck, groin, and armpits. Later fatigue, weakness, loss of appetite, weight loss, and shortness of breath develop. The spleen may swell, giving rise to a dragging sensation in the left abdomen.

Treatment. There is no cure yet for chronic lymphocytic leukemia; treatment is usually begun only when symptoms develop. Even then, overtreatment is more dangerous than undertreatment. Treatment consists of irradiation and anticancer drugs, with selective transfusion of blood cells if needed for bleeding or anemia, and antibiotics if infections develop.

Prognosis. The average survival of patients with chronic lymphocytic leukemia is about six years from the onset of symptoms. In certain types of this leukemia, the prognosis is much better and many elderly patients die of other, unrelated causes.

For more information, call the toll-free telephone number of the Cancer Information Service at 1-800-4-CANCER.

Disorders of the Bone Marrow

The marrow inside your bones is an active tissue that produces all of the cells that circulate in your blood. Normally the bone marrow produces just enough blood cells to keep you healthy, increasing production when needed to respond to infection or blood loss, for example. The disorders described here occur when inappropriate numbers of cells—either too many or too few—are produced.

Polycythemia Vera

Polycythemia vera is a disease in which the bone marrow produces an excess of all types of blood cells: red cells, granulocytes, and platelets. However, it is the excess red cells that are responsible for most symptoms of the disease.

Polycythemia vera is a disease of unknown cause and must be distinguished from *secondary polycythemia*, in which increased red cells are produced for well-understood physiologic reasons: lung disease (including excess smoking), heart disease, and certain tumors that secrete blood-stimulating hormones. Secondary polycythemia is reversed when the underlying condition is treated.

Symptoms. As the number of red blood cells in the circulation increases, headaches, dizziness, fatigue, weakness, shortness of breath, and a ruddy complexion develop. Often there is severe generalized itching. The liver and spleen may swell because they become engorged with blood. The blood tends to clot easily because of its thickness (increased viscosity) and the increased numbers of platelets. This may result in bone pain and other symptoms that are caused by clots forming within blood vessels.

Diagnosis. The chief problem of diagnosis is to distinguish between primary polycythemia (vera) and secondary polycythemia, since the treatments are completely different. This is done by measuring your total blood volume with radioactive markers and making certain that you don't have kidney disease or a tumor that excretes *erythropoietin* (the hormone that stimulates red blood cell production by the bone marrow). Lung studies will also be performed to rule out a condition that causes carbon dioxide to be retained. Carbon dioxide is a strong stimulator of red cell production. Blood tests and microscopic examination of the bone marrow are also essential tests

Treatment. The first goal of treatment of polycythemia vera is to lower the number of circulating red blood cells. This is done by removing blood *(phlebotomy)*. In fact, this is the only medical condition for which bloodletting is therapeutic. Anticancer drugs and radioactive isotopes may also be given to depress the marrow production of all types of blood cells.

Prognosis. There is no cure for polycythemia vera, but with proper treatment, many patients live with few symptoms for 7–15 years after diagnosis. No matter what kind of treatment is given, the bone marrow eventually gives out, leading to myelofibrosis, in which the marrow is replaced by fibrous tissue and there is a decline in the production of all types of blood cells (*pancytopenia*). In some patients, leukemia may eventually develop. However, since this is primarily a disease of older persons (average age at onset is 60 years), most people die of other causes.

Multiple Myeloma

Multiple myeloma is a cancer of the *plasma cells*, a type of white blood cell responsible for producing the antibodies that destroy invading bacteria and foreign cells. Normally plasma cells make up only a small portion of the bone marrow cells. In multiple myeloma, however, a single plasma cell undergoes a malignant transformation and begins to multiply out of control. Eventually the bone marrow becomes riddled with masses (tumors) of plasma cells that not only replace the normal marrow cells, but destroy the surrounding bone as well.

Symptoms. Because of the replacement of normal marrow, anemia results from the lack of red cell production, bleeding can result from the lack of platelets (*see* Thrombocytopenia *above*), and infections result from the loss of granulocytes. The anemia causes weakness, fatigue, and pallor. Often the first sign of disease may be a bacterial infection, such as pneumococcal pneumonia. Bone pain may also be an early symptom, especially in the back and chest. The plasma cell tumors weaken the bone so that the vertebrae collapse and *pathologic* fractures develop. A pathologic fracture is one that occurs with no, or only trivial, trauma, and usually results from structural weakening of the bone, especially by tumors that invade bone.

Treatment. Anticancer drugs and corticosteroids are given to reduce the uncontrolled growth of plasma cell tumors. Localized radiation and analgesics are given to relieve bone pain. Antibiotics are administered as necessary to combat infection.

Every effort should be made to be up and out of bed in order to avoid contracting pneumonia. It is important also to drink plenty of water, because the plasma cells produce a protein that can cause the kidneys to fail if dehydration develops.

Prognosis. With proper treatment and a good response to anticancer drugs, substantial relief of symptoms can be achieved. The average life span after the onset of symptoms is 2–3 years. However, many people live much longer than this. The disease is characterized by periods of relief followed by relapses. In many cases, several different anticancer drugs can be administered when previously successful drugs no longer prove effective.

For more information, call the Cancer Information Service: 1-800-4-CANCER.

Aplastic Anemia

In true aplastic anemia, there is diminished production of all elements of the bone marrow: red cells, white cells, and platelets. However, there are also conditions that result in diminished production of only a single type of cell, e.g., decreased production of granulocytes is known as *agranulocytosis.*

There are many causes of bone marrow depression, including radiation, toxins, and drugs. Several antibiotics, for example, can cause aplastic anemia in certain individuals. Often the cause cannot be determined, in which case the aplastic anemia is said to be *idiopathic.*

Symptoms. There are three main groups of symptoms, each relating to decreased production of the main cell types of the marrow. Decreased production of red cells causes anemia with its associated weakness, fatigue, and pallor. Decreased production of white cells increases susceptibility to infection. Decreased production of platelets can lead to easy bruising and bleeding (*see* Thrombocytopenia).

Treatment. When a drug is thought to be responsible for aplastic anemia, withdrawal of that drug may resolve the problem completely. Anemia and bleeding are treated with appropriate transfusions. Infections are treated with antibiotics. In some cases bone marrow transplantation carries the best chance for a cure, especially in younger people. In older people, infusions of equine antithymocyte globulin or cyclosporine may help stimulate the depressed bone marrow.

Disorders of the Lymphatic System

The lymphatic system consists of the lymph vessels that are distributed throughout the body, often running parallel to blood vessels, and the numerous lymph glands, which are connected to the lymph vessels. The lymph glands produce lymphocytes, the white blood cells responsible for producing antibodies that help fight infection and for ridding the body of foreign substances. Lymph glands also fight infection by trapping bacteria, thus preventing their spread. This is why lymph glands often become swollen during an infection. The spleen is also a part of the lymphatic system, since it is actually a large lymph gland.

Lymphangitis and Lymphadenitis

Lymphangitis is an infection of the lymph vessels, usually caused by the streptococcus bacterium that infects a wound, cut, or abrasion. The symptoms include rapid development of fine red streaks extending upward from the site of infection on the hand or foot. Usually, these streaks continue up to the armpit or groin, and the lymph nodes in these areas become enlarged and tender *(lymphadenitis)*. Generalized symptoms may include fever, chills, headache, malaise, and loss of appetite. In severe cases, the bacterium may reach the bloodstream, giving rise to septicemia (*see* p. 210). If lymphadenitis is not treated, suppuration along the lymphatic path can occur, although this is rare.

Treatment. Prompt treatment with antibiotics, usually penicillin, brings lymphangitis under control within several hours. Supportive measures include rest, limited use of the affected limb, and plenty of fluids. The prevention of lymphangitis includes the prompt care of wounds, as outlined in the First Aid section of this book, and meticulous care of skin infections, as discussed on p. 448.

Lymphomas

Lymphomas are cancers of the lymphatic glands. The most common are Hodgkin's disease and non-Hodgkin's lymphoma. Rarer lymphomas include Burkitt's lymphoma and mycosis fungoides.

Hodgkin's Disease

This cancer is caused by a malignant transformation of one of the lymph gland cells that then grows out of control, spreading to the spleen and lymph glands throughout the body. It is a disease primarily of young adults, and the cause is unknown.

Symptoms. The chief symptom is persistent swelling of the lymph glands, particularly in the neck, groin, or armpit. As the disease spreads, fever, night sweats, weight loss, and intense itching occur. The fever is often a Pel-Ebstein fever, which is characterized by a few days of high fever regularly alternating with a few days or weeks of normal temperature. If the tumors invade bone, pain may develop in the involved bones, particularly the vertebrae. An unusual symptom may be a clue to the presence of Hodgkin's disease, namely the onset of pain immediately after drinking an alcoholic beverage. The diagnosis of Hodgkin's disease is made by biopsy of one of the involved lymph glands.

Treatment and Prognosis. If the disease is discovered at an early stage, radiation treatments cure the disease in 80–90% of cases. If the disease is found at more advanced stages, a combination of radiation and anticancer drugs is used, with complete eradication of the disease in more than half of all patients treated.

Non-Hodgkin's Lymphoma

This is similar to Hodgkin's disease, except that different cell types are responsible for the tumor growth, and it is not as easily cured.

Symptoms. Often the first sign of disease is swelling of lymph glands in the neck, armpits, or groin. Loss of appetite, malaise, fatigue, weight loss, and night sweats also occur. The diagnosis is made by biopsy of an involved lymph node.

Treatment and Prognosis. Both radiation and anticancer drugs are used to treat non-Hodgkin's lymphoma. Cure can be expected in about 50% of those with early disease. In more advanced disease, cure can be expected in about 20–25% of patients.

For more information about lymphomas, call the toll-free number of the Cancer Information Service at 1-800-4-CANCER.

Cross-section of the respiratory system

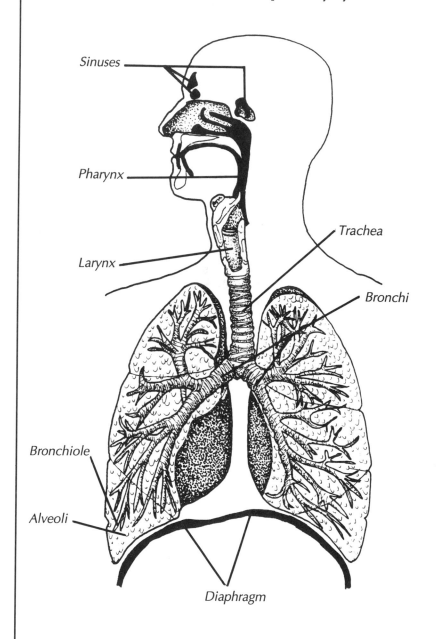

Sinuses

Pharynx

Larynx

Trachea

Bronchi

Bronchiole

Alveoli

Diaphragm

Your Respiratory System

The Common Cold, Influenza, and Allergies

The common cold produces a group of signs and symptoms that include a stuffy or runny nose, watery itchy eyes, and sneezing, all of which you normally also associate with flu and allergies. Often it is difficult to distinguish among them, except that colds and flu are often accompanied by fever, aching muscles, and *malaise* (a wonderful medical term for "feeling lousy"). Allergies, such as hay fever, on the other hand, are seldom accompanied by these flu-like symptoms. To help you make some sense of all of this and determine the most logical remedy for each problem, I will discuss in turn colds, flu, and common allergies.

Colds

That bane of all humankind, modern and ancient: the common cold. For relief of colds, the Romans recommended onions and water. In Colonial America cold sufferers were given a bewildering variety of herbal concoctions: bloodroot and buckthorn, cohosh and colts-foot, hyssop and yarrow, not to mention pennyroyal tea. Do they—or anything else—cure colds? The answer is no. Medical science still must confront that irksome taunt: "We can put a man on the moon, but you can't cure the common cold." This, however, doesn't mean that a great deal can't be done to ease a cold's miseries.

What Causes Colds?

In reality there is no such thing as the "common" cold. There are at least 200 different viruses that cause the symptoms we associate with a cold. Most of these are of a type known as rhinoviruses, which are chiefly responsible for summer and fall colds.

Because of the great variety of viruses, it is unlikely that a single vaccine could be developed to immunize us against all, or even most, of them. In fact, when several people in a group all contract colds, each is apt to be infected with a different virus!

How Do We "Catch" a Cold?

Under experimental conditions, spraying a rhinovirus directly into the noses of volunteers almost always produces a cold. The warm, humid environment inside your nose is an ideal culture site for these viruses. The natural transmission of colds has been debated. Some scientists believe that the hands are the principal means of contagion. It is likely that colds are often spread by handling a contaminated object and then touching your nose or eyes. Rubbing your eyes with contaminated hands can presumably give you a cold, because the tears containing the virus pass down the tear ducts directly into your nose. Coughing and sneezing can also transmit colds in tiny droplets through the air. Curiously, such oral contact as kissing is an inefficient means of transmission. Saliva appears to create an unfavorable environment for these viruses.

Avoiding Colds

Avoiding all contact with people having colds is effective in preventing them. This will pose few problems if you live in a monastery. But if you enjoy a robust social life, or if you are the parent of a young child, other measures are needed. Certainly you should avoid handling objects used by others who have a cold. Rhinoviruses can survive up to three hours outside the nose. Wash your hands regularly and avoid putting them to your face unless you have just washed them. Avoid using a handkerchief for your cold; use disposable tissues, and dispose of them so that they needn't be handled by others.

There is no good evidence, despite the widespread belief, that exposure to cold temperatures or getting your feet wet disposes you to a cold. Neither do sudden changes in the weather.

What about megadoses of vitamin C? Despite the recommendations of Nobelist Linus Pauling, no clinical study has ever shown vitamin C to prevent colds or to be of more than marginal value in reducing the severity of a cold once contracted. In the mammoth doses once recommended by Dr. Pauling (60,000 milligrams a day) vitamin C may give you diarrhea, and, because it is eliminated by the kidneys, is certain to result in expensive urine.

At this time there is no over-the-counter cold "preventive" that really prevents colds. In fact the Food and Drug Administration has ordered manufacturers to eliminate this claim from their advertisements unless it can be substantiated. Thus far none has been shown to be effective to the FDA's satisfaction.

Managing a Cold

You can treat most colds by yourself. There is little that a trip to the doctor can accomplish other than to enrich the doctor. Antibiotics, including penicillin, do nothing for the common cold and should not be taken unless a complication develops. (*See* Sore Throat, p. 247). Over-the-counter cold remedies usually lessen the symptoms of a cold, but do not reduce their duration. Here are some relief measures:

NASAL CONGESTION

Congestion in the nose, sinuses, and chest is caused by swollen blood vessels in the membranes of the nose and air passages. These blood vessels dilate in response to the release of histamine in the mucous membranes, which in turn are stimulated by nasal infection in the case of colds, or by allergens (e.g., pollen) in the case of an allergic attack. There are numerous decongestant preparations, both oral medications and nasal sprays, that are effective in relieving congestion. Typical oral decongestants include pseudoephedrine (Novafed, Sudafed), and phenylpropanolamine (Entex, Propagest). Nasal sprays contain phenylephrine (Neosynephrine).

Decongestants act by constricting blood vessels in the mucous lining of the nose, thus opening the nasal passages and making it easier to breathe. They also act to reduce nasal secretions, helping to dry a runny nose. After a few days use, nasal sprays can have a "rebound" effect, which *increases* swelling and makes it more difficult to breathe. You should limit the use of sprays that contain a decongestant to no more than three consecutive days.

Decongestants are chemically related to adrenalin, a natural decongestant, but also a stimulant. Their side effects include a jittery or nervous feeling, an inability to sleep, increased heart rate, and elevated blood pressure. If you suffer from an irregular heart rhythm, high blood pressure, heart disease, diabetes, glaucoma, or thyroid disease, you should take decongestants only on the advice of your doctor. Some men with swollen prostates experience difficulty urinating when taking decongestants (*see* Prostatic Enlargement, p. 380). Decongestants are often used in diet pills to curb appetite. If you are taking diet pills, don't add a decongestant.

ANTIHISTAMINES

These are included in many "cold" preparations, but are more effective against hay fever than colds. In fact they may act to thicken mucus, making it more difficult to cough up. In most people they cause drowsiness. Antihistamines are added to most over-the-counter cold preparations both for their drying properties and for their ability to counteract the stimulant effect of decongestants.

Some of the numerous combination antihistamine/decongestant preparations available include: Actifed, Chlor-Trimeton D, Contac, CoPyronil 2, Deconamine, Demazin, Dimetapp, Drixoral, Nolamine, Novafed A, Ornade, Sudafed Plus, and Triaminic.

In general, combinations should be avoided because then you usually end up taking one or more drugs for symptoms you don't have and risking unnecessary side effects. The most prudent approach to cold relief is choosing a drug specific to your symptom. To dry a runny nose, for example, you may try taking an antihistamine only at night when drowsiness is desirable and taking a decongestant alone during the day. Or you may take them together, increasing the antihistamine at night, while decreasing the decongestant dose, and doing the opposite during the day.

A relatively new antihistamine, terfenadine (sold under the trade name Seldane) has been reported to cause less drowsiness and to be just as effective as Chlor-Trimeton. It is expensive and requires a prescription, but may be worth trying. At this time two new nonsedative antihistamines, Hismanal and Claritin, are under review by the Food and Drug Administration. Ask your doctor about them.

Do not take antihistamines with alcoholic beverages because the combination increases drowsiness and decreases alertness and coordination. Avoid these drugs if you have asthma, glaucoma, emphysema, chronic pulmonary disease, shortness of breath, or difficulty urinating caused by an enlarged prostate, unless they are prescribed.

OTHER COLD SELF-TREATMENT MEASURES

If you prefer not to take pills and syrups, nasal congestion can be relieved by using saline nose drops (1/4 tsp of table salt in a glass of water) several times a day to clear your nasal passages.

Hot drinks, including the time-honored honey tea and chicken soup, help increase the flow of nasal secretions, probably because of the soothing effects of the inhaled vapors on your nose and throat.

Increasing the humidity in the air will make you feel better. Use a cold-mist vaporizer or humidifier, especially at night. *See box.*

Cough

Coughing is an important physiologic reflex that clears your air passages of excessive secretions and irritants. There are two types of cold-induced coughs—wet and dry—which should be treated differently. A wet, productive cough that clears your air passages should not be suppressed with anticough medicines, unless coughing inter-

---

HUMIDIFIERS

Humidifiers add moisture to dry air, which helps relieve nose and throat irritation and reduces the symptoms of colds, flu, and asthma. The best free-standing humidifiers are the ultrasonic variety that spray a fine, cool mist that stays suspended in the air without making the room damp. Never use hot steam vaporizers; they are dangerous, especially around children. If you have forced air heating, a humidifier can be attached directly to your heating unit. Follow the service directions carefully.

One problem with humidifiers is that they can serve as a growth medium for bacteria and fungus. People who are allergic to these microorganisms can be made worse, rather than better, by an infective mist blowing in their faces. To avoid this problem, change the water daily. Once a month clean the humidifier by adding a tablespoon of chlorine bleach to the water and running the humidifier for a few minutes. (Be sure to vent the slightly irritating fumes.) Then rinse the unit with plain water.

---

feres with sleep. Instead, try hot drinks (nonalcoholic), suck on hard candies, or inhale steam.

For a dry, unproductive cough, a cough suppressant can be tried. Cough suppressants inhibit the cough center in the brain. Most contain codeine or dextromethorphan. Codeine is a narcotic and is available only by prescription in most states. Dextromethorphan, a derivative of morphine, is just as effective as codeine, but it is not a narcotic. Cough syrups that contain a suppressant include among many others: Benylin, Congesperin, Pertussin 8 Hour, Romilar 8, and St. Joseph's Children's.

Cough suppressants should not be used for persistent or chronic coughs, such as those caused by smoking, asthma, and emphysema. In these conditions coughing is essential to clear the airways.

Cough syrups may also contain an *expectorant*, which is supposed to ease coughing by loosening secretions in the bronchial passages so that they may be more easily expelled. There is still controversy about whether expectorants really work, but probably they do no harm. The most widely used expectorant is guaifenesin.

Many cough syrups contain multiple ingredients, including a suppressant and/or an expectorant with a decongestant and/or anti-

---

WHEN TO SEE YOUR DOCTOR ABOUT YOUR COLD

You should see your doctor about your cold if:

1. You have a temperature over 100°F for more than two days.
2. You experience sudden pain or discharge from one or both ears.
3. You have general discomfort in your ears that lasts more than a few days.
4. Your runny or stuffy nose lasts more than 10 days.
5. Your cough produces a thick, foul-smelling yellow or greenish phlegm (caused by a bacterial infection).
6. You have a sore throat and pain with swallowing for longer than 48 hours (often a sign of strep throat, which should be treated with antibiotics).
7. You develop an unexplained skin rash (possibility of erysipelas caused by streptococcus bacteria).
8. You have a stiff neck, accompanied by a persistent headache (possibility of meningitis).
9. You have sinus pain, fever, and a yellow or greenish nasal discharge longer than 48 hours (possible sinusitis).

---

histamines. Most doctors do not recommend these combination preparations, (1) because many contain ingredients in doses that are less than effective, (2) because there is a greater chance of an unwanted side effect, and (3) because some contain drugs that may have competing effects.

Muscle Aches and Fever

Although muscle aches, headaches and fever are more characteristic of flu, they often develop in the early stages of colds as well. The use of a pain reliever, such as aspirin, acetaminophen (Tylenol or Panadol) or ibuprofen (Advil, Nuprin) can help you feel better. Remember that aspirin must not be given to children under 16 years of age because of the danger of causing Reye's Syndrome. Pregnant women should avoid both aspirin and ibuprofen.

About fevers, you should understand that the body's elevated temperature in response to bacterial and viral infections is a natural defense mechanism that is instrumental both in mobilizing the immune system to fight infection and to inhibit growth of the invading organisms. Many viruses, for example, cannot reproduce when the body temperature exceeds 100°F. Thus, there is no good physi-

---

WHEN TO CALL THE DOCTOR ABOUT YOUR CHILD'S COLD

Call your doctor when your child:
1. Develops a fever over 103°F.
2. Refuses to take liquids.
3. Becomes unusually irritable.
4. Is excessively sleepy.
5. Pulls at an ear.

---

ological reason to lower body temperature by means of drugs, unless it exceeds that level.

Drug Dosages for Children

The side effects of cold remedies can be much more severe in children. For example, decongestants may dry secretions to the extent that they actually block the nasal passages. In some children they act as a stimulant, making them more irritable. Indeed some children nearly go through the roof. Saline nose drops (1/4 tsp of table salt in 8 oz. warm water) are often effective in clearing the noses of young children who have difficulty breathing. Nose drops containing a diluted decongestant (1/8 of 1%) are appropriate for older children. Acetaminophen should be used only if a child complains of aches and pains or has a temperature above 100°F.

The expert panel established by the FDA to advise on the efficacy of over-the-counter cold remedies recommends:

- The dose for children 6 through 11 years old should be half the adult dose; for children 2 through 5 years old, it should be one quarter the adult dose. For infants up to 2 years of age, the panel recommends that the dosage be determined by your doctor.
- Asthma and cough preparations should not be given to children 2 through 5 years old in any amount except on the advice of your doctor.
- Any product with an alcohol content of more than 10 percent is not appropriate for children under age 6.

Colds vs Flu

Influenza is a contagious respiratory disease caused by a virus. There are three families of flu virus—A, B, and C. Types A and B are the most common. Within each family are several strains of virus; the strains of the A family generally cause more severe disease than those in B. About every 10 years, a flu strain develops that is different from other members of its family. When this occurs, there follows a world-wide epidemic because no one has immunity to this new strain. Such virus strains are named for the city in which outbreak is first reported, for example, Hong Kong flu or Moscow flu.

How do you know whether you have a cold or the flu? It may be difficult, but here are some differences:

Symptom	Cold	Flu
Fever	Low grade	Often high (102–104°F) Lasts 3–4 days
Headache	Mild	More severe
Muscle aches and pains	Mild	Common, often severe
Fatigue and weakness	Mild	Early and prominent
Nasal congestion	Common	Sometimes
Sneezing	Usual	Sometimes
Sore throat	Common	Sometimes
Cough	Mild to often severe, including moderate chest discomfort	

What Can Be Done for Flu Symptoms?

As with most viral infections, there is little to be done for flu other than get plenty of bed rest to avoid bacterial complications, particularly during the two to four days of fever. There is some evidence that the prescription drug, Symmetrel (amantadine), may be effective in treating influenza A when begun soon after the onset of the illness. Taken early, it can shorten the length and reduce the flu's severity, though there are some side effects, such as insomnia and nervousness, associated with the drug. Your doctor should decide whether amantadine is indicated for you.

For people with chronic illnesses, especially lung disease, antibiotics are often prescribed as prophylaxis against pneumonia. Should you develop a severe sore throat after flu symptoms have begun, consult your doctor to determine whether you need antibiotics to overcome or prevent a bacterial infection.

For congestion and cough, apply the same remedies as those used to treat colds (*see above*). Flu can often be prevented by vaccination. *See* p. 27 for specific indications of just when it may be warranted.

Allergies

Hay Fever *(Allergic Rhinitis)*

The term *hay fever* is actually a misnomer; it is neither caused by hay nor causes fever. It causes plenty of other symptoms, however, including nasal and sometimes chest congestion, running or itchy nose and eyes, sneezing, and often a chronic cough produced by post-nasal drip. All of these symptoms are rooted in allergy to airborne particles. In severe cases it can cause asthma, with audible wheezing and difficult breathing. Hay fever is often confused with a spring or summer cold. The absence of fever, headaches, and muscle aches are its usual distinguishing features.

What Causes Allergies?

An allergic reaction occurs when the body is invaded by a substance that is "recognized" by the immune system as foreign. In the case of hay fever, plant (e.g., pollen) and animal (e.g., dander, dust, etc.) substances enter the body through the membranes of the eyes, nose, or throat, setting off an immune reaction designed to counter the foreign "invader," which is known as an *allergen*. The immune system responds by producing an antibody known as immunoglobulin E (IgE), one of the many produced by the human body. When an individual who is thus sensitized encounters the allergen again, the antibodies combine with the allergen to initiate an "immune reaction." Ordinarily this is a beneficial and protective mechanism. However, in people who suffer from hay fever, the immune response is exaggerated, producing many unwanted symptoms.

There are several substances released into the bloodstream during an immune reaction, although histamine is the best known of these chemicals. Histamine causes dilation of the blood vessels in the eyes and the air passages. The results are itchy noses and eyes, tearing, watery nasal secretions, and sneezing. In asthmatics these substances cause the constriction of the air passages that leads to wheezing and labored breathing.

Early spring hay fever is usually caused by common tree pollens, such as those of elm, maple, willow, birch, beech, ash, oak, walnut, sycamore, and alder. Late spring and summer hay fever are more commonly caused by grasses (e.g., Bermuda, timothy, sweet vernal, orchard, and Johnson) and by weed pollens (e.g., sheep sorrel, English plantain). Fall hay fever is also caused mostly by weed pollens, and by ragweed in particular. Occasionally, seasonal hay fever is caused by airborne fungal spores. Most colorful and fragrant flowers have pollen that is too heavy to become airborne. Since such flowers rely on bees and other insects for pollination, these plants seldom cause allergy. Thus the term "rose fever," another name for hay fever, is also a misnomer.

Some people have year-round hay fever symptoms. Such allergies are most often caused by animal dander (cats, dogs, horses, wool, and feathers), cosmetics, molds, foods, and house dust. House dust is a complex mixture of fabric materials, molds, danders, and insect parts, especially those of dust mites, which are highly allergenic. People with dust allergy are usually worse in winter when indoor humidity falls.

What Can Be Done For Hay Fever?

GENERAL MEASURES

SEASONAL HAY FEVER

- Keep windows and doors closed during periods of heavy pollination. While driving, keep car windows closed.
- Change or clean air filters monthly in your heating and air conditioning system.
- Consider wearing a pollen mask when working outside. These are generally available at drugstores and paint shops.

YEAR-ROUND HAY FEVER

- Maintain your home as dust-free as possible.
- Use a humidifier in winter, but beware of possible mold growth in the humidifier (*see* p. 233).
- Change from feather pillows, woolen blankets, and woolen clothing to cotton or synthetic materials.
- Enclose your mattress and box springs in a plastic "barrier" cloth.
- Sleep with the head of your bed elevated (use multiple pillows or bricks under the bedposts) to minimize postnasal drip.
- If you become allergic to your pet (cats are highly allergenic), consider another animal; goldfish have never been known to cause allergies.

SPECIFIC MEASURES

1. *Antihistamines and decongestants* are the most frequently prescribed drugs for relief of the eye and nasal symptoms of hay fever. How-

ever, since decongestant nasal sprays like Neosynephrine and Afrin can become habit-forming, leading to a "rebound" phenomenon in which nasal congestion actually becomes worse, they probably should not be used for hay fever, or if used, never for more than three days.

2. *Corticosteroids.* When hay fever symptoms are severe, and are not adequately relieved by conservative measures, small doses of steroids are often very effective (e.g., 5 milligrams of prednisone taken every other day). Steroids must be prescribed and managed by your doctor, because their continued use can result in suppression of the normal functioning of your adrenal glands with serious consequences. The newer steroid nasal sprays (e.g., Vancenase, Beconase, Nasalide) often relieve allergies without risking the side effects of oral steroids.

3. *Cromolyn sodium.* This drug, administered as a nasal spray (under the brand name Nasalcrom) or as eye drops (under the brand name Opticrom), may also be effective when other measures fail. This is a drug used *to prevent* rather than to relieve, acute symptoms. It acts by blocking the reaction of allergens with tissue *mast cells*, which are responsible for releasing histamine and other substances that give rise to the symptoms of hay fever. They are more costly than other drugs and their effects are limited to the nose and eyes. Since they must also be started well before the hay fever season, relief may not become apparent for 2–4 weeks if symptoms have begun.

4. *Desensitizations.* Desensitization or 'immunotherapy' is frequently advised if you tolerate drugs poorly, if steroids must be administered to control your symptoms, or if asthma develops. In immunotherapy, the sensitizing allergen(s) are first identified by administering batteries of skin tests using a variety of allergen solutions that your history suggests are the likely causes of allergy. Alternatively, allergists may use the Radio-Allergo-Sorbent (RAST) test, which is a laboratory blood test that identies the specific allergens.

Once a diagnosis has been made, you will receive weekly injections of progressively more concentrated extracts of the allergens. The strength of the dose is increased until control of symptoms is achieved. This therapy requires several months to years and is usually begun after the end of your allergy season in anticipation of the next season. Often injections must be continued indefinitely.

The theory underlying immunotherapy is that the body responds to the injections by producing antibodies known as IgGs (immunoglobulin G). These in turn bind to the allergen before they can bind to the IgE that sets off the immune reaction described above. Nearly 80% of individuals allergic to pollens and dust achieve substantial relief, and about half of these are cured, i.e., their hay fever symptoms do not return when the shots are stopped. However, since a 50/50 chance is not very encouraging, many continue with the shots indefinitely. The success rate among those allergic to animal dander is even lower.

The field of immunotherapy is rapidly advancing. Several new developments that promise to increase the quantity of allergenic mixture administered and increase its specificity are now under development. New polymer substances that decrease the duration of treatment and have fewer side effects are being tested. Ask your doctor about these advances.

5. *Surgery.* In some cases surgical corrections are indicated, as in the case of nasal polyps, or a narrowed or deviated nasal septum. Such corrections can dramatically relieve breathing problems even though the allergy is unaffected.

Food Allergies

Unfortunate is the person who suffers from food allergies: the offending foods may be difficult to identify—and they change over time—the symptoms are often difficult to relate to the offending food—and they change over time!—the allergic condition is still very difficult to diagnose—and there is little that can be done short of avoidance even when the allergen is appropriately recognized.

Food allergies are common. In a recent study almost 50% of those who suffered from chronic allergic rhinitis tested positive for food allergies and suffered an aggravation of their symptoms when given those foods to eat.

What Foods Cause Reactions?

Any food can cause an allergic reaction in susceptible individuals; the commonest include milk, fish, shellfish, eggs, nuts, berries, chocolate, corn, wheat flour, legumes (green peas, soy beans, lima beans, peanuts), and such fresh fruits as peaches and citrus fruits. Some individuals react whenever they eat an allergenic food. Others have problems only during certain seasons when large quantities are consumed or when other allergies, such as hay fever, challenge the immune system. Some foods cause reactions only when taken with an alcoholic drink or on an empty stomach, presumably because they are then absorbed more rapidly. Thus you begin to understand how, in many people, the elements of the problem are murky indeed.

Unfortunately the variety of symptoms produced by food allergens is almost as lengthy as the list of allergy-causing foods. Migraine headaches, eczema, debilitating weakness, depression, diarrhea, abdominal pain, palpitations, sweating, dizziness, and fainting spells are but a few. No system in the body is proof against the affects of immune reactions. If the respiratory system is the principal target, symptoms include itching and runny nose, sneezing, stuffiness, and itchy, red, and watery eyes. Asthma manifested by coughing and wheezing may be dominant. If the intestinal tract is involved, symptoms include diarrhea, nausea or vomiting, and abdominal cramps (colic in infants). When the skin is involved, itching, hives (urticaria), and blotchy swelling (so-called 'angioedema') may develop. Eczema, a chronic skin disease found chiefly at the bends in the arms and legs, may be caused by food allergies.

Allergic reactions are of two types: immediate and delayed. The immediate type is usually sudden and dramatic, occurring within minutes of ingestion of the allergen. This kind of reaction is especially common in people allergic to such foods as nuts, eggs, and shellfish. The most serious of all allergic reactions, *anaphylaxis*, is of this type. Anaphylaxis is characterized by the explosive onset of itching, generalized flush, hives, respiratory distress, and vascular collapse (fainting, weak rapid pulse), and sometimes seizures and even death.

Delayed reactions to foods often occur several hours after eating and are more subtle, but may be just as varied as early reactions. It is thought that, in these cases, the allergen is not the whole protein found in the food, but rather a digestion product to which the individual is sensitive. Naturally, such allergies are difficult to identify correctly. Often allergic individuals are sensitive to several substances and their symptoms are frequently complex and bewildering. It is not surprising that some individuals have been labeled as neurotic or simply as "crocks."

The cause of immediate food reactions is usually obvious because of the short lapse of time between eating the food and suffering the consequences. Finding the cause of delayed allergic reactions is much more difficult and involves skin testing, laboratory tests (*see* Hay Fever Diagnosis *above*), and "elimination diets." In the latter, a food suspected of causing an allergy is eliminated from the diet for a week or two to see whether the symptoms disappear. Then the food is eaten in large amounts for some days to see whether the symptoms reappear. All such tests must of course be supervised by an allergist.

Treatment. Except for avoiding the offending foods, no specific treatment is yet available. Individuals who are severely allergic must carefully check packaging labels and consult restaurant personnel to make certain that a dish or product does not contain their "nemesis" food. Once a severe reaction has been experienced, it is prudent to have epinephrine (adrenalin) available at all times for use as prescribed by your doctor.

Hives usually disappear in 1–7 days. Treatment with an oral antihistamine, e.g., Benadryl (diphenhydramine, 50–100 mg four times daily), ordinarily relieves itching.

The development of severe asthma, choking (acute pharyngeal edema), and anaphylaxis are medical emergencies that require immediate medical attention. Get the victim (or yourself) to a doctor or hospital at once! One of the most common stories told of people who die of food allergies is that they delayed doing anything about their symptoms because they thought they would go away. In a recent study of those who had died of a food-induced allergic reaction (anaphylaxis) it was shown that victims most often:

- had taken alcohol, suggesting diminished alertness
- denied the severity of their symptoms
- relied on oral antihistamines alone
- were taking steroids for chronic asthma

These findings underscore the importance to food-allergic individuals who suffer an allergic attack of having the means to self-administer epinephrine (adrenalin).

Food Additives and Food Intolerance

Several substances added to foods to enhance their color, texture, or shelf life can cause systemic reactions that closely resemble allergies. For example, monosodium glutamate, often used to enhance food flavor, may produce flushing, anxiety, and pressure in the chest. This annoying reaction has been dubbed the "Chinese restaurant syndrome." The yellow dye, tartrazine, which is chemically similar to aspirin, often causes asthma in those who are sensitive to aspirin. Sulfite preservatives produce symptoms, in rare individuals, that resemble an acute allergic reaction, including itching, hives, nausea, diarrhea, dizziness, shortness of breath, asthma, and even death. Sulfites are found in numerous foods, wines, and drugs. Worse, their presence is often unlabeled. Until the Food and Drug Administration adopts a restrictive policy concerning sulfite use, sensitive subjects must use utmost caution to avoid innocent encounters with this deadly substance.

A food *intolerance* is an abnormal physical response to a food or additive that is not an immunologic reaction. A commonly cited example is milk (lactose) intolerance, manifested by cramps and diarrhea in people having a congenital absence of the enzyme *lactase* that is required to digest the lactose found in cow's milk. Similarly, lack of the enzyme that digests gluten, a protein found in wheat and rye, produces *celiac disease*, which resembles, but is quite distinct from, an allergy. Other food intolerance reactions may be caused by the natural drug-like chemicals contained in foods. Examples include the jitteriness caused by caffeine in coffee, tea, and many soft drinks. Natural amines found in chocolate and cheese may produce headaches in sensitive individuals. Here, too, avoidance is the only remedy.

For further information write to: Asthma and Allergy Foundation of America, 19 West 44th Street, New York, New York 10036; or to the American Lung Association, 1740 Broadway, New York, NY 10019, 1-212-315-8714.

Drug Allergy

Some drugs, such as penicillin, produce a true immunologic reaction. Most reactions, however, are caused by an unusual sensitivity to the drug. This is often called an *idiosyncrasy* to distinguish it from true allergic reactions. Examples include a ringing in the ears (tinnitus) associated with aspirin sensitivity. Such drugs as quinine, quinidine, sulfa drugs, and certain antibiotics and tranquilizers can produce severe anemia in doses that are well-tolerated by most recipients. Drug reactions vary widely and can seldom be anticipated. If, while taking any medication, you experience an unexplained symptom (headache, rash, palpitations, etc.), call your doctor to determine whether the symptom is expected, unrelated, or an idiosyncratic reaction that suggests the need to discontinue the drug.

Other Allergies

Insects

Several insects, including dust mites, fleas, and cockroaches, are known to cause hay fever symptoms or asthma. The mechanism of action is the inhalation of insect feces, eggs, or body parts contained in house dust. The sensitizing insect is identified by skin testing. Elimination of the insects is the best remedy. In the case of dust mites, however, this is nearly impossible. Since the mites live largely in pillows and mattresses, plastic covers can provide a partial barrier that may reduce symptoms. (*See* Hay Fever, p. 237).

The stings of a group of insects known as Hymenoptera may evoke unusually severe allergic reactions. Hymenoptera include bees, wasps, hornets, fire ants, and harvester ants. Reactions to these stings vary from simple discomfort to acute allergic reactions. Several deaths caused by insect stings are recorded each year. Sensitive individuals should undergo desensitization by an allergist. Your doctor may also recommend a kit containing adrenalin (epinephrine) for subcutaneous injection, a measure that can be life-saving in severely allergic people. For milder symptoms, such as hives and abdominal cramps, an oral antihistamine (e.g., Chlor-Trimeton) at double the usual dose may be effective in relieving symptoms. Whenever you are in serious difficulty and doubt, treat yourself with adrenalin or seek emergency medical care.

If, after being stung, the insect's stinger and venom sac are still attached to your skin, the venom sac should be carefully removed with your fingernail or a penknife, taking care not to compress the sac and thus inject yourself with more venom. Absorption of venom may be slowed by placing ice on the sting site or by applying a tourniquet if the sting is on the arm or leg. The tourniquet must be released for a minute every 15 minutes to maintain circulation to the limb. If you know yourself to be allergic, it is prudent to go to a doctor or hospital and remain there for an hour or so. If no reaction occurs, it is then safe to leave.

Toxic reactions may occur following multiple stings. As with snake bite, a sufficient quantity of injected venom will produce a poisoning effect, and prompt hospitalization is required.

People sensitive to insect stings generally know not to go barefoot in the park. Other rules of avoidance can be obtained from the Asthma and Allergy Foundation of America at the above address.

Heat, Light, Cold

Among the most baffling of all allergies are the *physical* allergies. Exposure to cold may induce rashes and angioedema (*see above*) and may even cause systemic reactions and shock. Sensitivity to sunlight most commonly results in a rash. All of these agents may aggravate asthma. The mechanism responsible for the allergic response is thought to be an alteration of your blood serum proteins, which then react with IgE immunoglobulins, setting off the immune reaction. Avoidance of known triggering stimuli is the only effective prevention. Otherwise, your symptoms should be treated much as are other immune reactions described above.

So-called "photic sneezing" may be an example of a physical allergy. Certain individuals, upon entering direct sunlight, respond by a series of sneezes. There appears to be a familial pattern to this phenomenon. In one case study, a man would sneeze twice upon entering sunlight. The father, a brother, and even a 6-month-old daughter also exhibited this behavior, each sneezing exactly twice.

The Nose and Sinuses

Loss of Smell

Loss of the sense of smell *(anosmia)* is a distressing symptom that can greatly diminish your pleasure in life. Many people lose all interest in food, for example. The causes of anosmia are complex and require careful examination by an otolaryngologist. In young people, head trauma and nasal obstruction are the most common causes. In older individuals, malnutrition, especially deficiencies of niacin, vitamin B_{12} and zinc are associated with loss of smell. Often a severe viral infection precipitates the symptom. About 10% of individuals who lose their sense of smell are found to have cancer, which emphasizes the importance of a careful examination by your doctor.

Unless a specific cause for diminished smell can be found, hopes for treatment are not encouraging. Increasing the variety of textures in your food may help. If there is some sense of smell (hyposmia), the flavor of foods can be amplified with commercially available odors.

Trauma to the Nose

Fractures

The nose is the most commonly fractured facial bone. It can be suspected whenever a blow to the nose results in bleeding. It is easily recognized if the nose is deviated, unstable, or makes a grating sound when moved.

A doctor should pack and splint a broken nose to ensure proper healing. A blood clot (hematoma) inside the nasal septum is a medical emergency and must be quickly incised and drained. Difficulty in breathing after a nasal fracture is common and may require surgical treatment.

Nosebleeds (Epistaxis)

Nosebleeds are common in children and most often result from trauma, especially from picking the nose or blowing it too hard. Frequently, nosebleeds occur spontaneously, especially during the cold weather months. They are usually caused by the erosion of blood vessels exposed to dry air. The site of bleeding is generally a small group of blood vessels in the nasal septum. Bleeding can be stopped by pinching your nose between your thumb and forefinger for 5–10 minutes. If this fails, try stuffing your nose, on the side of bleeding, with cotton that has been smeared with vaseline. If this fails, your doctor may have to cauterize your nose or investigate for more subtle causes of bleeding. There are a host of bleeding disorders known as *coagulopathies* that may underlie serious nosebleeds.

Sinusitis, Postnasal Drip, and Sinus Headache

The sinuses are air-filled spaces within the bones of your face that are extensions of the nasal air passages. They are lined with mucous membranes that continuously produce secretions needed to cleanse these airways. Normally these secretions are being constantly swept to the back of your throat and swallowed without you being aware of their presence. But when the sinuses become infected as a complication of colds, flu, or hay fever, you can readily become aware of them.

Postnasal Drip

When your nasal passages become irritated by allergies, air pollutants, colds, and the like, your sinus secretions increase to the point that you become aware of having to clear your throat frequently to handle the increased volume. They may also cause a persistent cough, especially when you lie down. If the air is dry, the secretions may become thick and sticky.

SIMPLE REMEDIES FOR POSTNASAL DRIP

1. Oral antihistamines and nasal spray decongestants (*see* p. 238) are usually effective in drying runny secretions. If the secretions become thick and sticky, however, they may be difficult to clear; antihistamines should then be avoided.
2. Use a humidifier when you have a cold, and sleep with the head of your bed elevated. These measures promote sinus drainage.
3. Avoid air pollutants, especially tobacco smoke.
4. If secretions become greenish or foul-smelling, you probably have an infection and should consult your doctor.

Sinus Headache

A headache in your face, cheeks, forehead, or around your eyes associated with a cold or nasal congestion, and often described as "splitting," is probably a *sinus headache*. They are caused by pressure from an infection in, or blockage of, one or more of the eight sinuses. Usually the pain is relieved by a decongestant and an analgesic, such as aspirin or acetaminophen. A decongestant spray is the most effective therapy (e.g., 0.25% phenylephrine every 3 hours). Oral decongestants are generally less effective. Remember that nasal sprays should not be used longer than 3 days. Antibiotics are required if the nasal secretions become greenish or foul-smelling, or if the headache fails to respond to conservative measures.

The Throat

Pharyngitis *(Sore Throat)*

Nearly one out of every 10 Americans develops a "strep throat" *(pharyngitis)* every year and 40 million adults will see a doctor for it at some time or another. But there are several causes of sore throat, most of which you don't need to see your doctor about.

Viral Sore Throat

Literally hundreds of viruses can cause the "flu" or the "common cold" and these are frequently accompanied by sore throat. When you get a stuffy or runny nose, sneezing, and generalized aches and pains accompanied by a sore throat, it is probably caused by a virus, especially if your fever measures less than 101°F. These infections are highly contagious and often several members of a household or community will exhibit the same symptoms. They heal themselves as the immune system begins to make antibodies against the virus.

Bacterial Sore Throat

The most common bacterial infection in the throat is caused by a particular strain of the streptococcus bacterium, giving rise to "strep throat." It is often accompanied by fever, a "beefy" red throat, as well as muscle aches and pains, fever, and swollen neck glands. This type of infection should be treated with antibiotics because it is associated with several serious complications, including damage to the heart valves and kidneys, tonsillitis, pneumonia, sinusitis, and ear infections. Throat cultures must usually be taken by your doctor because strep throat is not always obvious by examination alone. Because of

---

SELF-TREATMENT OF A MILD SORE THROAT

- Increase nonalcoholic fluid intake: warm tea with honey is soothing.
- Use a humidifier in your bedroom (*see* p. 233).
- Gargle with warm salt water (1/4 tsp salt to 1/2 cup water).
- Nonprescription throat lozenges are relieving.
- Take a mild analgesic, such as acetaminophen or aspirin for adults.

---

the highly contagious nature of streptococcus, some doctors treat all members of the family if one develops a strep throat.

Other Causes of Sore Throat

Sore throats are often associated with hay fever because the same pollens and allergens that affect the nose and eyes also irritate the throat. Mouth-breathing dries the throat, causing irritation. If you tend to breath through your mouth, you may have a nasal obstruction and you should see your doctor. Other irritants that may cause sore throat include smog, tobacco, and excessive strain on the voice (from singing, yelling, or reading out loud for a long time).

An occasional cause of morning sore throat is reflux of stomach acids up the esophagus and into the back of the throat. *See* p. 279 for a discussion of *reflux esophagitis*.

WHEN SHOULD YOU SEE YOUR DOCTOR FOR A SORE THROAT?

When a sore throat is severe, lasts longer than 5–7 days, and is not associated with an allergy or irritation, you should see your doctor. Any of the following signs and symptoms should alert you to the need for medical attention:

- Severe and prolonged sore throat
- Difficulty breathing
- Difficulty swallowing
- Joint pains
- Earache
- Rash
- Fever over 101°F
- Blood in your phlegm
- Frequently recurring sore throat
- Lump in the neck
- Hoarseness lasting more than two weeks

Tonsillitis

The tonsils and adenoids are small masses of lymph glands that lie in the back of the throat. They serve to trap bacteria and viruses. In becoming infected themselves, they form antibodies that then protect the rest of your body from subsequent invasion. However, the need for this protective function is over by age three. From then on, tonsils and adenoids serve little known function. And in some people they can be a source of recurrent sore throat and even interfere with breathing and swallowing. The symptoms of *tonsillitis* are thus similar to those of a flu: fever, headache, muscle aches, sore throat, chills, and fever.

Treatment. If you develop tonsillitis, your doctor will likely prescribe an antibiotic and an analgesic such as acetaminophen. In times past, removal—tonsillectomy and adenoidectomy—was often carried out to prevent later complications, such as ear infections, rheumatic fever, and repeated bouts of tonsillitis. However, it is now believed that such complications are relatively infrequent, and that the tonsils and adenoids may have other functions, such as the control of allergies. Complications of the surgery itself (bleeding and anesthetic deaths) limit the indications for removal to a relatively few conditions. Everyone agrees that interference with breathing and swallowing are sound indications for removal. Others advocate removal in children with two or three strep throats in a year for 2–3 years, but opinion varies. See your doctor for advice about the following signs and symptoms: recurrent sore throats, recurrent ear infections, mouth breathing, snoring, and sleep disturbances.

Laryngitis

Laryngitis, inflammation of the larynx (voice box) may be of viral, bacterial, or traumatic origin. Viral laryngitis is the most common. Hoarseness and unnatural voice changes, usually associated with a continual urge to clear your throat, are the most prominent symptoms. In severe viral and many cases of bacterial laryngitis, fever and muscle aches may also be present.

There is no specific treatment for viral laryngitis. Conservative measures include mild analgesics for pain if any exists (aspirin or acetaminophen), use of a humidifier in case of dry air, and resting your voice. If the laryngitis is severe, a culture should be obtained and antibiotics administered when medically important bacteria are identified.

Mechanical or traumatic laryngitis results from straining your voice. It is common among singers and others who develop hoarseness from vocal overuse. Rest your voice, avoid talking over background noise, and avoid changing your voice's pitch. If hoarseness persists more than a week or two, see your doctor to rule out the possibility of vocal cord polyps or vocal cord paralysis.

The most dangerous throat infection is called *acute epiglottitis*. This is a bacterial infection of the larynx. The swelling may close off the airway, especially in children, constituting a real emergency. When someone with a sore throat has difficulty swallowing or breathing, get them to the doctor or to an emergency room at once.

Hiccups

Hiccups occur from sudden, involuntary contractions of the diaphragm against a closed glottis, the upper opening of the voice box. Why hiccups occur is unknown, because—unlike such other spasmodic reflexes as coughing, sneezing, and gagging—hiccups have no known utility. In most people, they last from a few minutes to an hour or so. They are usually associated with overeating, eating too rapidly, and of course, drinking too much. The classic movie drunk always has hiccups.

Folk medicine is replete with hiccup remedies, and chances are your favorite is as good as any.

- You may sip water slowly, or if that fails, gulp it down.
- Try holding your tongue and pulling it forward.
- Put ice chips in your mouth.
- Bartenders recommend eating a lemon wedge saturated with Angostura bitters.
- Tickle the back of your throat.
- Have a friend slap your back.
- A physiologically sound remedy is to breathe for a few minutes in a paper (not plastic!) bag or hold your breath for 30 seconds. This raises the carbon dioxide level in your body and stimulates the phrenic nerve supplying your diaphragm.
- If you have an acid stomach, take two antacid tablets.

Hiccups that last longer than a day or two often have more serious causes. They are associated with pneumonia, kidney failure, ulcers, epilepsy, or brain tumors. They can be extremely fatiguing because they interfere with eating and sleeping. Naturally, you should see your doctor for prolonged hiccups. The *Guinness Book of World Records* claims that the record duration for hiccups, 60 years, is held by an Iowa man. His primary complaint was that his false teeth kept falling out. Finally, relief was attributed to prayers to St. Jude, the patron saint of lost causes.

Speech Problems

Speech and language disorders greatly affect the way we talk and understand. After all, the ability to communicate is one of our most human characteristics. Fluid communication is essential to learning, working, and all social interactions. Among the causes of speech and language disorders are: hearing loss, cerebral palsy and other neuromuscular disorders, head injury, stroke, viral diseases, mental retardation, drugs, physical impairments such as cleft palate, and inadequate speech models. Frequently the cause is genetic or is unknown. However, most speech and language problems can be overcome or greatly improved.

STUTTERING

There is a widespread misconception that stuttering results from tense, neurotic, or overweening parenting. This misconception often leads to parental guilt that their child's speech problem is their fault. Numerous studies, especially studies of stuttering among twins, suggests that stuttering is largely, if not entirely, genetically determined. Stutterers and their parents are no more neurotic than nonstutterers, nor does stuttering result from some misguided child-rearing practice. Neither are children who stutter more anxious than nonstutterers.

Stuttering is common; almost 5% of Americans develop a stuttering problem at some time in their lives. Syllable repetitions, especially on the first words of sentences, are the most frequent speech problems. Sound prolongations and tense pauses also occur.

Stuttering most often begins between ages 3 and 5. The incidence decreases until puberty, after which the onset of stuttering is rare. Some children stop stuttering after a few months with no treatment at all. In about 1% of individuals, the disorder becomes chronic, and signs such as avoidance and withdrawal indicate the need for professional care. As occurs with many developmental problems that begin during childhood, boys are affected more often than girls, and this sex ratio increases with age. The risk of stuttering among the close relatives of stutterers is more than three times that of the general population. If one identical twin stutters, there is a greater than 50% chance that the other twin will stutter.

Environmental factors do play a part in stuttering, but they are not related to parental interactions. For example, the most common cause of adult-onset stuttering is head injury or stroke. Children with brain injury are also more prone to stutter.

Several comparative studies have shown that intensive training in fluent speech skills can produce considerable improvement. In most cases, stutterers who have continued to work on maintaining fluency will stutter only rarely after two years of therapy and will no longer be handicapped by the problem. If your pediatrician cannot recommend a speech-language pathologist, contact the National Association for Hearing and Speech Action, Dept SLD, 10801 Rockville Pike, Rockville, MD, 20852, or telephone 1-800-639-8255.

Other Speech Problems

Voice disorders are characterized by inappropriate pitch (too high, too low, unmodulated) loudness, or quality (harsh, hoarse, breathy, nasal).

Articulation disorders fall mainly into one of three categories: omissions, substitutions, or distortions. Examples of omission are the use of "and" in place of "hand," or "at" for "hat."

Examples of substitution are the use of "th" for "s" and in "thun" in place of "sun," and "w" for "r" as in "wabbit." Such speech errors are usually corrected by the parents' serving as gentle and consistent role models. Of course if the parents say "at" in place of "that," so likely will the child (regional accents are not articulation problems unless they interfere with work or social integration).

Distortion occurs when, for example, a sound is said inaccurately, but approximates the intended sound: "bood" in place of "bird."

Most articulation problems clear spontaneously. Children should make all of the sounds of English by 8 years of age. Correct pronunciation of "p," "m," and "b" usually precede correct pronunciations of "s," "l," and "r." Persistent articulation problems can almost always be corrected by speech-language instruction. See the above address for professionals in your area.

Disorders of the Lungs

The lungs consist of a sequence of air passages starting with the large trachea (windpipe), which divides into the left and right main bronchi, and then into ever smaller air passages called bronchioles. Each bronchiole ends in a cluster of small air sacs called alveoli that are surrounded by a network of capillaries stemming from the pulmonary arteries. It is here that the venous blood from the body gives up its load of carbon dioxide and takes on a fresh supply of oxygen from the lungs.

Most disorders of the lungs arise from damage caused by breathing contaminated air, whether that contamination is from bacteria and viruses (pneumonia, bronchitis) or from chemical irritants (asthma, emphysema, lung cancer, and so on).

Acute Bronchitis

Bronchitis is an inflammation of the mucous membranes lining the lower respiratory passages, namely the bronchi and smaller bronchioles. This condition usually begins as a cold or flu (*see* p. 229) and spreads downward. Inflammation increases the production of mucus in the respiratory passages. Ciliary action sweeps the mucus upward through the trachea to the throat, triggering the cough reflex that brings the material up as a grayish or yellow phlegm. All of the symptoms of a cold or flu may be present before and during the stage of bronchitis. Burning and tightness in the chest is common as is wheezing.

Treatment. The treatment of cold and flu symptoms has been discussed on p. 230. For comfort you may also want to take a cough preparation, such as Robitussin. Use a vaporizer or humidifier to help loosen secretions. Drink plenty of water to loosen secretions and decrease the coughing effort necessary to bring them up. Call your doctor if your temperature goes above 101°F, if you cough up blood, or if your condition does not improve in a few days.

Chronic Bronchitis

Chronic bronchitis is a productive cough that fails to improve or that recurs many times, often leading to thickening and distortion of the mucous membranes of the bronchi and bronchioles. A chronic cough is much more likely to develop if you smoke or if you live in a contaminated atmosphere for prolonged periods. As time goes on, your cough worsens, and you may begin to wheeze.

Treatment. If you smoke, of course, you must stop; smoking is the single most common cause of chronic bronchitis. If you work or live in a polluted atmosphere, try to move to a cleaner, drier climate. Stay away from people with colds because your bronchitis only worsens when you develop a respiratory infection. Your doctor will most likely prescribe antibiotics to control infection and bronchodilating medications to ease the effort of breathing.

Asthma

Asthma is an often devastating condition that affects millions of individuals. The most common cause of asthma, especially in children and young adults, is an allergy to such allergens as pollen, dander, dust, foods, food additives, and so on. (*See* p. 237 for a general discussion of allergies.) In asthma the target organ is the lower respiratory passages, which respond by becoming inflamed, constricted, and producing excessive mucus. All of these factors obstruct air flow, causing wheezing and labored breathing. In severe cases, breathing may be so difficult that all other activity must be suspended just to have enough energy to breath.

Asthma is sometimes triggered by respiratory infections and may be associated with nasal polyps, but the symptoms remain the same. In some people strenuous exercise or emotional upset may induce an asthmatic attack. Asthma can begin at any age and its course is highly variable. Many children grow out of their asthma attacks, whereas others continue to have attacks for life.

Treatment. Research now shows that, besides constricting the lung's airways, lung inflammation plays a major role in producing the symptoms of asthma. For this reason, it is currently recommended that everyone with any but the mildest forms of asthma use anti-inflammatory drugs to prevent, as well as to treat, their asthma.

For most asthma victims, this means using one of the two major types of anti-inflammatory drugs, both of which are delivered via inhalers. The first type are the cortisone-like steroid medicines such as Decadron, Vanceril, Beclovent, Azmacort, and Aerobid. The second type is an anti-inflammation drug called cromolyn (Intal).

Another new concept in managing asthma is the frequent use of lung function tests to measure air flow capacity. This includes self-administered tests using simple devices known as *peak flow meters.* These meters measure air flow and allow you to monitor your breathing capacity from day to day. You simply take a deep breath and blow out forcefully into one of the devices. A small gage measures how fast your lungs are emptied. The results can then be compared with standards for someone of your age, height, and sex. Peak flow meters are for asthmatics what blood pressure cuffs are for hypertensives. They allow you to monitor directly how well your disease is controlled at any particular time.

Anti-inflammatory drugs are meant both to prevent asthma attacks and to keep them under control. In the event of an acute attack, however, more potent drugs, including steroid pills and bronchodilators—inhalers or pills—are needed to open up constructed air passages. The most frequently used bronchodilators, known as beta-2 adrenergic agents, are usually delivered by inhalers. These drugs include albuterol (Ventolin, Proventil) and metaproterenol (Alupent, Metaprel). These drugs act like adrenaline to relax bronchial muscles and expand the diameter of the airways. Unlike adrenaline, however, they do not raise your blood pressure nor increase your heart rate. Theophylline, a potent drug that relaxes bronchial smooth muscles, is usually given intravenously for acute attacks. Epinephrine can also be used in acute attacks to open constricted bronchi.

During an acute attack, the most comfortable position for breathing is sitting up and leaning forward with support for the elbows. If the usually prescribed remedies do not work quickly, call your doctor at once. Avoid taking more than the recommended dose of an inhaled bronchodilator since overuse may be dangerous.

Between attacks of asthma, the foundation of asthma prevention rests upon avoidance of allergens. (*See* p. 237 for a discussion of allergies.)

For more information, call the National Asthma Education Program of the National Institutes of Health, 1-301-951-3260; or write to: The Asthma and Allergy Foundation of America, 19 West 44th St., New York, NY 10036.

For a booklet of exercises *Breathing Easy*, write to: Asthmatic Children's Foundation, Box 568 Spring Valley Rd., Ossining, NY 10562.

For a booklet, *Your Child and Asthma*, write to The National Jewish Center for Immunology and Respiratory Medicine, 1400 Jackson St., Denver, CO 80206, 1-800-222-LUNG.

Excellent books include: *Asthma* by Allan M. Weinstein, MD, McGraw-Hill Book Co., 1987, and *Asthma: Stop Suffering, Start Living*, (Addison-Wesley, Boston, 1989), and *Living Allergy Free: How to Create and Maintain an Allergen- and Irritant-Free Environment*, Humana Press, 1992, both by M. Eric Gershwin, MD, and Edwin L. Klingelhofer.

Emphysema

Emphysema is almost always associated with chronic bronchitis, and the two conditions are known as chronic obstructive pulmonary disease, COPD. Bronchitis narrows the respiratory passages through thickened bronchial walls and excess mucus that plugs the respiratory passages. This, in turn, makes it difficult to expire air because of the increased resistance to air flow. Lung secretions cannot be cleared and this causes an inpouring of white blood cells. These cells release destructive enzymes that ultimately cause the alveoli to rupture. As the alveoli are damaged, the exchange of oxygen and carbon dioxide across the alveolar capillary membranes becomes less efficient.

The main symptoms of emphysema are shortness of breath, cough, and wheezing. In advanced cases the chest assumes a barrel-like shape as the lungs become overinflated. Even minor respiratory infections may be slow to clear up and greatly worsen the symptoms of emphysema. Many patients must sleep in a semi-sitting position because breathlessness (dyspnea) prevents them from lying down. In severe emphysema the skin and lips may take on a bluish appearance (cyanosis) because of the lack of sufficient oxygenated blood to maintain a pink complexion.

As emphysema progresses, other body systems become affected. The heart may enlarge because decreased blood oxygen constricts blood vessels within the lungs, requiring greater heart exertion to pump blood through the lungs. This condition is known as *cor pulmonale*. It is usually manifested as a type of heart failure (*see* p. 197) with swelling of the feet and increased fatigability as the earliest symptoms. Later, cardiac irregularity, distention of the veins in the neck, and even cyanosis (blue skin) may develop.

The number of red blood cells may increase (*polycythemia*). Reduced blood flow to the brain may lead to headaches, insomnia, confusion, and irritability. In severe emphysema, there is also increased risk of pneumothorax, a collapse of the lungs caused by their rupture, with air entering the pleural space between the lungs and the chest wall.

Treatment. Emphysema is treated by a variety of drugs and procedures aimed at increasing ventilation and ridding the lungs of excess secretions. Drugs include bronchodilators, antibiotics, corticosteroids (to control wheezing), and expectorants. In addition, your doctor may instruct you how to get rid of lung fluids by postural exercises and controlled coughing. If you suffer a chronic lack of oxygen in your blood, long-term oxygen administration may be required.

MANAGING YOUR EMPHYSEMA

- *Stop smoking.* Smoking is the single biggest factor in increasing the severity of emphysema. This includes pipes, cigars, and marijuana, all of which are dangerous.
- *Avoid atmospheric pollution.* Avoid the "secondary" smoke from other smokers. Consider moving to a cleaner, drier climate if you live in a city with high humidity and air pollution. Avoid excessive heat, cold, or very high altitudes. Even the pressure in some commercial airlines is low enough to cause discomfort in severe emphysema.
- *Avoid contact with those suffering respiratory infections.*
- *Stay well-hydrated* by drinking lots of water. This helps keep phlegm loose so that coughing will bring it up more easily.
- *Maintain a nutritious, high protein diet.*
- *Read more on the topics above,* if you suffer asthma or allergies.

Pneumonia

Pneumonia, or pneumonitis as it is sometimes called, is not a specific disease, but rather a general term for several types of inflammation of the lungs. It can be caused by many different bacteria, including pneumococcus, tuberculosis, and legionella, which is responsible for Legionnaire's disease. Pneumonia may be caused by a fungus, such as histoplasmosis, or by protozoa, such as *Pneumocystis carinii*, responsible for pneumocystis pneumonia so common in patients with AIDS. It can be caused by several viruses and even by toxic substances that cause chemical damage to the lungs when inhaled, e.g., chlorine and mustard gas. The lung inflammation that results from smoke inhalation is a type of chemical pneumonia.

The variability of pneumonia has led to several popular and medical descriptive terms. *Bronchopneumonia* refers to a distribution of inflammation within the lungs that is patchy and irregular. *Lobar pneumonia* means that an entire lobe of the lungs is inflamed. The left lung has two lobes; the right lung has three. If you are told that you have "double" pneumonia, it simply means that both lungs are involved.

The symptoms of pneumonia vary with the cause of the inflammation, but the most common symptoms include chills and fever, cough and lethargy. In severe cases, shortness of breath, bloodstained sputum, headache, and chest pain may develop.

The diagnosis of pneumonia is usually easy. Your doctor will listen to your lungs through a stethoscope and tap your chest to search for areas in the lung with absent air. Chest X-rays, blood tests, and sputum examinations may also be ordered.

Treatment. Again, the treatment depends upon the cause. Bacterial pneumonias are treated by appropriate antibiotics, determined by sputum cultures. Viral pneumonias, on the other hand, do not respond to antibiotics and are treated by general supportive measures to alleviate cough, fever, pain, and shortness of breath.

Pneumonia is often treated in the hospital because of serious complications that can develop. Pneumonia is the sixth leading cause of death in the United States. It especially attacks and is fatal to the elderly and those who are disabled by chronic diseases.

Complications of Pneumonia

The following are some of the complications of pneumonia, although they may result from other causes as well.

1. *Lung abscess.* An abscess is a walled-off area of infection filled with pus. Lung abscesses are relatively rare, because antibiotics are generally effective in arresting the disease before they develop, but if treatment is delayed or you are debilitated, an abscess may form. The symptoms are chills, fever, productive cough, and occasionally bloody sputum. A chest X-ray is generally necessary to locate the abscess. Lung abscesses can often be treated with antibiotics alone, although surgical drainage may be required.
2. *Empyema.* This term means an accumulation of pus in the pleural cavity, the narrow space between the lungs and the chest wall. Antibiotics and drainage through a needle or tube are usually effective treatments.
3. *Bronchiectasis.* This is a chronic condition resulting from repeated lung infections occurring over many years. The bronchi become enlarged and filled with secretions, resulting in chronic productive cough and debilitation. The most common cause of bronchiectasis is cystic fibrosis (*see* p. 262). The treatment of bronchiectasis is similar to that of emphysema (*see above*).
4. *Pleural effusion.* This is similar to empyema, only the fluid in the pleural cavity is clear serum, not pus. The usual cause is an irritation of the pleura, the membrane lining the chest cavity. Tumors also cause pleural effusion.
5. *Pleurisy.* Pleurisy is a sharp, lancinating chest pain usually made worse by breathing. The usual cause is an inflammation of the

pleura, caused by infection, trauma, or occasionally pneumothorax (air in the pleural cavity). There may also be a degree of pleural effusion associated with the inflammation. The pain subsides when the underlying cause of the inflammation is corrected.

Special Types of Pneumonia

TUBERCULOSIS

Until recently, cases of tuberculosis (TB) have been rare in the United States. The increased susceptibility of AIDS victims to *Mycobacterium tuberculosis*, the causative organism, is greatly increasing the incidence of this disease. Worldwide, it is still an important cause of death, taking more than 3 million lives each year. It is an especial threat to the elderly, the poor, alcoholics who are malnourished, and such immune-compromised individuals as those with chronic debilitating diseases and those on long-term steroid medications.

Tuberculosis is a contagious lung disease that is spread by close contact with infected persons' sputum or droplets from coughing. Though the disease chiefly affects the lungs, it may spread to other organs, mainly the bones and kidneys.

The earliest symptoms are cough, more pronounced in the morning, caused by material accumulated in the respiratory tract overnight. Night sweats are common. In later stages, bloody sputum, shortness of breath, and chest pain may occur. The diagnosis is suspected on the basis of chest X-ray findings and confirmed by microscopic demonstration of *acid-fast rods* in the sputum and by sputum culture.

Pulmonary tuberculosis requires prolonged treatment with multiple antibiotics. In severe cases, 4 drugs are advisable. These include INH, rifampin, streptomycin, and ethambutol. Recently, *M. tuberculosis* strains resistant to many of these antibiotics have developed, so that careful drug sensitivity testing is essential. Often several months of treatment are required.

HISTOPLASMOSIS

Histoplasmosis is caused by the fungus, *Histoplasma capsulatum*, which is prevalent in the Mississippi, Ohio, and Missouri river valleys. The fungus flourishes in regions where the soil is contaminated with bird, chicken, and bat droppings. The spores from the mature fungus become airborne, from whence they are inhaled to produce pneumonia-like symptoms. In most cases it is a mild disease characterized by headaches, cough, chills, and fever, and is often mistaken for viral pneumonia unless your doctor requests a sputum culture. The disease is usually self-limited and can be treated by such anti-fungal drugs as ketoconazole or amphotericin B.

In debilitated individuals, the fungus may become disseminated and produce widespread disease, or else a condition not unlike chronic tuberculosis with its deteriorating effects.

COCCIDIOIDOMYCOSIS

Coccidioidomycosis is an acute lung disease endemic to the south-western United Stated that is caused by inhalation of the fungus, *Coccidioides imitis*. The disease is most prevalent in the San Joaquin valley, where it is known as Valley Fever. The symptoms include fever, nonproductive cough, and weight loss. In some cases, lumps on the legs may develop. Most patients recover without treatment. In severe cases, amphotericin B may be prescribed.

CRYPTOCOCCOSIS

The fungus, *Cryptococcus neoformans,* is often spread through pigeon droppings. Inhaling the spores produces a simple form of pneumonia that usually clears by itself, but may become severe in debilitated and immune-compromised individuals, such as victims of AIDS. In these patients treatment with amphotericin B is required.

LEGIONNAIRE'S DISEASE

Legionnaire's disease was first identified in Philadelphia in 1976, when several delegates to an American Legion convention contracted a severe type of pneumonia—hence the name. The cause was eventually found to be a previously unrecognized bacterium that was immediately named *Legionella pneumophila.* Found worldwide, this bacterium seems to thrive in the warm, moist areas of air-circulation systems of large building, the source of the Philadelphia outbreak.

The disease is characterized by rapidly developing high fever, chills, headache, and malaise. A mild, dry cough begins early and worsens over several days. Many also cough up some blood in the mucus. This severe disease can be fatal in up to 15% of cases. The treatment is hospitalization and the use of such antibiotics as erythromycin.

Occupational Lung Diseases

There are several diseases of the lung caused by breathing various types of particles in the air, often associated with particular occupations that expose the victim to high concentrations of airborne particles. There are many factors that determine when an individual will be affected by breathing such particles. These include particle size, the number of particles in the air, the duration of exposure, and individual sensitivity to the particles. The most common disorders are:

1. *Pneumoconiosis.* This is a chronic lung disease caused by long exposure to high concentrations of dust particles. A common variant is "coal-miner's pneumoconiosis," or "black lung disease," caused by breathing coal dust.
2. *Silicosis.* This chronic lung disease is caused by inhaling crystalline silica (quartz dust). It was once common in such industries as metal mining, foundries, pottery making, and stone cutting.
3. *Berylliosis.* This is caused by inhaling dust or fumes containing beryllium compounds found in such industries as mining, electronics, chemical plants, and the manufacture of fluorescent light bulbs. Beryllium compounds are common in the aerospace industry.
4. *Asbestosis.* This disease results from the inhalation of asbestos dust.
5. *Byssinosis.* This disease, similar to chronic bronchitis and emphysema, is found among cotton, flax, and hemp workers, and has been known as "cotton mill fever" or "Monday morning fever."
6. *Farmer's lung.* This is caused by exposure to a certain fungus (aspergillus) that grows in moldy hay or grain. It affects only those who are allergic to the fungus.

Symptoms. The symptoms of these occupational lung diseases vary with the particle causing the disease, but most of the symptoms are similar to those found in asthma and emphysema. After many years of exposure, shortness of breath, wheezing, cough, and difficulty breathing develop. In many cases it is hard to separate the symptoms caused by occupational exposure from those caused by tobacco abuse.

Diagnosis. The diagnosis of these lung diseases depends on a history of exposure, chest X-rays, lung function tests, and often a biopsy and microscopic examination of lung tissue.

Treatment. Generally there is no reversal of the lung disease that has already taken place. Progression of the disease can be slowed by avoiding breathing contaminated air. Smoking worsens all of these diseases—Stop Smoking! If you work in a dusty environment, make certain your employer monitors air dust concentrations and takes appropriate measures to limit such concentrations. In many cases, exposure can be greatly reduced by wearing protective face masks. Drugs such as bronchodilators and corticosteroids may relieve symptoms to a variable degree.

Cyctic Fibrosis

Cystic fibrosis is an inherited disease that affects both the respiratory and digestive systems. It is common among white children, affecting nearly 1 in every 2000 infants. The disease seldom affects black, Asian, or Jewish children. It is transmitted by a *recessive* gene, which means that both parents must be carriers.

Cystic fibrosis affects the mucus and sweat glands of the body. It may first be detected when an infant develops intestinal obstruction because of thickened stools. As the infant grows older, chronic respiratory disease develops, including bronchitis, atelectasis (collapse of segments of the lung), pneumonia, and fibrosis of the lung. These conditions develop because the mucus in the child's lung is thick and sticky. Instead of acting as a lubricant, it clogs the respiratory system and provides a rich culture for bacteria and other microorganisms to grow on, and thereby add to the underlying problem.

The most common symptoms are chronic cough, shortness of breath, poor appetite, and exercise intolerance. The pancreas is also affected and may not provide sufficient enzymes to digest fats and proteins completely. This can cause chronic diarrhea and malnutrition, with the result that normal growth is retarded. Since the sweat glands are affected, the child's sweat may be extremely salty. In hot weather this contributes to salt depletion and heat exhaustion. The disease is ultimately fatal; currently, about half of affected individuals are dead by age 25.

Treatment. The treatment of cystic fibrosis entails a long-term process of promoting drainage of its thickened lung secretions and promptly attacking all respiratory infections to limit the havoc they wreak on the lungs. Frequent medical checkups are essential.

There are special exercises that parents can help their child perform to loosen and drain the mucus secretions. These include postural drainage techniques and controlled coughs that your doctor will demonstrate for you. One or more of these exercises should be performed daily. Inhaling an aerosol to help loosen secretions may also be recommended by your doctor.

Recently, significant advances in the development of two aerosol drugs offer the promise of more effective therapy. One, the drug Amiloride, appears to be effective in balancing the salt secreted in bronchial mucus, which may help prevent mucus from clogging the respiratory passages. A second drug, DNA-ase, is currently on extensive clinical trials to determine its efficacy in breaking down the DNA in bronchial secretions, also aimed at loosening mucus. At this writing, neither drug is available outside clinical research trials, but developments are fast-breaking. Consult your doctor for further details about these drugs.

Prevention of respiratory diseases is very important. Your child will need vaccinations against whooping cough (pertussis), measles, and a yearly flu shot. At the first signs of respiratory infection (fever, increased coughing, and labored breathing), consult your doctor.

If you have a child with cystic fibrosis, it means that both you and your spouse carry the cystic fibrosis gene. Therefore, each additional child will have a 25% chance of having the disease, a 50% chance of being a carrier, and a 25% chance of having normal genes. Ask your doctor for information about genetic counseling.

For more information about all aspects of cystic fibrosis, including the latest treatment modalities, contact the Cystic Fibrosis Foundation, 6931 Arlington Road, Suite 2000, Bethesda, MD 20814; 1-301-951-4422 or 1-800-Fight-CF.

Sarcoidosis

Sarcoidosis is a disorder of unknown cause that results in many small patches of inflammation in one or several parts of the body. Though the lung is the most frequent site of involvement, the lymph nodes, eyes, liver, skin, spleen, and heart may also be affected. When the lungs are involved extensively, shortness of breath and cough are the chief symptoms. The diagnosis is made by chest X-ray, skin tests, and biopsy of affected tissue.

Treatment. Sarcoidosis often clears spontaneously with no treatment at all. In problem cases your doctor may prescribe a steroid medication. Careful, long-term followup by your doctor is important to avoid permanent lung damage.

Lung Cancer

Although there are several types of lung cancer, *bronchogenic carcinoma* is by far the most common and this disease is predominantly caused by smoking. A certain small percentage of lung cancers are caused by occupational exposures (uranium mining, asbestos production, and so on) and exposure to environmental agents, such as the radioactive gas, radon. Lung cancer is the leading cause of cancer deaths in both men and women, and the incidence is rising in women, primarily because it became glamorous (tragically) for women to smoke during and after World War II. Since lung cancer develops only after years of smoking, the grim harvest that "glamor" sowed is now being reaped.

The first symptom of bronchogenic carcinoma is usually a cough that is more persistent than the usual smoker's cough. The sputum may be blood streaked, always a danger sign that should prompt you to see your doctor at once. In the rare cases in which the cancer invades blood vessels, bleeding may be copious. Since chronic bronchitis often accompanies a long history of smoking, wheezing may be common and increase as the lung tumor spreads. Chest pain and weight loss are usually late symptoms of lung cancer that occur after the cancer has spread beyond the lungs.

Lung cancer is diagnosed by a combination of X-ray examinations, sputum analysis, and lung biopsy, usually during an examination of the bronchial tubes by a procedure known as bronchoscopy.

Treatment. Surgical removal of the tumor is the first line of attack, although in about two-thirds of cases, the tumor cannot be completely removed by the time it is finally diagnosed. Radiation treatments and chemotherapy often relieve symptoms and may prolong life considerably. In a few cases cure is possible.

Prevention

The only preventive measure likely to help avoid the development of bronchogenic carcinoma is to stop smoking. Annual chest X-rays are no longer generally recommended as a cancer screening test because their value in detecting lung cancer early enough to treat effectively is low.

For more information about lung cancer, call the Cancer Information Center of the National Cancer Institute: 1-800-4-CANCER.

The Digestive System

Tongue

Epiglottis

Esophagus

Diaphragm

Liver

Gallbladder

Pancreatic
duct

Pancreas

Ascending
colon

Appendix

Ileum

Rectum

Bile
duct

Stomach

Transverse
colon

Duodenum

Jejunum

Descending
colon

Cecum

Sigmoid
colon

Your Mouth, Throat, and Gastrointestinal System

Your Mouth and Throat

Your Lips

Though the lips are a highly distinctive facial feature and serve as essential elements of speech-formation, they are best thought of as specialized features of the skin. The lips form the junction between the facial skin and the mucous membrane lining the mouth. Most disorders of the skin also affect the lips (*see* Skin, p. 437), and the conditions discussed here were chosen because they are particularly common and warrant attention.

Swelling of the Lips

Swelling of the lips is one of the many manifestations of allergic reactions and is called "angioedema" (*see* Allergies, p. 237). It is usually associated with wheezing, a rash, and other skin changes characteristic of allergic reactions. The swelling usually subsides after treatment with oral antihistamines, such as Chlor-Trimeton at a dosage of 4 milligrams every 6 hours. *See* p. 238 for a discussion of allergy treatment.

Cold Sores

Cold sores are small eruptions that occur along the vermillion border of the lips. They are usually caused by the *Herpes simplex* virus, type 1 (HSV-1). They are also known as "fever blisters" because they may appear following a febrile illness, but sometimes occur following an abrasion, sunburn, food allergy, or merely anxiety.

Cold sores typically begin after a few hours of burning or tingling sensation about the mouth. Later a red area appears near the border of the lips that then develops into a patch of small blisters. When these blisters break, they crust over and heal in the course of a week or so. In rare instances, the initial herpes infection may be accompanied by fever and sores inside the mouth. Cold sores are contagious during their early stages. They can be spread by direct contact, such as kissing, but not by sharing eating utensils or by shaking hands.

There is no cure for cold sores, but petrolatum or any of the lip balms available from your drug store are soothing and prevent cracking and bleeding. Keep the sores clean by washing gently with soap and water. Commercial blister medications do little except lubricate the skin; on the other hand they probably do no harm. Excessive makeup used to hide the sores may retard healing, so it is best to leave them exposed to air and suffer the mild embarrassment they may cause.

After blister formation, the HSV-1 viruses enter local nerve cells and remain dormant. However, they can and do emerge periodically, for example, when the area in which they are harbored is damaged or the immune system is challenged by a cold or flu. If cold sores tend to occur following sun exposure, use a sunscreen rated 15 or higher. If they are recurrent, multiple, or painful, your doctor may prescribe a topical or systemic antiviral agent, such as acyclovir. Corticosteroids should not be used because they promote the spread of lesions. Oral vitamins, consisting of equal parts of citrus bioflavonoids and ascorbic acid (e.g., 400-mg Mevanin-C capsules used three times daily for three days), may greatly reduce the duration of the lesions if begun with the first symptoms.

Cheilosis

Cheilosis (pronounced key-lo´-sis) is a fissuring and dry scaling of the skin along the vermillion border of the lips and at the angles of the mouth; it is often a sign of riboflavin (vitamin B_2) deficiency. They are also associated with sores in the mouth and around the eyes. The cause is a diet lacking in the proteins found in beans, milk, eggs, fish, and meat. Cheilosis may be confused with cold sores, except they are slow to heal (longer than two weeks). You should consult your doctor for treatment and diet recommendations.

Smoker's Patch

Smoker's patch is a firm, brownish, often scaly plaque that occurs on the vermillion border of the lower lip. It is most common among smokers who hold a cigaret or pipe in one place in their mouth. Such lesions must be biopsied to rule out the presence of skin cancer. Smoker's patch will disappear in time once smoking is stopped, but the condition must be carefully observed by your doctor until it is completely healed.

Lip Cancer

Cancer of the lip is almost always associated with a long history of smoking. *See* p. 472 for a discussion of skin cancer.

Your Mouth

The mouth is lined with a smooth, delicate, mucous membrane that is kept lubricated by saliva. There are three main pairs of salivary glands: the *sublingual glands*, located beneath the tongue; the *submandibular glands*, located beneath the floor of the mouth (which can be felt as smooth almond-shaped structures under your jawbone); and the *parotid glands*, located above the angle of your jaw.

Oral Thrush (Oral Candidiasis)

Oral thrush is caused by an overgrowth of the common fungus, *Candida albicans*. It usually causes creamy white patches in the mouth, on the tongue, and sometimes in the throat. If these patches are rubbed off, they leave a raw soreness beneath. Thrush is most common in the very young, the elderly, and the debilitated, who lose their immunity to this commonplace fungus. Thrush frequently occurs after a prolonged fever in Sjögren's disease, chronic illness and in some cases of iron-deficiency anemia.

The thrush itself is of little concern; usually it will disappear upon recovery from illness. Avoid hot liquids and spicy food, and pay special attention to good oral hygiene. If thrush causes mouth discomfort or persists for several days, see your doctor, who may prescribe such antifungal drugs as nystatin or ketoconazole.

Ulcers of the Mouth

- *Canker sores* are small painful ulcers that develop and often recur on the inside of the lips and cheeks, either singly or in groups. Their cause is unknown; they may represent one manifestation of an immune reaction. Deficiencies of vitamin B_{12} and folic acid appear to increase susceptibility. They begin as small, raised, reddish lesions that later become covered with a whitish or yellowish covering caused by secondary bacterial growth. Most canker sores heal within two weeks. No known treatment speeds healing. Symptomatic relief may usually be had by a topical anesthetic (e.g., Kank-A, Orajel, or Anbesol Gel) every four hours or before meals. A stronger prescription anesthetic is 2% lidocaine, used as an oral rinse. A dental protective paste (Orabase) helps prevent irritation by the teeth and oral fluids. If mouth ulcers don't resolve after 14 days, or if they recur frequently, see your doctor, who may prescribe a corticosteroid or a tetracycline solution and search for an underlying condition that may be promoting the sores.
- *Oral herpes* lesions are similar to canker sores, except that they usually occur as small fluid-filled vesicles on the hard palate or gums.

Minor lesions can be treated by a topical anesthetic (*see* preceding paragraph). Multiple or recurrent lesions should be treated by your doctor with antiviral drugs.

- *Oral lichen planus* is relatively rare, and is often associated with lichen planus on the skin. It most commonly begins as small pimples on the inside of the cheeks and sides of the tongue that later form a fine, white, lacy network or slightly raised patches. The usual symptoms include a slight soreness of the mouth, often accompanied by a metallic taste or dry mouth. The cause of lichen planus is not known. It may be brought on by emotional stress or chronic illness.

Treatment. If the condition does not clear in 10 days of maintaining scrupulous oral hygiene and an ample intake of liquids, see your doctor, who may prescribe a corticosteroid.

Dry Mouth

The most common cause of *dry mouth* is simple dehydration arising from excessive loss of body fluids, either from perspiration or urination *(diuresis)*. An important principle of exercise is to avoid dehydration by drinking plenty of fluids while exercising. If the reason for fluid loss is high ambient temperature, drink plenty of cool, non-alcoholic, unsweetened liquids, both to reduce core body temperature and to replace fluids. The most common causes of diuresis are consumption of such diuretics as: caffeinated beverages (coffee, tea, soft drinks), alcoholic beverages, and prescription drugs, especially diuretics and anticholinergic drugs. With caffeine and alcohol, dry mouth is resolved by reducing their consumption and drinking more plain water. With prescription diuretics, you may need to consume more liquids, but you should ask your doctor if the dosage may be reduced or an alternative drug tried. Persistent dry mouth may lead to painful stones formed in the salivary gland ducts.

Another rarer, more serious cause of dry mouth is an autoimmune disorder know as *Sjögren's syndrome.* It is similar in many respects to rheumatoid arthritis, although joint inflammation occurs in only a third of patients with Sjögren's syndrome. It is characterized by dryness of the mouth, eyes, and other mucous membranes, including the nose, throat, larynx, bronchi, vulva, and vagina. The diagnosis is made by salivary gland biopsy. Treatment is largely supportive.

Treatment. Sipping small amounts of nondiuretic fluids throughout the days alleviates dry mouth and helps prevent the serious dental decay and bad breath that accompany reduced salivary secretions. An "artificial saliva" of 2% methyl cellulose (e.g., Salivart) may be used as a mouthwash. Avoid drugs that reduce salivary secretions such as decongestants and antihistamines. Fastidious oral hygiene and frequent dental cleanings are essential. Recently, hydroxychloroquine has been used to treat the primary manifestations of Sjögren's syndrome. Ask your doctor about this drug.

For more information about Sjögren's syndrome, contact: Sjögren's Syndrome Foundation Inc., 382 Main St., Port Washington, NY 11050; 1-516-767-2866.

Mumps

Mumps is one of the common viral diseases of childhood, although it has become less common with widespread childhood vaccination programs. Mumps first affects the salivary glands, especially the parotid glands, located at the angle of the jaw. Swelling usually starts on one side and then affects the opposite side a day later. The swellings are often accompanied by fever, dry mouth, diarrhea, and a vague feeling of illness (malaise). Usually the infection clears after about 10 days.

Not infrequently, mumps will affect one or both testicles in a boy or the ovaries in a girl. After three or four days, a boy will notice pain and swelling in the testicles. Girls may experience only lower abdominal pain. In rare instances, mumps results in sterility, especially if they occur during adulthood. Also in rare instances, mumps may cause meningitis, characterized by a stiff neck and worsening of symptoms. The incubation period of mumps is 14–24 days, and permanent immunity results.

Treatment. Usually no treatment is necessary. Analgesics, such as acetaminophen, may be given for headache. *Do not give children and young adults aspirin.* Ice packs to the jaw (or scrotum) may be soothing. If pain or swelling is severe, consult your doctor. Mumps is prevented by a single vaccination that is recommended be given at 15 months.

Parotid Gland Swelling

Besides mumps, diseases of the parotid glands are relatively uncommon. Infections are accompanied by fever and painful swelling, usually unilateral, at the angle of the jaw. Painless swelling may indicate a salivary duct stone or one of several salivary gland tumors. See your doctor for any such swelling, since careful diagnostic tests are required to determine the cause.

Leukoplakia

Leukoplakia refers to white patches of thickened mucosa in the mouth or sides of the tongue. The usual cause is chronic irritation from dentures or a roughened tooth, or from smoking or chewing tobacco. Often your dentist is the first to notice the lesions, since they are usually not symptomatic, unless they become very thickened and ulcerate.

Treatment. Removing the source of irritation usually causes leukoplakia to disappear. Your dentist can correct ill-fitting dentures and smooth irregularities of the teeth. If you smoke or chew tobacco, stop at once because 5% of these lesions become cancerous. If the lesion does not disappear within several weeks, it should be biopsied to rule out the possibility of malignancy.

Tumors of the Mouth and Tongue

Both benign and malignant tumors can occur anywhere in the mouth, except on the teeth. Benign tumors are usually small, slowly growing painless lumps or nodules. Malignant tumors also begin as small, painless lumps, but then usually ulcerate and bleed. Any lump or ulcer in the mouth should prompt you to see your doctor at once.

The Tongue

Inflammation of the tongue (*glossitis*) has many causes, most of which reflect a more serious underlying disease such as anemia, vitamin deficiency (e.g., pellagra), or diabetes. Persistent inflammation that does not respond to such conservative treatment as gargling with warm salt water (one teaspoon per glass of water) should be investigated by your doctor.

Canker sores and herpetic lesions can usually be treated by a topical anesthetic (e.g., Anbesol gel, Kank-A); this relieves pain temporarily and encourages eating. Meticulous oral hygiene is essential. Smoking obviously aggravates any inflammatory condition. Persistent irritation, painful burning, or a slick, glazed tongue (*atrophic lichen planus*) should be treated by your doctor. The appearance of a painless ulcer on the tongue or lip may mean primary syphilis (chancre). See your doctor.

Hairy tongue is a benign, asymptomatic condition caused by a profuse overgrowth of the normal tongue taste buds following antibiotic therapy, a fever, or prolonged illness. Brown discoloration of the taste buds usually results from excessive smoking. Discontinuing antibiotics or smoking usually returns the tongue to normal. Brushing your tongue with a toothbrush improves tongue's appearance.

White patches on the tongue are often a sign of candidiasis, a type of yeast infection (*see above*). A precancerous lesion known as "leukoplakia" may also appear on the tongue, lips, or gums. Your doctor will prescribe an antifungal drug, such as nystatin, for candidiasis (*see* Oral Thrush, p. 269). A biopsy is required to diagnose leukoplakia (*see* previous page).

Grooved or *geographic tongue* is a relatively common condition associated with prominent lines or fissures on the tongue. This condition is thought to be hereditary and is of no medical significance.

Changes in Taste

Distortions of taste (*dysgeusia*) are often associated with loss of smell (*see* p. 245). There may be several causes, including vitamin deficiencies, recent viral infection, trauma, or cancer. Several antibiotics may cause taste distortion, one example of which is tasting something, usually unpleasant, when nothing is in the mouth (*phantogeusia*). This problem is one for your doctor to try to solve.

Bad Breath

Bad breath (*halitosis*) may result from disorders in the esophagus, stomach, or lungs, but usually the cause lies in the mouth. Dry mouth is a common cause of bad breath in the morning. Saliva contains a natural antibiotic that keeps bacteria in check. During the night, salivary secretion diminishes, and in the morning an unpleasant odor may be detected. Usually brushing and flossing is effective in eliminating this odor for the rest of the day. Mouth washes are very temporary at best and are seldom needed.

Short-term bad breath may occur as the after-aroma of eating such foods as onion, garlic, and alcoholic beverages. These are more difficult to mask because the odor passes into the bloodstream, from there to the lungs, and then exhaled in the breath. Smoking also may leave an odor in the breath that is unpleasant to some people. This can be masked by mouthwash, sprays, or mints, but the only long-term solution is to stop smoking.

Chronic bad breath may be caused by inflammation of the gums (*see* following page). Your dentist can provide the best counsel for its optimal remedy. Chronic bad breath is also associated with some systemic diseases. Liver failure is sometimes accompanied by what has been called a "mousy" smell known as *fetor hepaticus*. Diabetics whose disease is not under control may have a sweetish, slightly cloying breath smell because of *ketoacidosis*. These problems must be addressed by your doctor.

Adult Rumination

It is not uncommon for infants involuntarily to regurgitate small amounts of food from the stomach, chew, and then reswallow them. This behavior is rare in adults and, when found, may result from stress or some emotional disorder. Rarely, an esophageal disorder may underlie the problem and appropriate diagnostic tests would then need to be undertaken. In some cases the drug metoclopramide, a stimulant of intestinal activity, is useful. If repeated spitting is observed, psychiatric consultation is probably indicated.

Inflammation and Bleeding of the Gums

Inflammation of the gums (*gingivitis* or *periodontitis*) is character-ized by redness, swelling, soreness, and bleeding. This condition is chronic and, if not treated, leads to receding gums and tooth loss. The most common cause is poor dental hygiene, which encourages bacte-rial growth known as "plaque" on the tooth surfaces These bacteria give off toxins that inflame the gums and provide a focus for second-ary infection.

Some dentists believe there is also a component of autoimmune disease associated with chronic periodontitis. According to this theory, the bacteria stimulate the body's own immune system to mistake the normal gum tissue for a foreign invader and send white cells to attack normal tissue.

The best remedy for common gingivitis is daily brushing and floss-ing of the teeth, as well as periodic cleaning (every 6–12 months) by your dentist. Bleeding during brushing your teeth is not normal. If you have no other evidence of gum disease, such as redness or sore-ness, try a different brush, preferably one with soft bristles. Use one of the antiplaque toothpastes (e.g., Tartar-Control Crest) and brush at least twice daily, holding the brush at an angle pointed towards the junction of tooth and gums. Floss once daily. If bleeding persists, you should consult your dentist.

Other causes of sore or inflamed gums include misalignment of the teeth (*malocclusion*), food impaction, poorly fitted dentures, and mouth-breathing. These problems should be treated by your dentist.

A special case of gingivitis, known as *pericoronitis*, occurs around the gingival flap of a partially erupted tooth, most commonly the third molar. Treatment is local irrigation of the area with water. For some sufferers, a few drops of carbamide peroxide in glycerol 10% (e.g., Gly-Oxide) applied directly on the inflamed gum is beneficial. The problem usually disappears when the tooth has fully erupted. Severe infections may require antibiotics. See your dentist.

Trench mouth is an acute inflammation causing painful, bleeding gums, salivation, and a foul breath. Swallowing and talking may be difficult. If secondary infection occurs, fever and malaise are characteristic. It is also known as *Vincent's infection* and is caused by a fusiform bacillus and a spirochete *(fusospirochetosis)*. It is most frequently seen in young adults and is associated with poor oral hygiene, stress, nutritional deficiencies, and chronic illness. Treatment consists of gentle, but thorough, brushing of the gums and rinsing the mouth with warm saline (one teaspoon of salt in a glass of water or 1.5% peroxide solution), repeatedly for the first 2–3 days. Avoid smoking and hot or spicy foods. Analgesics (aspirin or tylenol), good nutrition, high fluid intake, and rest are all essential supportive measures. Antibiotics are unnecessary and should be avoided unless a fever greater than 101°F is present.

During pregnancy, a mild inflammation of the gums, a so-called *gingivitis of pregnancy*, may develop. This usually disappears after the first trimester. Occasionally overgrowth of the *interdental papillae* occurs during pregnancy, a condition known as *pregnancy tumors*. If these do not subside after pregnancy, they may require dental excision. Occasionally malnutrition or other chronic debilitating diseases give rise to gingivitis.

Receding Gums

Chronic gingivitis leads ultimately to the formation of pockets of infection between the gums and the teeth known as *periodontitis*. The gums then lose their attachment to the teeth and recede below the dentine–enamel junction. This induces further loss of supporting bone and is the most common cause of tooth loss. Pain is usually not a feature unless secondary infection develops. Gum recession can be halted and even reversed by good dental hygiene and proper dental care. In advanced cases, surgery is required to close the pockets. See your dentist. In some cases gum recession is caused by *overbrushing*. Only brush your teeth until they are clean; then give your mouth a rest.

Your Teeth

Tooth Decay and Toothaches

Tooth decay begins when dental "plaque" appears. This is a rough layer of food particles, mucus, and bacteria that forms between the teeth and along the gum lines. The bacteria break down sugars, liberating acid and, in turn, dissolving the calcium and phosphate in the tooth enamel to form a "cavity" or dental caries. If the caries becomes deep enough, it will reach the tooth pulp, inflaming the nerves to produce a toothache.

Prevention of Tooth Decay

Pain that is localized to a particular tooth or is provoked by eating sweets or by cold or heat is usually caused by dental caries and you should see your dentist as soon as possible. In fact, pain is one of the dental emergencies.

The best approach to toothache is the prevention of tooth decay. The underlying principles of preventive care should be taught to every young child to instill life-long habits of proper dental hygiene. These include:

- Regular brushing with a fluoride toothpaste
- Drinking fluoridated water
- Flossing
- Periodic plaque removal
- Dietary discretion

The contribution of cooked starches and sugars to tooth decay is well documented, especially when they are eaten between meals without brushing afterward. Avoid sugary snacks, sugared chewing gum, and refined sugars in general to reduce your trips to the dentist … and make your clothes fit better as well!

Tooth Discoloration

There are several causes of tooth discoloration, beyond the slight yellowing that normally occurs with age. Smoking and excessive use of tea and coffee can cause a brownish staining. The death of a tooth's pulp causes it to turn gray. Certain drugs, such as tetracycline, and some illnesses, such as whooping cough and measles at particular stages of tooth development, can cause mottled discolorations.

Treatment. Superficial stains from smoking and coffee are removed by your dentist during polishing. The discoloration caused by death of the pulp can usually be corrected by a bleaching process during a root canal procedure. Deeper discolorations can generally be corrected only by bonding a porcelain or plastic crown to the tooth or by recently developed bleaching techniques. See your dentist for advice.

Missing Tooth

Probably the last thing you are apt to remember if someone or something knocks out one of your teeth is to look for the tooth. But dentists now know that the tooth can be saved by reimplantation. And time is of the essence; the best results are achieved when the tooth can be fixed in the socket within 30 minutes or so of its dislodging. Here's what to do:

- Find the tooth and rinse it off with tap water or saliva.
- Call your dentist to tell him you are on your way.
- Gently place the tooth back in its socket. Bite down firmly on a tissue or handkerchief to hold the tooth in place and get to the dentist as quickly as possible.
- If you can't reinsert the tooth, put it in your mouth, or cup of water, while on the way to the dentist. Do not let it dry out.

If reimplantation is timely, you have about 50% chance of saving the tooth, which will serve you much better in the long run than a crown and bridge.

Wisdom Teeth

In the distant past, the human jaw was apparently large enough to accommodate three sets of molars. But today the third molars, or wisdom teeth, frequently cause problems: crowding, infection, and painful impaction (incomplete eruption). Wisdom teeth also promote fractures of the jaw in athletes who engage in such contact sports as football and boxing. As a consequence these teeth are often removed.

But do you need to have wisdom teeth removed if they are causing no problems? The consensus among dentists today is that it is best to leave wisdom teeth alone if they are not impacted, infected, painful, cavity-filled, or crowding the second molars. If you engage in contact sports, seek your dentist's advice.

Your Jaw

Temporomandibular Joint Syndrome

The temporomandibular joint (TMJ) holds the jaw flexibly attached to the skull. True disorders of the TMJ generally are related to previous trauma. Pain in the joint, a popping noise when opening or closing the mouth, or joint dislocation after yawning are the usual symptoms. The cause may be arthritis of the joint or a displacement of the articular disk in the joint. The diagnosis and differentiation of true joint disease from the more common TMJ syndrome (also known as *Myofascial Pain Dysfunction syndrome,* MPD) must be made by a dentist. Usually there is no specific therapy for TMJ arthritis. In rare cases, surgery may be indicated for dislocation of the TMJ disc.

The TMJ syndrome is one of the bugaboos of medicine in that the causes are hard to define and the treatment is highly debated. The syndrome consists of dull, aching pain usually centering around the ear on one side and extending to the jaw, back of the head, and often to the neck and shoulder muscles as well. Pain is often brought on during or after eating or yawning. There is also limited jaw movement; the normal jaw should open the width of your first three fingers. Most patients report a popping or clicking sensation with jaw movement. In some patients, the jaws may lock if opened too widely. These symptoms vary greatly and come and go for little apparent reason.

TMJ syndrome is more common among women and is thought to be the result of nervous stress. The cause of the pain is thought most often to be tension-relieving jaw clenching or tooth grinding *(bruxism)*. Another cause may be altered tooth alignment *(malocclusion)* brought on by losing a tooth and not having it replaced. In some cases, the chewing muscles overpower the teeth, causing the molar behind to tip into the space left by the lost tooth. The result is stressed chewing muscles, cramps, and spasm. Good dental hygiene and regular dental care will usually prevent this scenario.

Treatment. Treatment for TMJ syndrome is highly variable and often unsatisfactory. Many people who suffer from it have been to many doctors or dentists, all of whom have a different recommendation, because of differing experience with what does or does not work with their patients. Among the choices of therapy are analgesics (e.g., two aspirin tablets four times daily), anti-inflammatory drugs (such as ibuprofen), tranquilizers, a fitted biteplate for tooth-grinding, psychologic counseling, biofeedback, diet alterations, and surgery.

My advice is to avoid surgery if possible. More than 80% of TMJ cases are relieved through conservative measures. Sometimes severe tooth or jaw misalignment may be a factor that can be relieved by orthodontia or surgery. The best place to start if you are one of the unfortunate sufferers of TMJ syndrome is with a good (conservative) dentist. If surgery is advised, by all means seek a second opinion, preferably from a TMJ specialist from the nearest university with a dental or medical program.

There are several things you may be able to do yourself. Since stress is the usual cause, try spending a few weeks in Bermuda, or a similar stress-free resort. If this is unrealistic, pinpoint the pressure points in your life and try to relieve them. Regular exercise is an excellent way to relax. Make more time for friends and low-stress activities.

Try to become aware of your facial habits. If you bite your nails, or chew the inside of your cheek, try to stop these habits. Think about your habits of tooth grinding and jaw clenching, and break them. If you wake up with jaw pain, you are probably grinding your teeth during sleep. See your dentist about a biteplate that will reduce tooth wear. If pain develops during eating, try a softer diet and cut your food in smaller pieces. Your jaw needs a rest. Ask your doctor about biofeedback and hypnosis techniques.

If pain persists for more than a few days, see your dentist. If you have headaches, dizziness, ringing in your ears, eye pain, or blurred vision, see your doctor.

Your Esophagus and Its Disorders

The esophagus is the muscular tube that connects the back of your throat (the pharynx) with your stomach. Most disorders of the esophagus cause either heartburn or difficulty in swallowing. Both symptoms are distressing, and there is rather a lot you can do to achieve relief should you develop one of the following problems.

Hiatus Hernia and Heartburn
(Gastroesophageal Reflux; Reflux Esophagitis)

Hiatus hernia is an abnormal protrusion *(hernia)* of the upper stomach through the opening *(hiatus)* in the diaphragm through which the esophagus passes to join the stomach. The cause appears to be a weakening of the muscles of the diaphragm. This condition is quite common and, fortunately, most people have no symptoms whatever. In others, particularly those who take liberties with their health, the consequence is heartburn, a deep-seated, burning chest pain that is sometimes mistaken for angina or heart trouble. These symptoms are usually made worse by lying down. Belching and reflux of the acidic stomach contents into the throat are also common symptoms. In severe cases you may experience coughing or difficulty breathing at night if the refluxed materials are aspirated into your lungs.

Heartburn is caused by the failure of the esophageal sphincter (a kind of checkvalve) to prevent the flow, or reflux, of the acidic stomach contents back into the esophagus. Hence the name *gastroesophageal reflux*. The acid reflux in turn irritates the delicate lining of the esophagus, and hence the other name given to this condition, *reflux esophagitis*, which is the name most doctors use. Many people with reflux esophagitis have no hiatus hernia, but merely a poorly functioning esophageal sphincter. However, the number of people with hiatus hernia increases with age. It is estimated that by age 65 nearly half of all people have it, and by age 85, some 85% of people develop hiatus hernia.

Treatment. There is little you can do about a hiatus hernia if you have one, but there are several things you can do to prevent heartburn, and the hernia from enlarging:

- *Don't overeat,* and avoid such foods as fats and chocolate, which slow stomach emptying. You will probably discover other foods that consistently cause heartburn, and thus should also be avoided. Many people find that caffeine, peppermint, tomatoes, and citrus fruits and juices cause heartburn. Contrary to popular belief, spicy foods *per se* do not cause heartburn and usually need not be avoided.
- *Certain drugs can promote heartburn,* including birth control pills, antihistamines (found in many cold remedies), valium, and many nonsteroidal anti-inflammatory drugs (NSAIDs), such as ibuprofen (Advil). If you are taking prescription drugs, ask your doctor whether one of them may be causing your heartburn.
- *Eat at least two hours before napping or retiring* to give your stomach time to empty before lying down.
- *Stop smoking.* As well as causing cancer and a hundred other adverse health problems, nicotine slows stomach emptying and promotes gastroesophageal reflux.
- *Avoid alcohol before bedtime.* Extra wine taken at supper and after-dinner drinks are among the most common offenders.
- *Avoid tight clothing,* especially waist-pinching belts.

- *Lose weight* if you are overweight. Excess poundage increases abdominal pressure, which promotes reflux and heartburn.
- *Increase your dietary fiber* to prevent constipation. Straining at stools promotes reflux.
- *Make use of gravity* by elevating the head of your bed 5–6 inches. This is accomplished by putting books or bricks under the upper bedposts.

Antacids

Probably the first remedy most people turn to for heartburn is an antacid. Antacids work by neutralizing stomach acid and making reflux less irritating when it does occur. Antacids are usually rapid-acting, especially liquids and powders; tablets act more slowly unless well-chewed. Antacids are quite effective in relieving the pain and burning sensations of heartburn. However, they should be thought of only as "quick fixes" and not relied upon for long-term use, especially those containing sodium bicarbonate (plain baking soda, Alka-Seltzer, Bromo Seltzer) because they have high sodium contents and thus can interfere with kidney function. These compounds may also provoke "rebound," i.e., increased acid production a few hours later, necessitating more antacids.

Calcium carbonate is both cheap and effective (e.g., Tums, Titralac, Amitone); however, these compounds also tend to promote acid rebound. Calcium-containing antacids are often taken by postmenopausal women to increase dietary calcium; this intake should be limited to 1000–1500 milligrams of calcium a day, and aluminum-based antacids, which actually deplete body calcium, should be avoided. Thus, if you take calcium-containing antacids, don't take calcium supplements too.

Magnesium hydroxide (milk of magnesia) is also quick-acting and effective, although it may induce diarrhea in the large doses favored by some.

Aluminum compounds (e.g., Amphogel, AlternaGel) are less effective as antacids and in high doses may cause constipation. These compounds are not recommended if you need to increase your calcium intake, if you are over 65, or if you have kidney problems, unless they are prescribed by your doctor.

Aluminum–magnesium combinations (e.g., Maalox, Digel, Mylanta, Riopan, Wingel) are often the best choices because they carry a low risk of either diarrhea or constipation.

No matter which antacid you use, do not depend on it for long-term heartburn control. If you are on a salt-restricted diet, avoid antacids that contain sodium. If you are pregnant, have stomach ulcers, or kidney disease, consult your doctor before using any antacid.

Other medications. Your doctor may prescribe sucralfate (Carafate), a compound that forms a protective coating over inflamed mucosa and speeds healing.

Such drugs as Tagamet, Pepcid, Axid, and Zantac are so-called "H$_2$-receptor antagonists" (*see* p. 286). They act to inhibit the production of stomach acids and thereby prevent esophagitis (and gastritis, which has similar symptoms). A very potent inhibitor of stomach acid, omeprazole (Prilosec), turns off acid production almost completely. So far, it is only used in very severe esophagitis, in erosive esophagitis, and with the acid-producing tumor, gastrinoma.

A new class of drug, metoclopromide (Reglan), acts by increasing the tone of the esophageal sphincter and by increasing intestinal motility to empty the stomach faster. In truly intractable cases, surgical procedures can be performed to control reflux.

Difficulty Swallowing

Painful swallowing and difficulty in swallowing (*dysphagia*), such as when foods and liquids seem to "stick" in the esophagus, can be caused by several conditions. Pain is often associated with the types of esophagitis discussed above; alternatively, it may be caused by spasms of the esophagus, a condition also associated with reflux.

Both pain and difficulty swallowing are also associated with a condition known as *achalasia*, a disorder of the nerves that control the muscles of the esophagus. In achalasia, the muscles do not contract in the proper sequence, thus creating a functional block to the passage of food. Often people with achalasia have difficulty swallowing even plain water. Aspiration of food or fluids into the lungs may then cause choking, especially at night.

Other causes of difficulty in swallowing include esophageal stricture or cancer of the esophagus, both fortunately rare. Their diagnosis must be made by a gastroenterologist, who examines the esophagus by means of a tube (*endoscopy*) and measures pressures at various places in the esophagus and stomach (*manometry*). Barium X-rays also identify strictures and incoordinate swallowing. The treatment for these problems may be surgical repair or mechanical dilatation of the

esophagus, depending upon individual differences. In some cases drugs are effective in reducing esophageal spasms.

Your Stomach and Duodenum and Their Disorders

Indigestion *(Dyspepsia)*

Indigestion is a vague term that generally refers to abdominal discomfort, bloating, or merely a prolonged feeling of fullness that is experienced after eating. Other common symptoms include heartburn, nausea, and belching. Often there is an element of dietary indiscretion: drinking a bit much, indulging in greasy foods or foods that are known to "disagree" with you, eating too fast, or chewing inadequately. Several foods, including cabbage, cucumbers, beans, and onions are especially prone to cause indigestion.

Indigestion is nearly universal; everyone has it now and then. In this respect, it is relatively harmless. It is only when indigestion recurs often, without known cause, or in ways that interfere with the quality of your life that medical attention should be sought.

Treatment. You can usually avoid indigestion by limiting alcohol intake, stopping smoking, and avoiding foods and drugs that you have learned cause you indigestion. Eat smaller, more frequent meals. Avoid emotional stress at mealtime. The use of antacids is frequently all that is required to relieve symptoms (*see* p. 281). If indigestion is accompanied by abdominal pain, prolonged nausea, and vomiting, vomiting of blood, or fever, consult your doctor. Indigestion is a common and often persistent complaint in such serious medical problems as gallbladder disease, duodenal ulcer, and stomach cancer.

Nausea and Vomiting

Everyone experiences nausea at some time or another, and most people have vomited on occasion. Usually you do not know the cause, since nausea and vomiting are common symptoms associated with more than a hundred different conditions and diseases. Often, however, the cause is benign, such as simple indigestion, and disappears spontaneously.

Treatment. The best approach to nausea is to take nothing by mouth until the nausea passes. Sometimes eating a cracker or other dry food is relieving. It is a myth that carbonated beverages relieve nausea. The carbonation more likely than not will bloat an already upset stomach and *cause* vomiting. Drinking colas or ginger ale may be a good way of replenishing fluids after an episode of vomiting, but they should be flat, at room temperature, and taken in small sips at a time.

Gastritis

Gastritis literally means an inflammation of the lining of the stomach. Inflammation can be caused by bacteria or viruses, or by irritating drugs, such as aspirin, steroids, and many of the nonsteroidal anti-inflammatory drugs, or NSAIDs (ibuprofen, naproxen, etc.). However, by far the most common causes of gastritis are alcohol and tobacco, when used to excess.

The symptoms of gastritis include all of the symptoms of indigestion listed above. In addition, a burning pain may develop in the pit of your stomach, which, when it occurs, is a sign that something must be done.

Treatment. Mild symptoms of indigestion are usually handled adequately by limiting alcohol, caffeine, and tobacco use, and prudent eating habits. Antacids frequently relieve symptoms (*see* p. 281). If pain develops, it can usually be controlled by not eating for a day. Instead, take small amounts of liquids, such as milk or water, at frequent intervals. Avoid aspirin and NSAIDs, which may cause erosions and bleeding of the stomach lining. After a day or two, you can begin to take small amounts of relatively bland foods that you know won't disagree with you. If pain persists, or if you vomit blood (or what looks like coffee grounds), or if you develop black, tarry stools (indicating the presence of blood), see your doctor at once.

Peptic Ulcer

Peptic (stomach)ulcers are a major health problem, affecting more than 4 million people each year in the United States. They occur in the stomach and duodenum (the first part of the small intestine) as raw areas or erosion in the gastrointestinal lining (the *mucosa*). It is thought that excessive secretions of stomach acids and digestive enzymes overcome the natural protective barriers of the mucosa and quite literally digest away the gastrointestinal lining. Why this occurs is not known, although recent research suggests that a certain bacterium, *Helicobacter pylori*, may play a role in ulcer formation.

Duodenal ulcers occur more commonly in men, although in recent years, the women's rate regrettably appears to be drawing even. Duodenal ulcers tend to occur in younger and middle-aged individuals, whereas stomach ulcers generally occur in older people.

It is difficult to distinguish stomach from duodenal ulcers by their symptoms. Both types of ulcer cause nausea and vomiting, belching, bloating, and pain. Ulcer pain occurs deep in the pit of your stomach, often waking you in the middle of the night, and is commonly relieved by eating or by taking antacids. In some cases, only a sharp sense of hunger will be felt when your stomach is empty. In serious cases, when blood vessels beneath the ulcer erode, bleeding may occur with vomiting of "coffee ground-like" material or with black, tarry stools. Obviously these are causes for immediate medical attention.

The usual methods of diagnosing peptic ulcers are by an "upper GI series," a group of X-rays of the stomach and intestines taken after swallowing a barium-containing liquid, and by *endoscopy*, in which a long flexible tube made of optical fibers is passed down the throat and into the stomach and duodenum. X-ray studies outline the ulcer crater, whereas endoscopy allows the doctor to directly examine the ulcer. Endoscopy is also effective in diagnosing stomach cancer, which may be difficult to distinguish clinically from peptic ulcer. Analysis of gastric juices may also be useful, especially in diagnosing hypersecretion of acids that occurs in the Zollinger-Ellison syndrome, caused by an enzyme-secreting tumor of the pancreas, a gastrinoma.

Treatment. *Diet.* It used to be recommended that bland foods (an "ulcer diet") be taken to promote the healing of ulcers, although much less emphasis is placed upon diet today. More important is that you eat several small meals each day to buffer the stomach acid and avoid prolonged periods of an empty stomach. Avoid coffee, tea, and alcohol, all of which stimulate gastric acid and do little to buffer it. Taking frequent glasses of milk is no longer recommended, because milk causes a "rebound" effect: initially the milk's calcium buffers stomach acid and promotes relief; however, the fats and protein in milk later stimulate acid secretion and indigestion may become worse. Foods that make peptic ulcer symptoms worse vary among individuals. You will quickly discover what these are and will do well to avoid them, especially before bedtime.

Stop smoking. Nicotine increases the secretion of gastric acid, retards healing, and increases the risk of serious complications, such as bleeding.

Antacids. These are simple acid-neutralizing drugs that are quite safe and effective treatment for ulcer symptoms. See p. 281 for a description of the most common types. Antacids seem to be most effective when taken 1–2 hours after meals and at bedtime. Whether you take antacids in liquid or tablet form seems to make little difference, although tablets should be well chewed to speed their neutralizing effect.

Remember that antacids can interfere with the absorption of certain medicines. Review these with your doctor if you are taking any other medicines. Avoid aspirin and nonsteroidal anti-inflammatory drugs (e.g., ibuprofen, naproxen, etc.), which are known to worsen peptic ulcers.

Acid suppressors. Four drugs, cimetidine (Tagamet), ranitidine (Zantac), nizatidine (Axid), and famotidine (Pepcid) are powerful inhibitors of stomach acid and pepsin secretion. They are known as H_2-receptor blockers. Cimetidine is usually taken four times daily, ranitidine is taken twice daily, and famotidine and nizatidine are taken once daily. All of these drugs have side effects, may interfere with the metabolism of other drugs, and must be monitored by your doctor.

Ulcer coaters. A relatively new prescription drug, sucralfate (Carafate), works by forming a thick gel within the stomach and coating the ulcer to prevent contact with stomach acids and enzymes. This drug has almost no side effects.

Once peptic ulcers have healed, recurrence is very common unless medication is continued. This is most often accomplished by continuing to take one of the above H_2-receptor blockers at bedtime. Ulcers heal more slowly for smokers, and smokers also have a higher recurrence rate after initial healing.

The many new ulcer-fighting drugs have made the management of peptic ulcers much less vexing, and there are several new drugs, such as omeprazole (Prilosec), that almost completely eliminate stomach acid secretion.

Today it is much less common to have to resort to surgery to treat ulcers. However, when such complications as bleeding, obstruction, or perforation (erosion into the peritoneal cavity) occur, or in the case of severe, recurrent ulcers, surgery may be required. In such cases, portions of the stomach or duodenum may be removed, or the vagus nerve may be severed *(vagotomy)* to reduce acid secretion. Bleeding ulcers are treated by endoscopy, using either a laser beam or electrocautery to "weld" the blood vessel shut. But remember that most ulcers can be treated by conservative means and by prudent lifestyle (including exercise). The sober life pays off again.

For more information on peptic ulcer disease, write to: National Digestive Diseases Information Clearinghouse, Box NDDIC, Bethesda, MD 20892; 1-301-468-2162.

Pyloric Stenosis

The pylorus is the muscular ring that controls the flow of food from the stomach into the duodenum. In rare cases, particularly as a result of peptic ulcers, the pylorus becomes narrowed and obstructed. The symptoms include bloating, vomiting, and belching of foul-smelling gas. The diagnosis is easily made by endoscopy (*see* description above). The treatment usually involves a surgical widening of the pylorus.

Cancer of the Stomach

Although stomach cancer is common in Japan, Chile, and parts of Eastern Europe, it is relatively uncommon in the United States. It occurs more frequently in men, and the average age of onset is 55 years.

Stomach cancers often have the same early symptoms as benign ulcers: persistent indigestion, bloating, slight nausea, and heartburn. Later the cancers may bleed, causing blood in the stools, anemia, and weight loss.

Diagnosis and Treatment. The diagnosis of stomach cancer is made by endoscopy (passing a fiberoptic tube into the stomach) and by biopsy. If the tumor is discovered early, the cancer may be cured by surgical removal (partial gastrectomy). If the cancer has spread, treatment with anticancer drugs (chemotherapy), or occasionally with X-rays, may be recommended.

For additional information, write to the: Office of Cancer Communications, National Cancer Institute, Bethesda, MD 20892, or call 1-800-4-CANCER.

Gastroenteritis

Gastroenteritis is an inflammation of the mucosal lining of the digestive tract that gives rise to nausea, vomiting, diarrhea, and sometimes fever and cramping abdominal pain, depending on the cause. The most common cause is one of several viruses that result in the 24- or 36-hour attacks of vomiting and/or diarrhea usually called "intestinal flu" or "stomach flu."

However, there are numerous other causes of gastroenteritis. The table on p. 290 lists several causes of gastroenteritis and food poisoning, their symptoms, and means for their prevention.

Your Intestines and Their Disorders

The small intestine is the principal digestive tube extending from the stomach to the colon. It measures about 16 feet long and is the organ from which most nutrients are absorbed into the bloodstream.

The large intestine, or colon, is about 5 feet long and is chiefly responsible for the reabsorption of water and the storage of undigested food materials until they are conducted to the rectum and excreted from the body. A wide variety of problems affects the intestines, and none more commonly than "functional" disorders, i.e., alterations in such bowel functions as diarrhea, constipation, and excessive gas.

Functional Bowel Problems

Diarrhea

Few bodily functions are subject to more variation than is defecation. In urban civilizations, the normal frequency of bowel movements ranges from 2–3 per day to 2–3 per week. I suppose that you have diarrhea when your frequency of bowel movements increases noticeably above your usual pattern and when the water content increases beyond usual experience, i.e., your stools become "loose." Notice that both features must be present because of the wide variation in frequency. Of course, the simultaneous occurrence of nausea and vomiting, cramping abdominal pain, and fever will also influence your decision to treat your symptoms.

Diarrhea has numerous causes. The most common are the various types of gastroenteritis (*see* chart, p. 290). Other causes include alcohol abuse; food allergies or intolerances (*see* p. 240); certain medications, such as colchicine, used to treat gout; toxins, such as certain wild mushrooms, and shellfish exposed to the so-called "red tide"; radiation; and irritable bowel syndrome (*see* p. 296).

Treatment. For the occasional bout of mild diarrhea, treat with diet, water, and fiber. Foods that add bulk to the stool include bananas, rice, applesauce, and whole grain cereals. Drink plenty of fluids to compensate for the increased loss with diarrhea. Fruit juices and soft drinks are better than water because they contain more minerals, which are also lost with diarrhea. If diarrhea is severe, you may try a homemade solution to replace fluid and minerals: dissolve one teaspoon salt, one teaspoon baking soda, and four teaspoons sugar in a quart of water. You may wish to add a flavoring agent to make the drink more palatable. A commercial preparation containing similar ingredients is marketed as Pedialyte. One quart of this rehydration formula per 24 hours while diarrhea lasts should be sufficient replacement for most adults as long as total fluid intake equals 8–10 glasses per day. For infant diarrhea, consult your doctor.

Fiber adds bulk to loose stools by absorbing and binding water. Try two tablespoons of wheat bran or a psyllium preparation, such as metamucil, with your breakfast.

See your doctor if diarrhea lasts more than a few days, if you develop a fever, if you have severe abdominal pain, or if you notice blood in your stools. Remember, if nausea and vomiting accompany diarrhea and you cannot keep fluids down, you may be in serious danger of becoming dehydrated.

Effective over-the-counter antidiarrhea medications include: activated attapulgite (Kaopectate, Rheaban), polycarbophil (Fiberall), and loperamide (Imodium). Take as directed on the package.

Your doctor may prescribe one or more of the following prescription drugs:

- Antispasmodic drugs, such as diphenoxylate (Lomotil) three or four times daily, atropine, or propantheline. These drugs may also cause dryness of the mouth and sluggishness of the bladder.
- Opiates include codeine, 15–30 mg two to three times daily and paregoric (camphorated opium tincture), one teaspoon every four hours. These tend to be sedating and should not be taken if you drive or operate machinery.
- Tranquilizers may be advised if periods of increased stress clearly worsen your symptoms.

Note that none of these drugs should be given to children without specific directions by your doctor.

Constipation

Constipation is defined medically as "difficult or infrequent passage of stools" and is usually accompanied by a mild discomfort or feeling of incomplete evacuation. Constipation has many causes: diet, change of exercise habits, sedentary lifestyle, emotional problems, medications, laxative abuse, dehydration, and simply putting off going to the bathroom until elimination becomes difficult. Some people believe they are constipated merely because they failed to have a bowel movement at the expected time.

Common Causes of Gastroenteritis

Disease and organism that causes it	Source of illness	Symptoms	Prevention methods
Salmonellosis *Salmonella* (bacteria; more than 1700 kinds)	May be found in raw meats, poultry, eggs, fish, milk, and products made with them. Multiplies rapidly at room temperature.	Onset: 12–48 hours after eating. Nausea, fever, headache, abdominal cramps, diarrhea, and sometimes vomiting. Can be fatal in infants, the elderly, and the infirm.	• Handling food in a sanitary manner • Thorough cooking of foods • Prompt and proper refrigeration of foods
Staphylococcal food poisoning Staphylococcal enterotoxin (produced by *Staphylococcus aureus* bacteria)	The toxin is produced when food contaminated with the bacteria is left too long at room temperature. Meats, poultry, egg products; tuna, potato, and macaroni salads; and cream-filled pastries are good environments for these bacteria to produce toxin.	Onset: 1–8 hours after eating. Diarrhea, vomiting, nausea, abdominal cramps, and prostration. Mimics flu. Lasts 24–48 hours. Rarely fatal.	• Sanitary food handling practices • Prompt and proper refrigeration of foods
Botulism botulinum toxin (produced by *Colostridium botulinum* bacteria)	Bacteria are widespread in the environment. However, bacteria produce toxin only in an anaerobic (oxygen-free) environment of little acidity. Types A, B, and F may result from inadequate processing of low-acid canned foods, such as green beans, mushrooms, spinach, olives, and beef. Type E normally occurs in fish.	Onset: 8–36 hours after eating. Neurotoxic symptoms, including double vision, inability to swallow, speech difficulty, and progressive paralysis of the respiratory system. **Obtain medical help immediately!** **Botulism can be FATAL!**	• Using proper methods for canning low acid foods • Avoidance of commercially canned low-acid foods with leaky seals or with bent, bulging, or broken cans • Toxin can be destroyed after a can is opened by boiling contents hard for 10 minutes—**Not recommended!**
Perfringens food poisoning *Colostridium perfringens* (rod-shaped bacteria)	Bacteria are widespread in the environment. Generally found in meat and poultry and dishes made with them. Multiply rapidly	Onset: 8–22 hours after eating (usually 12 hours). Abdominal pain and diarrhea. Sometimes nausea and vomiting. Symptoms last a day	• Sanitary handling of foods, especially meat and meat dishes and gravy • Thorough cooking of foods, especially eggs and chicken

Common Causes of Gastroenteritis *(continued)*

Disease and organism that causes it	Source of illness	Symptoms	Prevention methods
	when foods are left at room temperature too long. Destroyed by cooking.	or less and are usually mild. Can be more serious in older or debilitated people.	• Prompt and proper refrigeration
Shigellosis (bacillary dysentery) *Shigella* (bacteria)	Food becomes contaminated when a human carrier with poor sanitary habits handles liquid or moist food that is then not cooked thoroughly. Organisms multiply in food stored above room temperature. Found in mild and dairy products, poultry, and potato salad.	Onset: 1–7 days after eating. Abdominal pain, cramps, diarrhea, fever, sometimes vomiting, and blood, pus or mucus in stools. Can be serious in infants, the elderly, or debilitated people.	• Handling food in a sanitary manner • Proper sewage disposal • Proper refrigeration of foods
Campylo-bacteriosis *Campylobacter jejuni* (rod-shaped bacteria)	Bacteria found on poultry, cattle, and sheep and can contaminate the meat and milk of these animals. Chief food sources: raw poultry, meat, and unpasteurized milk.	Onset: 2–5 days after eating. Fever, abdominal cramping, and sometimes bloody stools. Lasts 2–7 days.	• Thorough cooking of foods • Handling food in a sanitary manner • Avoiding unpasteurized milk
Gastroenteritis *Yersinia enterocolitica* (nonspore-forming bacteria)	Ubiquitous in nature; carried in food and water. Bacteria multiply rapidly at room temperature, *as well as* at refrigerator temperatures (4–9°C). Generally found in raw vegetables, meats, water, and unpasteurized milk.	Onset: 2–5 days after eating. Fever, headache, nausea, diarrhea, and general malaise. Mimics flu. An important cause of gastroenteritis in children. Can also infect other age groups and, if not treated, can lead to other more serious diseases (such as lymphadenitis, arthritis, and Reiter's syndrome).	• Thorough cooking of foods • Sanitizing cutting instruments and cutting boards before preparing foods that are eaten raw • Avoidance of unpasteurized milk and unchlorinated water
Cereus food poisoning	Illness may be caused by the bacteria,	Onset: 1–18 hours after eating. Two	• Sanitary handling of foods

(continued)

Common Causes of Gastroenteritis *(continued)*

Disease and organism that causes it	Source of illness	Symptoms	Prevention methods
Bacillus cereus (bacteria and possibly their toxin)	which are widespread in the environment, or by an enterotoxin created by the bacteria found in raw foods. Bacteria multiply rapidly.	types of illness: (1) abdominal pain and diarrhea, and (2) nausea and vomiting. Lasts less than a day.	• Thorough cooking of foods • Prompt and adequate refrigeration
Cholera *Vibrio cholera* (bacteria)	Found in fish and shellfish harvested from waters contaminated by human sewage. (Bacteria may also occur naturally in Gulf Coast waters.) Chief food sources: seafood, especially types eaten raw.	Onset: 1–3 days. Can range from"subclinical" (a mild uncomplicated bout with diarrhea) to fatal (intense diarrhea with dehydration). Severe cases require hospitalization.	• Sanitary handling of foods • Thorough cooking of foods
Parahemolyticus food poisoning *Vibrio parahaemolyticus* (bacteria)	Organism lives in salt water and can contaminate fish and shellfish. Thrives in warm weather.	Onset: 15–24 hours after eating. Abdominal pain, nausea, vomiting, and diarrhea. Sometimes fever, headache, chills, and mucus and blood in stools. Lasts 1–2 days. Rarely fatal.	• Sanitary handling of foods • Thorough cooking of foods
Viral Gastrointestinal disease enteroviruses, rotaviruses, parvoviruses	Viruses exist in the intestinal tract of humans and are expelled in feces. Contamination of foods can occur in three ways: (1) when sewage is used to enrich garden/farm soil, (2) by direct hand-to-food contact during the preparation of meals, and (3) when shellfish growing waters are contamined by sewage.	Onset: After 24 hours. Severe diarrhea, nausea, and vomiting. Respiratory symptoms. Usually lasts 4–5 days, but may last for weeks.	• Sanitary handling of foods • Thorough cooking of foods • Use of pure drinking water • Adequate sewage disposal
Hepatitis	Chief food sources: shellfish harvested	Jaundice, fatigue. May cause liver damage	• Sanitary handling of foods

Common Causes of Gastroenteritis *(continued)*

Disease and organism that causes it	Source of illness	Symptoms	Prevention methods
hepatitis A virus	from contaminated areas, and foods that are handled a lot during preparation then eaten raw (such as vegetables).	and death.	• Thorough cooking of foods • Use of pure drinking water • Adequate sewage disposal
Mycotoxicosis mycotoxins (from molds)	Produced in foods that are relatively high in moisture. Chief food sources: beans and grains that have been stored in a moist place.	May cause liver and/or kidney disease.	• Checking foods for visible molds and discarding those that are contaminated • Proper storage of susceptible foods
Giardiasis *Giardia lamblia* (flagellated protozoa) **Amebiasis** *Entamoeba histolytica*	Protozoa exist in the intestinal tract of humans and are expelled in feces. Contamination of foods can occur in two ways: (1) when sewage is used to enrich garden/farm soil, and (2) by direct hand-to-food contact during the preparation of meals. Chief food sources: foods that are handled a lot during prepration.	Diarrhea, abdominal pain, flatulence, abdominal distention, nutritional disturbances, "nervous" symptoms, anorexia, nausea, and vomiting. Tenderness over the colon or liver, loose morning stools, recurrent diarrhea, change bowel habits, "nervous" symptoms, loss of weight, anemia, and fatigue.	• Sanitary handling of foods • Avoidance of raw fruits and vegetables in areas where the protoza are endemic • Proper sewage disposal

Source: FDA Consumer, 1991.

Probably the most common cause of occasional constipation is a diet low in fiber. One of fiber's main effects is to absorb water and carry it into the colon, where it softens and adds bulk to the stools. Diets high in refined grains, protein, fats, and processed foods tend to produce small, dry stools that are difficult to eliminate. This became painfully clear to the early astronauts who consumed mostly artificial foods low in fiber.

There are many drugs that cause constipation as a side effect: opiates; antidepressants; anticholinergic drugs used to treat Parkinson's disease and other disorders; painkillers, codeine, and nonabsorbable antacids containing aluminum hydroxide or calcium carbonate. Many drugs used to lower blood pressure are also constipating. Often a change in dosage, a shift to an alternative drug, or just increasing fluid intake can eliminate constipation.

Laxative abuse is also a common cause of constipation. Prolonged use of laxatives causes the colon to become "lazy," thus accentuating the problem that the laxative was originally taken to cure. Most doctors believe that more than four doses of a laxative in two weeks is an overuse if you are not bedridden. The way to wean yourself from laxatives is to switch to a bulk expanding laxative, such as psyllium or methylcellulose (Metamucil, etc.), and to increase dietary fiber and fluid intake. Then you can gradually wean yourself off the bulk laxative.

Treatment. Here are some measures to adopt to end constipation and prevent its recurrence:

- *Maintain a high-fiber diet* that includes ample whole grains, bran, potatoes, nuts, fresh fruits and vegetables, and avoids fat and refined foods.
- *Get plenty of exercise.* Take at least a half-hour walk each day.
- *Drink plenty of fluids:* 8–10 glasses of water per day. Add prune juice, if you wish; it really works.
- *Don't put off the "urge";* the longer the stool remains in the bowel, the more water will be absorbed and the harder it will become to eliminate. There is a wise adage: "When nature calls, don't try to bluff her, but haste away without delay or you will surely suffer."
- *Avoid stimulant laxatives* such as castor oil, cascara, and bisacodyl, which act by irritating the intestinal lining. Rather, try a laxative, such as Metamucil or Effersyllium for a few days. Plain wheat bran also works well and is wonderfully inexpensive. If this strategy fails, and if constipation lasts more than a week, see your doctor.

A word about enemas. Enemas are useful in preparing patients for surgery and occasionally in the elderly and bedfast for breaking up impacted stool. Otherwise they should not be used without the advice of your doctor. An habitual reliance on enemas will create a dependence upon them, just as laxatives do. Do not use soapsuds; they are irritating to the colon. The so-called "high colonic" enema recommended to rid your body of "poisons," and in which large amounts of water and additives are passed through a tube high in the colon, is not only a fraud, it can cause serious medical complications.

Some causes of constipation that require professional care include: mechanical bowel obstruction; adynamic ileus, which often accompanies inflammations such as peritonitis or diverticulitis; megacolon, a disease of infants and children in which the colon expands like a balloon; and hypothyroidism.

Excessive Gas

Gas—the type passed rectally, known as *flatus*—has always been a problem for us as social animals. The Romans even passed laws forgiving its passage in public. In small amounts it causes little problem. Everyone passes gas: the average is about a pint of gas per day (more if you are a vegetarian). But excessive gas can be embarrassing.

Gas comes primarily from two sources: swallowed air and bacterial fermentation of undigested food, which produces the gases hydrogen, carbon dioxide, and methane. All these are odorless. Trace amounts of fermentation gases are responsible for the characteristic odor of the fart. Some foods are well known to be more "flatulogenic" than others: beans, bran, broccoli, Brussels sprouts, cabbage, raw apples, cauliflower, onions, and milk in the lactose intolerant.

Treatment. Though there are numerous products on the market that are hinted to be useful in reducing flatulence, few are really effective. The FDA has approved simethicone for relief of gas, although many experts find no good scientific evidence proving its efficacy. Activated charcoal may be useful, but it must be taken in large quantities: one gram orally before an offending meal and one gram four hours afterward. It is probably just as easy to avoid the "offending" meal than take the charcoal. Be aware also that charcoal may bind other drugs you may be taking, thus interfering with their action. If you have developed flatulence shortly after increasing bran in your diet, try cutting back on the bran and then increasing the amount slowly to your desired level of intake. If you sleep with a partner, sleep with your backside to the outside.

Much of the gas that is formed by bacterial fermentation results from eating complex carbohydrates known as *oligosaccharides*, for which humans lack a digestive enzyme. The bacteria that inhabit the colon, however, have this enzyme in abundance and set upon these carbohydrates in a feeding frenzy, and in the process generate plentiful hydrogen and carbon dioxide. Recently a commercial product, called Beano appropriately enough, that contains the missing enzyme has been marketed. The manufacturer claims that a dose of Beano before your *frijoles rellenos* will spare you the usual postprandial embarrassment. Maybe yes; maybe no.

For the abdominal pains sometimes associated with gas, there are a few things you can do to get the gas "moving" and thus reduce the spasms. If the pain is on one side of your abdomen, lie down on the floor or on a bed on the same side that hurts. Rock back and forth or knead your abdomen with your free hand to move the gas along in the colon. It is the stretching of the colon under pressure from the gas that causes the spasms and pain.

Irritable Bowel Syndrome (Spastic Colon, Mucous Colitis)

This is a common and highly annoying condition that affects about 15% of all adults (two-thirds are women) at some time or another. The most common complaints are cramping abdominal pain along with irregular bowel movements, although some have chronic diarrhea without pain. Irregularity may run from simple constipation to formidable diarrhea, and the two may alternate from week to week for no apparent reason. Accompanying these major symptoms are various other minor ailments: excessive gas, abdominal fullness or bloating, passage of mucus, and a veritable symphony of inner gurglings, known as "borborygmi."

There is no known cause of irritable bowel syndrome. Symptoms seem to wax and wane, often in concert with one's pattern of emotional stress. The diagnosis of irritable bowel syndrome is usually made after your doctor has ruled out all of the many other causes of chronic diarrhea, i.e., it is a "diagnosis of exclusion."

Treatment. Review the discussions of diarrhea and constipation above for a general approach to the treatment of problems with bowel functioning. One of the first things your doctor will most likely advise will be to increase your dietary intake of fiber. Foods that are high in fiber include legumes (peas, beans, lentils), cereals, fruits, and vegetables. You will probably want to supplement this with one or two tablespoons of wheat bran before breakfast and gradually increase the amount if necessary. Many doctors prefer one of the psyllium preparations, such as Metamucil or Effersyllium. Paradoxically, dietary fiber helps whether you have diarrhea or constipation. This is because fiber absorbs intestinal water, firming up a soft stool, and softens a hard stool by drawing water from the body into the bowel.

There is much controversy whether drugs are of any use in treating the irritable bowel syndrome. Most of those who suffer from it are sufficiently miserable to keep trying the antispasmodic drugs used to combat diarrhea and constipation described above.

Inflammatory Bowel Disease
(Regional Ileitis and Ulcerative Colitis)

Inflammatory bowel disease (IBD) is the collective term for two separate, but similar, diseases. Crohn's disease, also known as *regional ileitis* or *regional enteritis*, can involve any part of the gastrointestinal tract, but most frequently manifests in the lower small intestine and colon, whereas *ulcerative colitis* involves only the colon. Inflammatory bowel disease may also be so mild as to result in only occasional bouts of diarrhea, or it can be so devastating that it completely controls one's social, career, and sex life to the extent that one's existence revolves around the bathroom.

Ulcerative colitis is an inflammation of the mucous membranes lining the colon. This causes fever; bouts of diarrhea, usually bloody and often at night; muscle aches; cramping abdominal pain; poor appetite; and weight loss.

Crohn's disease affects both small and large intestines. Abdominal pain and diarrhea are the most common symptoms. In severe cases, fever, loss of appetite, weakness, and weight loss occur. Complications include abscess, fistula, bowel obstruction, and bleeding. Half of all patients eventually require surgery for such complications.

The cause of IBD is not known. It may be one of the "autoimmune diseases," in which the body literally forms antibodies against itself, in this case against the intestinal tissues. The disease is intermittent; it is more common among Jews, least common in blacks and Orientals, and it seems to run in families, suggesting a genetic cause. It is mostly a disease of young and middle-aged adults. In IBD there may be inflammation in other parts of the body, including swelling and redness of the ankles, knees, wrists, and other joints; mouth sores; tender nodules over the lower leg *(erythema nodosum)*, and inflammation of the eyes *(uveitis)*. The diagnosis of IBD is made by direct visualization of the bowel by endoscopy, by intestinal biopsy, and by X-rays. Bowel infections that can resemble IBD are ruled out by appropriate stool cultures.

Treatment. Drug therapy consists of anti-inflammatory drugs, including corticosteroids and, in the case of ulcerative colitis, sulfasalazine and mesalamine. These drugs have potential side effects, so they must be taken exactly as prescribed. Ask your doctor what side effects you may expect and report them promptly so that the drug dosage may be adjusted if necessary.

Sometimes the disease becomes so severe that drugs do not work and surgery becomes necessary. Surgeons then remove the colon (*colectomy*) and create an *ileostomy*—an opening in the surface of the abdomen to which the end of the small intestine is attached, and then fitted with an ileostomy bag to catch feces. Although this sounds like a drastic procedure, patients quickly learn to cope and generally experience only mild inconvenience. In some cases, an *internal ileostomy* can be created, in which a segment of small intestine is used to create a colon substitute to collect wastes inside the body, which are then passed normally through the anus. Colectomy cures ulcerative colitis, but not Crohn's disease.

Other surgical procedures may be required to relieve intestinal obstruction and *fistulas*, abnormal openings that can lead from the bowel to the peritoneum, bladder, or vagina.

Here are some things you can do to help cope with IBD:

- This is a debilitating disease, so maintain proper nutrition by eating sufficient calories, protein, vitamins, and minerals supplied by a balanced diet. You will probably find that some foods worsen diarrhea, and these should be avoided. Frequent offenders are high-fiber foods such as seeds, nuts, and corn; fried and greasy foods; and caffeine. For some, the lactose in milk products worsens symptoms. Such patients can switch to milk substitutes, predigested milk, or commercially available lactase that can be added to milk to predigest the lactose.
- Eat foods slowly, chew them thoroughly, and try to eat small, frequent meals, rather than large, irregularly spaced meals.
- Remember that a common cause of weight loss in IBD is avoidance of eating for fear of aggravating symptoms. The problem to be overcome is discovering which foods have no or only a minimal effect upon your symptoms. Ask your doctor about the necessity of vitamin and mineral supplements, especially if you must maintain a highly restricted diet.
- Get plenty of rest and exercise. Avoid stress to the extent possible. Stress aggravates IBD symptoms.

For more information about IBD, write to:

American Digestive Disease Society Inc., 7720 Wisconsin Ave., Bethesda, MD 20814.

National Digestive Diseases Information Clearing House, Box NDDIC, Bethesda, MD 20892.

National Foundation for Ileitis and Colitis Inc., 444 Park Avenue South, New York, NY 10016.

United Ostomy Association Inc., 36 Executive Park, Suite 120, Irvine, CA 97214.

Malabsorption Syndromes

Most nutrients are absorbed into the bloodstream through the mucous membrane lining the small intestine. If this membrane is injured, as it is in Crohn's disease, there may be sufficient interference with the absorption of nutrients to cause debilitation. Another cause of malabsorption is the lack of an enzyme, as in *lactase deficiency*, where the enzyme, lactase, is congenitally missing. In celiac disease (sprue), the intestine becomes inflamed by the presence of gluten, a protein found in wheat and other grains. Severe liver and pancreatic diseases offer further examples of malabsorption syndromes.

The symptoms of malabsorption syndrome vary with the particular defect and the nutrient that is deficient. Commonly, there are abdominal discomfort, bloating, and flatulence; loose, greasy-looking, malodorous stools; weight loss; weakness; and fatigue.

Often fats are not absorbed and this results in the malabsorption of the four fat-soluble vitamins, A, D, E, and K. Vitamin K deficiency results in a tendency to bleed easily. Malabsorption of vitamin D impairs the ability to use calcium and magnesium, and thus bone pain may be a symptom of severe malabsorption. Impaired absorption of iron, folic acid, and vitamin B_{12} all result in anemia, weakness, and weight loss (*see* Anemias, p. 212).

Treatment. Your doctor's approach to malabsorption will depend upon its cause, which must be determined by blood and stool tests and often a biopsy of the intestine. Treatment of the underlying condition usually results in cure or lessening of the malabsorption and its symptoms. Often a high-protein, high-calorie diet with vitamin and mineral supplements are also recommended. In celiac disease, foods containing gluten (flour and many cereal products) must be scrupulously avoided. In lactase deficiency, which is present in about a quarter of all adults, avoiding milk and milk products cures the diarrhea and flatulence. In tropical sprue and Whipple's disease (both diagnoses made by intestinal biopsy), antibiotics may be recommended. In pancreatic diseases malabsorption may be corrected by oral administration of pancreatic enzymes.

Meckel's Diverticulum

This is a congenital disorder in which a pouch forms near the lower end of the small intestine containing displaced acid-secreting gastric tissue. In a small number of individuals, mostly men, the pouch may rupture or bleed, causing abdominal pain and maroon-colored blood in the stool. If intestinal contents enter the abdominal cavity, *peritonitis* with fever and often severe abdominal pain may result. This condition is often confused with appendicitis *(see below)*.

Treatment. Bleeding and rupture of a Meckel's diverticulum are surgical emergencies. Removal of the abnormal pouch and treatment of peritonitis is curative.

Appendicitis

The appendix is a small, worm-like sac extending into the abdomen from the first (ascending) section of the colon. Although the appendix plays an important role in digestion in rabbits, it does nothing in humans, except become diseased. Inflammation usually occurs when the appendix becomes blocked by food or foreign particles, leading to infection and, if untreated, rupture into the abdomen causing peritonitis or abdominal abscess. The symptoms are abdominal pain, often localized to the lower right side of the abdomen, nausea, and vomiting.

Treatment. This is a surgical emergency. Removal of the inflamed appendix (appendectomy) and treatment of peritonitis is curative. If an abscess is found at the time of surgery, the abscess will be drained and treated with antibiotics. In this case removal of the diseased appendix will often be delayed until the abscess has healed.

Diverticular Disease *(Diverticulitis; Diverticulosis)*

Diverticula are small sac-like bubbles that form in the wall of the colon when increased colonic pressure forces their tiny balloon-like projections out through weakened sections of the colon wall. The presence of these diverticula is known as *diverticulosis*, which occurs in 30–40% of persons over 50 and increasingly every decade thereafter. In most people the diverticula cause no symptoms at all; or they may result in cramps and tenderness in the lower abdomen relieved only when you pass gas or move your bowels.

The two chief complications of diverticulosis are bleeding and inflammation *(diverticulitis).* Bleeding from diverticula results in bright red blood in the stool, your cue to see your doctor at once. Inflammation results in acute abdominal pain, most often in the lower left abdomen. Rupture of the diverticula can result in life-threatening peritonitis.

Treatment. Bleeding is a medical emergency. The site of bleeding can usually be localized by a fiberoptic tube inserted into the colon (endoscopy) or by X-rays. If the bleeding does not stop spontaneously, removal of part or all of the colon (colectomy) may be required.

When pain is the prominent symptom, the usual treatment is conservative hospitalization, bed rest, and taking nothing by mouth until the symptoms subside. If high fever suggests peritonitis or abscess formation as a consequence of rupture of the diverticula, antibiotics and pain medications are usually prescribed. In severe cases, surgical drainage of abscesses or colectomy may be required. In some cases diversion of the fecal stream through a colostomy may be necessary until the inflammation subsides.

If you previously had diverticulitis, or if your doctor discovers in routine sigmoidoscopy that you have diverticula, you should adopt a diet high in fiber (plenty of whole grain cereals, bran, fruits, and vegetables) and sufficient fluid intake to keep stools soft and bulky, to prevent future trouble. Remember—This diet is for life!

Tumors of the Small Intestine

Tumors of the small intestine are relatively rare and most are benign. Cancers of the small intestine are even rarer and cause few symptoms until they have spread—weight loss, tiredness, and, occasionally, black or bloody stools.

A rare small intestinal tumor, the *carcinoid* tumor, produces hormones that can cause sudden flushing, swollen and watery eyes, wheezing, and explosive diarrhea.

Treatment. Surgical removal and chemotherapy is the best current treatment regimen for small intestinal tumors.

Cancer of the Colon and Rectum

Colon cancer is the third most common cancer in the United States and the second most common cause of cancer deaths. In men and women over 40 years of age, it is the most common cancer. Most cancers originate in polyps, which are small growths in the mucous membranes lining the colon, particularly the lower colon and rectum. These cancers bleed easily, and hence blood in the stool is often the first sign of their presence. In rare cases, cancer obstructs the colon, causing constipation and bloating.

The chance of surviving colon cancer depends greatly upon how early the cancer is found and removed. With localized cancers, the chance of living 5 years after discovery is about 85%. If even minimal spread has occurred, this 5-year survival rate, is only about 37%. Thus, a program for early detection is important. *What can be done?*

1. *Digital rectal examination.* This test is a part of every physical examination and can detect low rectal cancers. It is recommended every year after age 40.
2. *Tests for blood in the stool.* These are chemical tests to detect small amounts of blood in the stool (called "occult blood," because the blood is not visible). Stool from three successive bowel movements should be tested. Such tests are recommended annually after age 40 (earlier if you have a family history of colon cancer). You can perform this test yourself using a home test kit currently marketed under the names HemoQuant, Hemoccult, and Early Detector. If you perform the test yourself, be sure to send the results to your doctor for his records.

   Note that certain substances can cause "false positive" test readings. Before collecting stool samples for testing, you should avoid red meat, turnips, horseradish, and high doses of vitamin C. Some evidence suggests that the HemoQuant test is less likely to give false positive readings. Follow the manufacturer's directions carefully. If blood is found, consult your doctor for further diagnoses, because many other conditions besides cancer can give positive results, including peptic ulcers, inflammatory bowel disease, diverticulitis, benign polyps, and hemorrhoids.
3. *Sigmoidoscopy.* The chief problem with stool blood tests is that they may give "false negative" results in some cases. A false negative result is a negative test when a cancer is present. The reason for this is that many early cancers do not bleed. Therefore, periodic sigmoidoscopy is recommended if you are over 50 years of age, or if you have a family history of colon cancer, or have previously had a polyp removed. A sigmoidoscope is a flexible tube that is used to directly visualize most of the lower colon and to biopsy any suspicious tissue. An examination every 3–5 years is recom-

mended. Only mild discomfort is involved, although the test is moderately expensive, your insurance may not pay for it, and the detection rate is not well established.

4. *Colonoscopy.* The colonoscope is a longer flexible tube that can visualize the entire colon. Colonoscopy is much more complicated than flexible sigmoidoscopy, may require anesthesia or sedation, and is quite expensive. It is recommended only for persons at high risk of having colon cancer:

- Anyone who has had active ulcerative colitis for 10 years or more.
- Anyone who has already had a bowel cancer or polyp removed. If you have had a rectal or lower colon polyp, there is a 20–35% chance of having another polyp elsewhere in the colon.
- Anyone with two first-degree relatives (parents, sibling, child) who have had bowel cancer or polyps.

Treatment. Surgical removal of the cancer is the first line of therapy. Radiation therapy and chemotherapy may be recommended if the cancer has spread.

For additional information about colon cancer, call the National Cancer Institute Cancer Information Service, 1-800-4-CANCER.

Disorders of the Anus

The *anus* is the short channel that leads from the rectum down through the ring of muscles of the anal sphincter, to the anal opening. Most of the medical problems of the anus stem from improper bowel habits and are thus preventable.

Hemorrhoids (Piles)

Hemorrhoids are like varicose veins in your anus. The anus is surrounded by a network of blood vessels that may become enlarged and swell outward under pressure. Such pressure comes from constipation and straining during bowel movements. Hemorrhoids may be either internal or external. External hemorrhoids protrude outside the anal opening and can easily be felt as small, smooth lumps. Internal hemorrhoids are not so easily felt, although if they protrude into the anal canal, they may give the sensation of having an incomplete bowel movement.

Distention of these veins slows blood flow and this in turn favors blood clot formation *(thrombosis).* Clotting causes further swelling and pain, especially during a bowel movement. If a swollen blood vessel ruptures, bleeding occurs, sometimes copiously. As the hemorrhoids heal, itching is usually a prominent feature.

Treatment. The most time-honored treatment of thrombosed hemorrhoids is sitting in a warm bath several times each day. Keep the anus clean and free of fecal matter by gently washing with warm soap and water. Such over-the-counter anal wipes as Tucks or cleansing creams, such as Balneol, may be soothing.

Suppositories are not clearly helpful and should be avoided. To prevent hemorrhoids, keep your stools soft in order to minimize trauma during bowel movements (*see* Constipation, p. 289).

If home treatment does not promptly relieve an acutely inflamed hemorrhoid, a surgeon can open the thrombosed vessel and remove the clot, which brings prompt relief. Internal hemorrhoids can be treated by banding, in which a tiny rubber band is slipped over the protruding vessel and left in place until it spontaneously sloughs off. The vessels can also be injected with a sclerosing agent, thus sealing off the distended veins. This is known as sclerotherapy. Laser beams and cryosurgery (freezing) have also been used to seal distended vessels. If these measures fail, surgical removal is a last resort.

Anal Itching

The skin around the anus is delicate and seems to have a natural readiness to itch. There are many causes of anal itching, including allergic reactions, oral antibiotics, fungal infections, parasites, hemorrhoids, and poor anal hygiene. The last is probably the most common cause.

Treatment. After a bowel movement, cleanse the anal area with absorbent cotton, moistened, if necessary, with plain water. Avoid using soap, as this tends to dry out your skin and aggravate itching. Apply talcum powder (never corn starch) between the buttocks if excessive moisture is a problem. Wear loose, absorbent underwear and nightwear.

In children, anal itching may be caused by pinworms. Children usually contract pinworms by swallowing the eggs shed by another child or an infected pet. The tiny white worms then hatch out in the intestine, mature, and lay eggs around the anus that cause intense itching, especially at night. The presence of eggs can be discovered by dabbing a strip of scotch tape over the child's anus in the morning before a bowel movement and examining for the presence of the tiny white eggs. If your doctor confirms the presence of pinworms, your whole family will have to be treated with medication to eradicate the worms. You will also have to thoroughly wash all of the child's clothing and bed linens. Pets should be treated by a veterinarian.

Anal Fissure and Fistula

An anal fissure is a crack in the delicate skin of the anal canal, usually from passing constipated stools. The fissures then become infected, causing pain and itching. Self treatment is the same as for hemorrhoids (*see* p. 303).

An anal *fistula* is a tiny tube-like communication between the anal canal and the skin around the anal orifice. Drainage of pus may cause anal irritation and itching. An underlying anal abscess may be quite painful. See your doctor. The fistula will probably have to be opened and drained.

Pilonidal Sinus

A pilonidal sinus occurs when hairs become trapped beneath the skin between the buttocks, usually just below the tip of the sacrum (the coccyx). When these hairs becomes infected, a small abscess forms, which then drains through a sinus to the surface of the skin. Usually the sinus will heal with warm sitz bathes and careful cleansing two or three times daily. If the sinus persists or recurs, it may have to be removed surgically.

Disorders of Your Liver and Gallbladder

The liver is the largest internal organ of the body and by far the most complex organ metabolically. Some of the many functions of the liver include:

- Clearing and neutralizing toxins from the blood.
- Forming bile, an important element in digestion.
- Storing iron for the bone marrow to be used in forming new red blood cells.
- Regulating carbohydrate metabolism.
- Manufacturing fats and cholesterol.
- Manufacturing essential enzymes and proteins.
- Breaking down and detoxifying drugs.
- Clearing bacteria and other particles from the blood.

Bile is a waste substance formed by the liver and collected by the gallbladder, which is essentially a bile reservoir. When you eat, the gallbladder contracts and empties the bile into the duode-num, the first section of the small intestine. Bile plays an important digestive function by helping to digest fats. Most of the bile is reab-sorbed in the small intestine, but some is eliminated in the stool and is responsible for its brown color.

The pancreas is also an important digestive organ. It manufactures digestive enzymes that help convert the food we eat to products eas-ily used by the body. Disorders of the pancreas are discussed later.

Jaundice

Jaundice is a condition in which the skin and whites of the eyes become yellow from excess bilirubin in the blood. Bilirubin is formed in the liver as a breakdown product of hemoglobin, the oxygen-car-rying molecule found in red blood cells. There are two main causes of jaundice: excess formation of bilirubin and impaired excretion of bilirubin from the liver and gallbladder so that the concentration of bilirubin in the blood rises. The most common cause of excess forma-tion is an abnormal destruction of red blood cells, known as hemolytic anemia (*see* p. 216). Common causes of impaired excretion of biliru-bin are liver cell diseases, such as hepatitis and cirrhosis, or else obstruction of the gallbladder or of the bile ducts within the liver leading to the gallbladder.

Often there are no other symptoms associated with jaundice than the skin and eye discolorations. If jaundice is severe, the stools may be pale, the urine may be dark (owing to bile excretion by the kid-neys), and generalized itching sometimes occurs.

Treatment. Jaundice must always be investigated by your doctor, who will carry out tests to discover the underlying cause. The most common causes of jaundice are described in the sections below.

Cirrhosis of the Liver

This is a chronic disease in which the internal architecture of the liver gradually becomes altered, and many of the normal liver cells are destroyed and gradually replaced by nonfunctioning tissue fibers in a process known as fibrosis. Gradually the ability of the liver to perform the many functions listed above becomes compromised. Cir-rhosis is the third leading cause of death, after heart disease and can-cer, in the United States in the 45–65-year-old age groups. Though there are many causes of cirrhosis, alcohol abuse is by far the most common. Malnutrition, toxic chemicals, chronic heart failure, obstruc-tion of the bile ducts, and hepatitis are other causes of cirrhosis.

Many people with cirrhosis show no symptoms at all until extensive liver damage has already occurred. Night sweats and heart irregularities may be early signs that cirrhosis is developing (*see* Alcohol and the Heart, p. 188). As liver damage progresses, tiredness, loss of appetite, weight loss, malaise, indigestion, and loss of libido are common. Men may notice enlargement of their breasts, as well as impotence. There is a tendency to bruise and bleed easily; nosebleeds may be common. Women may stop having menstrual periods. A characteristic skin feature is the appearance of numerous *spider nevi*, small red blood vessel clusters on the face, arms, and trunk that blanch when pressure is applied and then fill again when pressure is released.

As cirrhosis becomes severe, jaundice develops (*see* previous page). The abdomen may swell with fluid (ascites) and the feet and lower legs may swell with standing. In very advanced stages, mental confusion, and ultimately coma, are signs of *hepatic encephalopathy*. The latter is caused by a buildup of blood toxins the liver is incapable of neutralizing. Life-threatening bleeding into the esophagus may result from enlarged veins around it (esophageal varices).

Treatment. Regardless of cirrhosis' cause, alcohol is especially poisonous, even in small quantities. If you have difficulty stopping drinking, see your doctor and discuss the problem frankly. There are many effective alcohol abuse programs, and they can save your life.

Several other drugs may result in liver damage, and these should be discussed with your doctor. Maintain a nutritious diet high in protein, carbohydrates, and vitamins, and low in fats and salt.

The serious complications of cirrhosis, such as bleeding and encephalopathy, are treated in the hospital. In the case of hepatitis, treatment may include corticosteroids and immunosuppressive drugs.

Hepatitis

Hepatitis is an inflammation of the liver that has numerous causes. The most common are the hepatitis A, B, and C viruses, and alcohol. Less common causes are other viruses (Epstein-Barr, yellow fever, cytomegalovirus), bacteria (tuberculosis, streptococcus), fungi (histoplasmosis), protozoa (amebiasis, malaria, toxoplasmosis), worms (schistosomiasis), spirochetes (leptospirosis, syphilis), and drugs. Hepatitis may be either acute or chronic.

Acute Hepatitis A

This is a highly infectious disease and is responsible for regional epidemics of "infectious jaundice." It is contracted by coming in contact with contaminated feces and is usually spread through contaminated food or water. Eating contaminated raw shellfish is often responsible. The incubation period is from two to six weeks. The infectious period lasts two to three weeks before, and ends shortly after, hepatitis symptoms develop.

Hepatitis varies from a minor flu-like illness to overwhelming, fatal liver failure. During any acute bout of hepatitis, you may experience weakness, loss of appetite, malaise, fever, nausea, and vomiting. Jaundice, light-colored stools, and dark urine may also be present if bile drainage is impaired because of liver swelling (*see* Jaundice, p. 306). Interestingly jaundice often peaks after other symptoms have subsided. Jaundice usually lasts from two to four weeks. Hepatitis A does not cause chronic hepatitis, nor does it result in a chronic carrier state (prolonged period of infectiousness).

Treatment. As with any serious illness, if you suspect you have jaundice, you should see your doctor, who will order blood tests to diagnose viral hepatitis. Though there is no specific treatment for viral hepatitis, it is important to rule out other causes of jaundice that can be treated. You should limit your activities as long as you feel weakened; however, there is no good reason for bed rest. You should not go to work until jaundice has cleared and you are no longer infectious.

You must be meticulous in your cleanliness to avoid spreading infection to others in and outside your household. Do not share dishes or a bathroom with others if possible. You must avoid all alcohol during your illness and should only resume moderate drinking when your doctor so advises (usually three months after disappearance of all symptoms). Recovery is complete in most cases, and your subsequent immunity will be life-long.

Hepatitis B

The transmission of hepatitis B virus is thought to be primarily through contamination with the blood of infected individuals, hence its frequent occurrence among intravenous drug abusers and individuals with multiple sexual partners. Transmission through blood transfusions is now rare in developed countries, because of universal testing of banked blood. The incubation period is 6–25 weeks.

This is a much more serious disease than hepatitis A, because 5–10% of cases do not resolve spontaneously, but go on to fester as chronic hepatitis (*see* following page). The symptoms are the same as in hepatitis A, although they tend to be more severe and last longer. It is also possible to be infected without having any symptoms, a condition known as the "chronic carrier state." If you are a carrier, ask your doctor for recommendations about how to avoid transmitting hepatitis to others.

Treatment. Treatment of hepatitis B is the same as for hepatitis A. It is possible to be vaccinated against hepatitis B, and all high-risk individuals should be so protected. *See* p. 28 for a description of individuals at risk of contracting hepatitis B.

Hepatitis C

Formerly known as "non-A, non-B hepatitis virus," hepatitis C virus has now been characterized. It is transmitted by blood contamination or by sexual contact. Transmission through blood transfusions is now rare, because new testing methods reliably detect the virus in donated blood. The symptoms are similar to those of hepatitis B, but often milder, and may not include jaundice.

Chronic Hepatitis

In 5–10% of cases with hepatitis B and almost half of cases of hepatitis C, infection with the virus persists in the liver, giving rise to chronic hepatitis, which may take two forms: chronic persistent hepatitis and chronic active hepatitis. In chronic persistent hepatitis, there may be no, or only vague, symptoms; the disease eventually resolves; and no treatment is usually necessary.

In chronic active hepatitis, the inflammation of the liver is more serious and often goes on to cause liver failure, cirrhosis, or liver cancer. The symptoms vary from person to person. Intermittent bouts of symptoms similar to acute hepatitis may occur, along with jaundice and joint pains.

Treatment. In rare individuals, chronic hepatitis may be caused by drugs (e.g., methyldopa, isoniazid, acetaminophen); stopping the drugs usually stops the progression of the hepatitis. In those cases caused by viral infection, treatment with corticosteroids or the immune-suppressing drug, azathioprine, may be effective. Some recent studies suggest that alpha-interferon can slow, or even halt progression of chronic hepatitis.

Cancer of the Liver

There are two general types of liver cancer, metastatic and primary. Metastatic cancer results from spread to the liver from cancers elsewhere in the body, most often from the breast, lungs, and colon. Primary liver cancers arise from cells within the liver. The most common of these, hepatocellular cancer, frequently develops in those with long-standing cirrhosis. The symptoms of liver cancer are loss of appetite, weight loss, and general debility.

Treatment. Some liver cancers may be successfully treated by surgical removal. Most are treated by chemotherapy. The outlook is poor in all types of liver cancer.

For more information about liver cancer, call the Cancer Information Center of the National Cancer Institute: 1-800-4-CANCER.

Gallstones (Cholelithiasis)

Bile is a waste product formed by the liver and stored in the gallbladder until food entering the duodenum stimulates gallbladder contraction, emptying the bile into the common bile duct that connects to the duodenum. Bile principally aids in the digestion of fats.

Bile contains large amounts of cholesterol, which becomes greatly concentrated in the gallbladder, where much of the water is removed. In some people this concentration results in oversaturation, so that cholesterol crystals precipitate out to form gallstones. If these stones enter the bile duct and obstruct it, the result is severe abdominal pain as gallbladder and bile duct contractions increase to try to overcome the obstruction. Typically the pain (known as *biliary colic*) is located in the right upper abdomen, sometimes radiating backward to the right shoulder blade. Usually the pains last for several hours, rising to a crescendo and then subsiding. Nausea and vomiting are common, but there is no fever. Episodes of biliary colic may be separated by pain-free intervals of days or months. Many persons with gallstones also complain of indigestion after eating, including belching, bloating, and nausea, although these symptoms may also be caused by peptic ulcer (*see* p. 284).

Gallstones are common; 20% of persons over age 65 in the United States have them. They are more common in women by 4 to 1. Factors that dispose to gallstones include obesity, a Western diet high in fats and cholesterol, and a family history of gallstones. Interestingly, some people develop their first gallstone symptoms following a crash weight-loss diet. So-called "silent" gallstones are those that give rise to no symptoms and are discovered incidentally while investigating other conditions.

The diagnosis of gallstones is made principally by ultrasound, which accurately localizes both the gallstones and the dilated bile ducts in the liver that usually accompany symptomatic stones.

Treatment. Some people describe certain foods that tend to precipitate biliary colic. Avoidance of such foods and resisting overeating can greatly reduce your number of attacks. If pain does develop, go to bed and take a painkiller. Do not eat, but take sips of water. If the pain lasts longer than 3–4 hours, call your doctor.

There are several ways your doctor may treat your gallstones. The most common is surgical removal of the gallbladder (cholecystectomy) through an incision made in the upper right abdomen. In some cases the gallstones can be removed by means of laparoscopy, in which a small tube is passed through tiny incisions that heal quickly and avoids the three- to four-week recovery period involved with cholecystectomy. Removal of the gallbladder usually ends the pain and may also reduce symptoms of indigestion. Cholecystectomy does not result in any nutritional problem, since bile simply enters directly into the duodenum. In rare cases, stones can form in the bile duct, even after cholecystectomy, and result in renewed symptoms.

Gallstones can also be treated by taking bile salts orally. Over a period of time the bile salts tend to dissolve the stones, thus preventing symptoms. Similarly, gallstone formation during dieting can be prevented by taking bile salts. The chief disadvantage of this form of treatment is that the gallstones often recur when the bile salts are discontinued.

Biliary *lithotripsy* can be used to "blast" the stones into tiny fragments that can be passed without causing symptoms. This technique is similar to kidney stone lithotripsy (*see* p. 330). It uses high-intensity sound waves focused on the stones to literally break the stones apart. With current techniques about 20% of persons with gallstones may be candidates for biliary lithotripsy. Of course, as with bile salt therapy, the stones have a tendency to reform because you still have a gallbladder.

Another new technique is to dissolve the stone with solvents. A delivery tube is either passed from the duodenum up the bile duct and into the gall bladder, or inserted through a large needle passed through the rib cage and liver and into the gallbladder. The solvent, a type of ether, is then instilled, dissolving the stones in a matter of hours. This procedure carries several risks and is probably most appropriate only for those in whom surgery is risky.

Cholecystitis

This is an acute inflammation of the gallbladder, most often caused by obstruction of the gallbladder's duct by a gallstone.

The symptoms include severe pain in the upper abdomen, similar to the pain caused by gallstones, which most patients with acute cholecystitis have experienced at some time in the past. Nausea, vomiting, and low-grade fever are also common.

Treatment. The pain of acute cholecystitis usually subsides in 2–3 days with bed rest and intravenous fluids to avoid stimulating the gallbladder. Painkillers and antibiotics are also given as needed. If radiographic tests show that the gallbadder is obstructed, cholecystectomy is usually recommended.

Hemochromatosis

This is an uncommon disease caused by iron overload in the body. In most cases it is caused by a genetically determined error in which too much iron is absorbed from a normal diet. It can also be caused by repeated transfusions of blood (*see* Thalassemia, p. 217). Hemochromatosis is primarily a disease of older individuals because it takes many years to accumulate excess iron.

Most of the excess iron is stored in the liver, where it eventually causes liver enlargement and a type of cirrhosis. There is often a peculiar bronzing of the skin because of iron deposited in the skin. Other symptoms include arthritis, impotence in men, cessation of menstruation in women, and diabetes mellitus. Once the diagnosis is suspected, it is easily proven by a blood test that reveals excess iron in the blood. This is then usually confirmed by a liver biopsy, which stains blue from the presence of iron.

Treatment. The treatment is literally bloodletting. Removal of a pint of iron-rich blood per week causes the bone marrow to draw upon the body's stores of iron. After about a year of this treatment, the iron stores are returned to normal, and then only occasional bleeding is required.

Disorders of Nutrition and Metabolism

Nutritional disorders involve primarily eating too much or too little food or vitamins. Metabolic disorders, on the other hand, are chiefly genetic problems that alter the way some nutritional element is utilized in the body. Although metabolic disorders are relatively rare, nutritional disorders are widely prevalent. By far the most common nutritional disorder is obesity.

Obesity

More than 34 million people in the United States are obese. This makes obesity one of the most prevalent health problems in the nation. Obesity is defined as excessive accumulation of body fat. But what is excessive? What is pleasingly plump, and what is obesity? The most common criterion that doctors use to determine whether you are obese says that you are obese when you are 20% or more over your "desirable" weight. See the *box on the following page* to find the desirable weight range for your height and sex. These ranges are based on the Metropolitan Life Insurance Company tables, which define the weight ranges that are compatible with the longest life. In other words, insurers of people's lives clearly recognize that you are likely to live less long if you are beyond a certain weight range.

Note that the ranges in this table are rather wide. This is because there is broad variability in the weight of such other tissues as bone and muscle. There is also a general tendency to gain weight with age without necessarily having adverse health consequences. As a first approximation in determining whether you are more than 20% above your desirable weight, use the average of the range. For example, if you are a woman of 5 ft, 6 in. height, the average of 118–150 is 134 pounds. Twenty percent more than this is about 161 pounds. Unless you have exceptional muscle development, it is likely that you are mildly obese if you weigh more than 161 pounds, and you may want to consider a weight-reduction program. If you have any doubt, consult your doctor.

Another way of determining desirable weight that many doctors use is to calculate your body mass index (BMI). You get this figure by dividing your weight in kilograms by the square of your height measured in meters. To do this:

1. First convert your weight to kilograms by dividing your weight in pounds by 2.2.
2. Convert your height in inches to height in meters by dividing by 39.4. Then square this number. A calculator helps.
3. Divide (1) by (2) to determine your BMI.

For men, a desirable BMI is 22 to 24. Above 28.5 suggests mild obesity. Above 33 indicates serious obesity.

For women, a desirable BMI is 21 to 23. Mild obesity occurs above 27.5 and serious obesity begins above 31.5.

Desirable Weight Chart
1990 Dietary Guidelines for Americans

Height (without shoes)	Weight (without clothes)	
	Age 19–34*	35 and older*
5'0"	97–128	108–138
5'1"	101–132	111–143
5'2"	104–137	115–148
5'3"	107–141	119–152
5'4"	111–146	122–157
5'5"	114–150	126–162
5'6"	118–155	130–167
5'7"	121–160	134–172
5'8"	125–164	138–178
5'9"	129–169	142–183
5'10"	132–174	146–188
5'11"	136–179	151–194
6'0"	140–184	155–199
6'1"	144–189	159–205
6'2"	148–195	164–210
6'3"	152–200	168–216

*Women or men.

Note: These weight guidelines have been published jointly by the US Department of Health and Human Services and the US Department of Agriculture and generally replace the old Metropolitan Life Insurance tables issued in 1959. The most important differences between this and older "ideal" weight charts is that frame size and sex are no longer considered, but age is.

Obesity is far from a mere cosmetic problem, and fat people delude themselves in believing that their weight is only a matter of personal preference. In fact excess fat affects more body organs and disorders than almost any other health factor. Here are the most important consequences of obesity:

- *Diabetes.* Diabetes can be brought on by obesity in adults and worsens the severity in those who already have it (*see* p. 168). The reason is that insulin is required to store excess sugar in the form of fat. As fat cells become overloaded, they become more resistant to the action of insulin. This causes blood sugar levels to rise, resulting in diabetes. The process usually reverses as weight is lost.
- *Cardiovascular disease.* Obese people have larger hearts, presumably because of the increased energy needed to drive blood through the extra blood vessels supplying fatty tissue. Obesity raises blood pressure, which increases the risk of heart attacks and stroke. Obesity also tends to raise blood cholesterol, another risk factor in heart disease and stroke.
- *Bone and joint disorders.* Excess weight places greater stress on both bones and cartilage, worsening the degenerative joint disease known as osteoarthritis (*see* p. 409). The weight-bearing joints—the hips, knees, and ankles—are most affected.
- *Cancer.* Obese women have a higher death rate from cancer of the gallbladder, breast, cervix, endometrium, uterus, and ovaries. Obese men tend to have higher death rates from cancer of the colon, rectum, and prostate.
- *Other problems.* Obesity has been shown to contribute to the seriousness of such diverse disorders as cirrhosis of the liver, gallstones, kidney stones, varicose veins, and blood clots.
- *Early death.* Obesity, especially that developed early in life, tends to shorten lifespan; the greater its degree, the higher the excess death rate. In extreme obesity, when weight is twice normal, a condition known as *Pickwickian* syndrome may result. Here obesity is so great that respiration is affected, threatening death by asphyxiation.

Treatment. The reason you add fat to your body is that you expend through exercise and metabolism fewer calories than you consume. Thus there are two ways of taking fat off: eat less and exercise more. Naturally this is simplistic and fails to recognize that any weight reduction program worth the hunger and sacrifice must not only take fat off, it must keep it off.

There are literally hundreds of diets you will find in books, magazines, and television. Each year another celebrity announces a "new" diet and practically every chic suburb in America has its diet: Beverly Hills, Southampton, Scarsdale. Most of these will work as well as any other if you are "mildly" obese, i.e., less than 40% above your desirable weight. *But you should avoid diets that:*

- Emphasize one particular food (for instance, yogurt or grapefruit) above all others.
- Omit one particular food group, e.g., the high-protein, low-carbo-hydrate diets that may take off pounds tend also to take off muscle as well as fat—just what you don't want.
- Advise megadoses of vitamin and mineral supplements. The diet you select should provide all of the nutritional elements that you need in the foods you eat.
- Advance fanciful theories of weight reduction, such as the need for a special "cleansing" regimen to eliminate body toxins.
- Recommend that you take fewer than 1200 calories per day, unless you are under medical supervision. Very low-calorie diets can cause severe disability and even death, unless carefully monitored by a doctor experienced in weight management. Remember, too, that on a diet of less than 1200 calories per day, you will lose muscle as well as fat.

WHAT TO LOOK FOR

If you are dieting on your own, *select a diet that:*

- Emphasizes low-calorie, highly nutritious foods, such as fruits, whole grains, and vegetables.
- Is geared to slow weight loss, rather than a "take-pounds-off-fast" diet. Though less dramatic, a diet that takes off 1 or 2 lbs. per week will be easier to stick to and live with over the years. Crash diets have a very poor track record of winning long-term adherents.
- Provides variety to avoid the boring experience of eating the same thing week after week. The diet should also offer advice about what to do when you eat out or travel.

A pound of body fat equals 3500 calories. To lose a pound of fat in a week, you must on average consume 500 calories less each day, or burn 500 calories more each day, than when you were just keeping your weight even.

The number of calories you gain from alcoholic beverages can be calculated using the following formula (for one double martini):

Number of ounces × proof × 0.8 = 2 × 80 × 0.8 = 128 calories

Most drinks contain sugars and other carbohydrates that also add to your caloric intake. If you drink excessively, your alcoholic drinks add greatly to your total caloric intake.

DIET STRATEGIES THAT WORK

- Adopt a regular exercise or sports program. For most people, this is the key to keeping weight off once you have reached your weight-reduction goal.
- Eat slowly. Eating is pleasurable, so extend the pleasure without gorging yourself. A diet that emphasizes more frequent, but smaller, meals is often more successful than the standard three meals per day.
- Limit your intake of butter, ice cream, cheese, salad dressings, and oils. Dieting is a life-long necessity, so it is essential that you change your eating habits. In this way eating will seem much less like dieting, for which we all have unpleasant associations.
- Bake, broil, and poach foods instead of frying or sautéing in fat.
- Seek diet counseling and join a support group. They work because overeating is much like an addiction. Falling off a diet is much like a smoker's relapse. But if you keep at it, you will adopt healthier eating habits that gradually replace your old inclination to eat whenever and whatever you wanted. You won't have difficulty finding plenty of company. At any given time, 65 million Americans are on some sort of diet.
- Reduce your alcohol intake. Alcohol represents "empty" calories, i.e., the alcohol goes straight to fat and provides no other nutritional value.

For information on choosing a nutritionist, write for the booklet of the American Dietetic Association, 430 N. Michigan Ave., Chicago, IL 60611.

PILLS AND POTIONS

Many products are sold in drugstores, health food stores, clinics, and salons that are promoted to help you lose weight. These should be used with caution. Some of the many include:

- *Amphetamines.* These are prescription-only appetite suppressants. Their use in treating obesity is severely limited because of their addiction potential. They are also stimulants and raise blood pressure.
- *Phenylpropanolamine.* This is a decongestant preparation that also suppresses appetite. It is the principal ingredient in such over-the-counter preparations as Dexatrim and Accutrim. In combination with a reduced-calorie diet they are effective for many people. These

preparations should be used with great caution in those with high blood pressure, diabetes, thyroid or kidney problems. Common side effects include nervousness, sleeplessness, headaches and irregular heart rhythm.

- *Benzocaine.* This is an anesthetic that is added to dietary candies and gums. It numbs the tongue and blunts the sense of taste. These may be for you if you think you are deriving too much pleasure from eating!
- *Others.* A host of other unproven dietary preparations includes the amino acids, arginine, ornithine, and phenylalanine. Phenylalanine is supposedly the active ingredient in spirulina, a pond algae that some health food stores promote. There is no good scientific evidence that any of these is effective in weight reduction.

Especially avoid diet aids that contain guar or gum arabic that swell upon contact with water and produce a nondigestable mass in the stomach that quickly makes you feel full. These masses can result in dangerous intestinal obstruction.

Even if a diet pill works for you temporarily, the weight will come right back on unless you adopt permanent dietary habits to limit your calories and an exercise program to burn more calories.

Your body will quickly accommodate to any diet pill so that its effect will be gradually neutralized.

Surgery for Obesity

Surgical procedures such as stapling a portion of the stomach closed, or banding to narrow the entrance to the stomach, or bypass procedures that reroute food past the stomach can be effective, but because of their many possible complications, they are only appropriate for seriously obese people for whom dieting has failed and who are in danger of medical complications of obesity *(see above).*

Liposuction, the insertion of tubes under the skin to suck out fat, is a cosmetic procedure that has little to do with correcting obesity.

Anorexia Nervosa and Bulimia

These are two of the most common eating disorders. Anorexia nervosa is characterized by compulsive starvation, often to the point of emaciation. Bulimia, on the other hand is more common among obese women who alternate binge eating with self-induced vomiting. These are primarily psychological and psychosocial disorders and will not be discussed. However, there are a variety of resources from which to learn more about causes and treatments of eating disorders:

American Anorexia Nervosa Association Inc., 133 Cedar Lane, Teaneck, NJ 07666.

National Anorexia Aid Society Inc., PO Box 29461, Columbus, OH 43229.

Anorexia Nervosa and Associated Disorders, Suite 2020, 550 Frontage Rd., Northfield, IL 60093.

Why Are They Starving Themselves? Understanding Anorexia Nervosa and Bulimia, by Elaine Landau, Stein & Day, 1984.

Porphyria

There are actually several different types of porphyria, all of which are genetic (missing gene) disorders involving an enzyme deficiency that results in a buildup of chemicals in the body called *porphyrins.* These chemicals are in fact the building blocks of hemoglobin, the oxygen-carrying molecule in red blood cells. Porphyrins accumulate in the liver, brain, and skin, where they can do harm and cause a wide variety of symptoms.

The symptoms of porphyria depend upon the exact type of porphyrin that occurs in excess. They include episodes of vomiting, abdominal pain, weakness, muscle cramps, itching, and psychological disturbances. Symptoms usually begin in early adulthood and may be precipitated by taking certain drugs, such as barbiturates or birth control pills, by alcohol, pregnancy, or even exposure to too much sunlight. Obviously these are all quite nonspecific symptoms, which is why porphyria is difficult to diagnose early in the course of the disease.

Treatment. At this time there is no cure, such as gene replacement, that can restore the functioning of the deficient enzyme. The principal management of porphyria relies on preventing attacks by avoiding those factors that are known to precipitate them. Certain drugs and a high carbohydrate diet may also limit attacks. Specific recommendations must be supplied by your doctor according to type of porphyria.

Deficiencies of Vitamin and Minerals

Vitamins are chemical compounds found in foods that do not supply energy, but are essential to the smooth functioning of the body's numerous metabolic processes. Many are needed to transform the food we eat into the energy the body uses in all its life functions. Most vitamins are needed in only minute quantities, and some, like vitamin D and niacin, can be manufactured by the body. However, when essential vitamins, i.e., those not made by the body, are lacking from our diet, symptoms of vitamin deficiency gradually develop.

Minerals are simple, naturally occurring elements that the body requires for normal functioning and to maintain electrolyte balance. They are found in adequate quantities in a balanced diet.

Vitamin and mineral deficiencies are uncommon in this country because of the varied and abundant foods we eat, because many food products are vitamin-fortified and because nourishing foods are almost everywhere available year-round. When deficiencies do occur, they usually result from faulty eating—such as the faddish, highly restricted diets so widely promulgated in our society—or from alcoholism, extreme poverty, malabsorption (*see* p. 299), kidney disease, or prolonged illness.

Tables 1 and 2 show the essential vitamins and minerals, their sources, the effects of deficiency, and their recommended daily allowances (RDA).

How do you know whether you need to take vitamin or mineral supplements? Everyone knows that these supplements are overpromoted. Furthermore, it is generally recognized that healthy men and women, including the elderly, who eat balanced diets do not need vitamin and mineral supplements. There are some individuals, however, who may consider taking these supplements:

- *Vegetarians.* Infants and children on a strict vegetarian diet may become deficient in vitamins B_{12}, D, and riboflavin. Intake of these vitamins will be adequate if appropriately fortified soy formula or fortified soybean milk drink is used. Intake of vitamin B_{12} may be inadequate in adult vegetarians unless their diets include milk or milk products (lactovegetarian diet) or eggs.
- *Dieters.* Even with supervised dieting, it may be difficult to meet recommended vitamin intakes on diets of 1000 calories or less. This merely reinforces the fact that all individuals on very low-calorie diets should be periodically evaluated by their doctors.
- *Eating disorder sufferers.* Those who struggle with such eating disorders as anorexia nervosa or binge–purge syndrome (bulimia) may

suffer vitamin deficiencies. Naturally more comprehensive treatment is needed for such people than mere vitamin supplements.

- *Pregnant women.* If you are pregnant or nursing an infant, your need for many vitamins and minerals increases. Ask your doctor whether you need supplements.
- *Menstruating women.* Particularly heavy menstrual bleeding may require iron supplements for iron-deficiency anemia (*see* p. 213). Remember that vitamin C enhances iron absorption, so that all menstruating women should include plenty of such foods as citrus fruits, tomatoes, potatoes, cabbages, and green peppers.
- Alcoholics should consider supplements of vitamin C (an antioxidant) and magnesium.

Drug Interactions

Several drugs interfere with vitamin absorption when taken for prolonged periods. Some common examples are:

- Cholestyramine, used to treat high serum cholesterol interferes with the absorption of the fat-soluble vitamins, A, D, E, and K.
- Mineral oil, taken daily by some who abuse laxatives, also interferes with the absorption of vitamins A, D, E, and K.
- Vitamins A and E, taken in large doses, can interfere with vitamin K absorption.
- Sulfasalazine, used in the treatment of regional enteritis and ulcerative colitis, may necessitate supplements of folic acid.
- Antibiotics taken for prolonged periods may necessitate supplements of vitamin K and some B vitamins.
- Dilantin, used in the treatment of seizures, may necessitate supplements of vitamins D and K and folic acid.
- Isoniazid, used in treating tuberculosis and some other infections, may require supplements of pyridoxine.

If you take vitamins, keep in mind that you should take them with meals to aid in the absorption of the fat-soluble vitamins. Megadoses of vitamins are never appropriate unless prescribed by your doctor. Large doses, especially of vitamins A and D, may have severe toxic effects. Though both vitamin A and vitamin C appear to have a protective effect against certain cancers, there is no evidence that supplements are superior to a well-balanced diet. Magnesim supplements should not be taken by people with kidney failure.

Table 1
The Principal Vitamins

Vitamin	Principal sources	USRDA Adults	Pregnant/ lactating	Deficiency symptons
A	Liver, butter, egg yolk, fortified and milk and derived products	M: 1000 µg F: 1200 µg	1200–1300 µg	Dryness of eyes, loss of night vision, blindness, dry skin and mucous membranes, diminished resistance to infection
(Carotene)	Green and yellow vegetables, carrots, tomatoes, cantaloupe, and other colored fruits and vegetables	(1 µg = 6 µg beta-carotene)		
D	Manufactured in human skin exposed to sunlight, fortified milk and related products, fish oils	M: 400 IU (6–24 yr) (all others) 200 IU (400 IU = 10 µg cholecalciferol)	400 IU	Inability to absorb calcium from the diet. Rickets in infants and children, osteomalcia in adults.
E	Eggs, fish, dairy products, fruits, vegetables, and grains	M: 10 µg F: 8 µg	10–12 µg	Never been observed in normal persons. In cystic fibrosis and disorders of the digestive system, damage to blood cells and to the nervous system may occur.
K	Green leafy vegetables, soy beans, eggs, dairy products, fruits, and grains	M: 80 µg (25+ yr) F: 65 µg		Bleeding from defective clotting of the blood.
Thiamine	Green vegetables, cereals, beans, milk, pork, beef, fortified flour and derived products	M: 1.2–1.5 µg (11+ yr) F: 1.0–1.1 µg	1.5–1.6 µg	Beriberi, a disease characterized by weakness, fatigue, loss of appetite, apathy, depression, constipation, memory loss, disordered function of the heart, nerves, and brain.

Table 1 *(continued)*

Vitamin	Principal sources	USRDA Adults	Pregnant/ lactating	Deficiency symptons
Niacin (Nicotinic acid)	Meat, poultry, dairy products, fortified flour and derived products	M: 15–20 µg (11+ yr) F: 13–15 µg	17–20 µg	Pellagra, a disease characterized by weakness, depression, insomnia, and the "3Ds": dermatitis, diarrhea, and dementia.
Riboflavin	Dairy products, meat, eggs, vegetables, enriched flour and derived products	M: 1.5–1.8 µg (11+ yr) F: 1.2–1.3 µg	1.6–1.8 µg	Sore throat, inflammation of face, lips, and tongue, anemia.
B_6 (Pyridoxine)	Whole grains, fruits, vegetables, dried beans, eggs, nuts, meat, poultry	M: 1.7–2.0 µg (11+ yr) F: 1.4–1.6 µg	2.1–2.2 µg	Convulsions may occur in infants totally deprived of vitamin.
Biotin	Milk, eggs, cereal	30–100 µg		Dry and inflamed skin, loss of hair.
Pantothenic acid	Whole grains, dried beans, milk, eggs, fruits, vegetables, meat	4–7 µg		Not clearly defined.
B_{12}	Milk, eggs, meat, fish	2.0 µg	P: 2.2 µg L: 2.6 µg	Anemia, nerve damage, behavioral disturbances.
Folic acid (Folate, Folacin)	Whole grains, green leafy vegetables, beans	M: 200 µg (15+ yr) F: 180 µg	P: 400 µg L: 260–280 µg	Anemia, behavioral disturbances, complications of pregnancy.
C (Ascorbic acid)	Citrus fruits, vegetables, and other fruits	60 mg	P: 70 mg L: 90–95 mg	Scurvy, a disease characterized by abnormal bleeding, defective connective tissue with possible loss of teeth, weakness, death.

µg = micrograms; IU = international units; mg = milligrams; P = pregant, L = lactating.

Table 2
The Principal Minerals*

Mineral	Principal sources	USRDA (mg) Adults	Pregnant/ lactating	Deficiency symptons
Calcium	Milk products, meat, eggs, fish, cereals	M: 800–1200 F: 1200	1200	Bone loss and fractures; tetany
Phosphorus	Milk products, meat, eggs, ceareals, nuts	800–1200	1200	Uncommon
Magnesium	Seafood, vegetables, cereals	280–350	340	Neuromuscular tremors, growth failure
Iron	Meat, eggs, cereals, beans	10–15	30	Tiredness, pallor, anemia
Iodine	Seafood, iodized salt, milk	0.15	0.175–0.25	Enlarged thyroid gland
Zinc	Seafood, meat, nuts, vegetables	12–15	19	Poor wound healing
Copper	Shellfish, nuts, cereals, liver	1.5–3.0	1.5–3.0	Uncommon
Chromium	Milk, meat, cereals	0.05	0.05	Worsens diabetes
Selenium	Meats, vegetables, cereals	0.05–0.07	0.05	Uncommon
Manganese	Vegetables, cereals	2.0–5.0	2.0–5.0	Uncommon
Fluoride	Vegetables, cereals, water supply supplement	1.5–4.0	1.5–4.0	Tooth decay

*Source: Recommended Dietary Allowances, Revised 1989, Food and Nutrition Board, National Academy of Sciences—National Research Council.

Some doctors, either unscrupulously or through misinformation, give patients vitamin B_{12} shots (sometimes called "liver shots") to "pep" them up. For practical purposes, the only condition that requires B_{12} shots is pernicious anemia (see p. 214). If you have not been specifically diagnosed with this disorder, you probably don't need B_{12} shots.

Another vitamin myth concerns the so-called "stress vitamins." These are high-potency formulas that usually contain vitamins C,

E, and B-complex. They are often advertised as "the vitamins for people living in the fast lane," especially students and business executives. Such special formulas are quite unnecessary since all of these vitamins are adequately contained in any balanced diet and there is no evidence at all that they help those facing psychological stress in any way.

Despite many claims made for it, vitamin E doesn't heal wounds, retard aging, affect heart disease, or enhance sexual performance. It is an antioxidant, like vitamin C and beta carotene, and may have a role in cancer prevention. However, this role has yet to be clearly defined.

Finally, a word of caution: Never attempt to treat yourself for what you believe may be a vitamin deficiency, since appropriate diagnosis and treatment may thereby be delayed. Always see your doctor.

For a list of the US Department of Agriculture's nutrition pamphlets, write to the Human Nutrition Information Service, Room 325A, 6505 Belcrest Road, Hyattsville, MD 20782.

Cross-section of the urinary system

Kidneys

Cortex

Medulla

Renal pelvis

Ureter

Bladder

Urethra

Your Urinary Tract

Introduction

The body can be thought of as a small, but complex chemical factory, energized by the food we eat and constantly producing chemical byproducts to serve growth and metabolism. Like any chemical factory, there are wastes to be disposed of and this is the kidney's chief function.

The kidney consists of millions of tiny units, called *glomeruli*, that continuously filter the blood, remove wastes and water, and excrete them in the form of urine. Urine is drained through the narrow tubular ureters to the bladder. From the bladder, the urine is expelled through another narrow tube, the urethra. The entire system of kidneys, ureters, bladder, and urethra is known as the urinary tract.

The primary medical disorders of the urinary tract can be grouped under infections, obstruction, vascular disorders, stone formation, tumors, and trauma.

Infection and Inflammation

Pyelonephritis

Normally the urine is sterile, containing no bacteria. When bacteria do enter the urinary tract, it is usually from below, i.e., up the urethra to the bladder and/or kidneys. More rarely, bacteria reach the kidneys from other parts of the body through the blood. When the kidneys become infected the condition is known as *pyelonephritis*, which may be either acute or chronic.

During acute pyelonephritis, you may experience chills, high fever, nausea, vomiting, and back pain that often spreads around to the groin. If the bladder is also infected, you may additionally experience frequent and burning urination. Acute pyelonephritis is more common in women, because of their shorter urethras.

Treatment. Your doctor will treat you with antibiotics as soon as the type of bacteria has been determined by urine culture. Bed rest, a bland diet, and increased fluid intake are important supportive measures. In children and adults who have frequent infections, additional X-rays and possibly direct visualization of the bladder through a tube inserted into the urethra, a procedure called *cystoscopy*, may be recommended.

Chronic Pyelonephritis

Repeated bouts of kidney infection occurring over several years can lead to gradual scarring and destruction of the kidneys. This condition is often associated with urinary reflux, wherein the normal valve action of the ureters that prevents backward flow of urine from the bladder to the kidneys is impaired. Ultimately kidney failure (*see* pp. 332) and high blood pressure may develop.

Treatment. Antibiotics are prescribed to eliminate infection. Sources of obstruction, such as kidney stones (*see below*) must be treated. If reflux of urine from the bladder into the kidneys occurs, valve action can be restored by surgical correction of the ureters. Your doctor will recommend that you drink plenty of fluids and avoid large quantities of proteins and salt in your diet.

Glomerulonephritis

Glomerulonephritis is a term used to describe several different diseases that effect the glomeruli, the tiny filtration units that produce the urine. Often it is caused by the attachment of blood proteins to the glomeruli, with the result that they become inflamed and cease functioning properly. If enough of the glomeruli become involved, kidney function as a whole is disrupted and kidney failure and high blood pressure result. The symptoms vary with the severity of the disease. In the mildest form, there are no symptoms. As the disease progresses, fatigue and a general feeling of being unwell (malaise) develops.

The diagnosis of glomerulonephritis is usually made by examining the urine and by kidney biopsy, in which a needle is inserted into the kidney, and a small core of tissue is extracted and examined under a microscope to determine the specific cause.

Treatment. The treatment depends on the biopsy results. Often the only effective treatment is corticosteroids to decrease the inflammatory process long enough for the condition to resolve spontaneously. If the disease does not resolve, kidney failure results, necessitating dialysis or kidney transplant.

Cystitis *(Bladder Infection)*

Cystitis is caused by bacterial infection of the bladder. Bacteria usually enter the bladder from the urethra. Consequently bladder infections are much more common in women because of their shorter ure-thras. It is thus not surprising that bladder infections commonly are caused by intercourse because pressure on the urethra may force bacteria upward into the bladder, and also often arise during pregnancy, when the pressure of the fetus on the bladder causes temporary obstruction. In men bladder infections are rare, and when they do occur, are most often associated with infections of the prostate gland (*see* p. 379) or with the presence of bladder stones.

The symptoms of bladder infections are pain or burning with urination (*dysuria*) and a frequent urge to urinate in small quantities. Often you will experience a dull or burning pain just below the naval where the bladder is located. Fever and bloody urine are uncommon and are signs that you should consult your doctor at once.

Treatment. Drink large quantities of water and empty your bladder as completely as possible. It may help to alkalinize your urine by taking one-half teaspoon of baking soda in a half glass of water every 3–4 hours. Do not continue this treatment longer than 48 hours. Your doctor may prescribe antibiotics, which quickly relieve the symptoms. Your doctor may also prescribe a urinary analgesic to be taken only as long as dysuria persists. Bladder infections in men should prompt tests to discover the underlying cause of the infection.

Prevention. Women should always wipe themselves from front to back after a bowel movement to avoid introducing fecal material into the vagina. Women should also try to empty their bladders soon after intercourse to wash out any bacteria that may have entered the urethra.

Trauma to the Kidney and Bladder

The kidney is well protected from injury by the ribs and back muscles. However, it may be injured by a blow to the body, especially during an automobile accident or contact sports. The most common symptoms are back pain and blood in the urine (*hematuria*). Usually, injuries to the kidney and ureter heal themselves. You will probably be hospitalized for observation to make sure you do not bleed internally. In the unlikely event that healing does not occur, the kidney may require removal. You can lead a normal, healthy life with only one kidney because the remaining kidney enlarges in compensation.

Trauma to the bladder is also rare, because it is very well protected by the pelvis. Surgical repair is required in cases of rupture of the bladder. Trauma to the urethra usually resolves by itself.

Cysts, Stones, and Tumors

Kidney Cysts

Cysts are fluid-filled sacs that have no outlet and so continue to enlarge over time. There are two types, single and multiple. Single cysts are benign, unless a tumor develops within the cyst. They usually cause no symptoms, except when they become large enough to bleed or press on surrounding organs.

Multiple cysts are known as *polycystic disease* and are congenital. These cysts also do not cause symptoms, unless they become so extensive as to cause obstruction of the kidney *(hydronephrosis)* or become infected.

Single cysts are most often discovered coincidentally during tests for other conditions. Because of the slight risk of malignancy, your doctor may perform an ultrasound examination to determine the cyst's size and consistency. In some cases it may be decided to aspirate fluid from the cyst through a long needle to examine the cells within the cyst fluid. If these cells are normal, nothing further need be done.

Treatment. Single cysts may be removed if they are large enough to cause discomfort or if malignant cells are found. There is no specific treatment for polycystic disease. If the disease progresses to the point of kidney failure, kidney transplantation or chronic dialysis may be required to prevent uremia and death.

Kidney Stones

Kidney stones form in the urine collecting system of the kidneys. They begin as small crystals that precipitate out of the urine when certain substances become too concentrated to remain dissolved. There are several types of kidney stones, although most are formed of calcium oxalate. Kidney stones are more common in men and are more common in whites than in blacks.

Small stones may pass out the ureter without symptoms. Stones larger than about five millimeters (about 1/5-inch) are too large to pass through the ureters and grow gradually over several years. If they become too large, they may obstruct the kidney, causing it to swell *(hydronephrosis)*. They may also erode the kidney, causing bleeding into the urine.

Intermediate-sized stones may pass through the ureter, distending and abrading it during passage, and causing acute bleeding and

---

MANAGING YOUR KIDNEY STONES

- Drink lots of water, at least 10 glasses per day. This dilutes the urine, preventing precipitation of calcium into stones.
- Avoid eating large quantities of meat, which contains high levels of uric acid found in many kidney stones.
- The role of dietary calcium in contributing to stone formation is controversial. Ask your doctor for a diet appropriate for you.
- Restrict the use of vitamin C to less than 1000 milligrams daily. A byproduct of vitamin C metabolism is oxalic acid, found in most kidney stones.
- Avoid foods high in oxalic acid, such as spinach, rhubarb, black pepper, and nuts.
- Depending upon the type of stones you form, your doctor may prescribe medications, such as allopurinol or thiazide diuretics, to prevent stone formation.

---

excruciating pain. This pain, known as "renal colic," has been called one of the severest pains humans are called upon to bear. The intermittent, stabbing pain begins in the back and, during passage of the stone down the ureter, gradually travels around the hip, and into the groin. The pain almost always occurs on one side of the body at a time, but if you are subject to stone formation, a subsequent attack may occur on the other side.

Treatment. During passage of the stone, treatment consists of controlling pain with analgesics or narcotics, depending upon the severity of pain. Large quantities of fluids should be drunk to facilitate passage of the stone. If the stone becomes trapped in the lower ureter, it may be removed under anesthesia by passing a cystoscope into the ureter and snaring the stone.

If the stone is too large to pass through the ureter, it may require surgical removal. Recently, *shockwave lithotripsy* has been developed to break up the stone while it is still in the kidneys. This device generates powerful sound waves and focuses them on the kidney stone. When they strike the stone, it is fractured into pieces sufficiently small to pass through the ureter.

Prevention. If you have had a kidney stone, you may be suffering a type of metabolic disease. Though there is not a great deal of scientific evidence for support, there are a number of measures generally recommended to reduce the number of symptomatic episodes of renal colic; these are outlined in the box on the previous page.

Kidney Failure

Kidney failure (renal failure) may be either acute or chronic. In acute kidney failure, the kidneys suddenly stop functioning, or more often, slow down their functioning. There are numerous causes, but most often the failure relates to some toxic substance or poison, an immune reaction to drugs, or as a response to some another disease, such as an infection. A massive bodily injury or a sudden drop in blood pressure, as during a heart attack, can also lead to kidney damage that results in acute kidney failure.

The symptoms of acute kidney failure are often markedly decreased urine output, weakness, fatigue, loss of appetite, and nausea. If the condition is not treated, drowsiness, confusion, delirium, coma, and death may ensue.

Treatment. Acute kidney failure will almost always be treated in the hospital. In most cases the underlying cause is addressed and the kidney repair takes care of itself. A diet of restricted protein and fluid allows the kidneys to rest as they are healing. In some cases, temporary kidney dialysis is require to take over the kidney function until healing occurs.

Chronic Kidney Failure

A much more serious condition occurs when damage to the kidneys occurs over a long period of time, resulting in irreversible kidney disease. The usual causes are chronic kidney infections, chronic glomerulonephritis, and polycystic disease. The symptoms may be similar to acute kidney failure, although often the output of urine increases, even though the chemical wastes of the body are not removed. If you know you have kidney disease, see your doctor when you notice any change in your symptom pattern.

Treatment. Usually the only treatment possible is chronic kidney dialysis or kidney transplantation. In either case chronic kidney failure need not be the swift passage to death that it once was.

Dialysis

In kidney failure, the kidneys are unable to filter excess salts and metabolic waste products from the blood. In a short time these substances build up to toxic levels that will threaten life unless they are removed by some other means, such as dialysis. There are two general types of dialysis: peritoneal dialysis and hemodialysis.

In *peritoneal dialysis* a soft silicone rubber catheter is inserted into the abdomen and a specially formulated solution, the *dialysate* is infused. Waste products from the bloodstream diffuse across the peritoneal membrane that lines the abdominal cavity and are picked up by the dialysate, which is then drained and discarded. This procedure is usually performed three times daily and requires 30–45 minutes at each session. Alternatively, an automated cycler machine can be attached to the catheter at bedtime and dialysis performed during the night. In many cases long-term peritoneal dialysis can be done at home. Complications that can occur during peritoneal dialysis include infection (peritonitis or abdominal abscess), occlusion of the catheter, bowel perforation, and bowel obstruction.

In *hemodialysis* an access to the bloodstream is inserted into the arm or leg. Arterial blood is pumped into a dialysis machine, where waste products are removed by means of an artificial membrane and then returned to the arm or leg vein. Persons on dialysis require 8–12 hours of dialysis per week, divided into several sessions. Most people elect to undergo dialysis in hospital outpatient centers, although in some cases hemodialysis can be performed at home. Complications of hemodialysis include infections, stroke, heart attack, and blood vessel occlusion (thrombosis).

Kidney Transplantation

In most cases, the medical complications and the psychological toll of being dependent upon machines associated with chronic dialysis makes kidney transplantation the preferred option. Approximately 60,000 kidneys are transplanted each year. Because of this demand and because of the need to match donor tissue types with those of the recipient, there is often a long wait for a suitable donor kidney to become available. During this time, the patient must depend on dialysis to take over kidney function.

Generally, healthy relatives, such as a parent, brother, or sister, are the most suitable donors because tissue compatibility is more likely. When a relative is not available as a donor, tissue-typing centers throughout the country are called upon to help locate an acceptable donor from among accident victims and others who have offered to donate their kidneys after their death. This is known as a cadaver transplant. Newer drugs, such as cyclosporine, have increased the likelihood of overcoming the body's natural tendency to reject a "foreign" kidney.

Not everyone with end-stage kidney disease is a suitable candidate for kidney transplantation. Those with coronary artery disease, infections, glomerulonephritis, and chronic diseases may not be in good enough condition to undergo the rigors of transplantation. However, when successful, kidney transplantation usually guarantees a more trouble-free life than long-term dialysis.

For more information about chronic kidney diseases and kidney transplantation, contact the National Kidney Foundation Inc., 30 East 33rd St., New York, NY 10016, 1-800-622-9010. Ask for a brochure entitled "Kidney Transplantation—A New Lease on Life."

Cancer of the Kidneys

There are two kinds of kidney tumors, both of which are malignant. *Wilm's tumor* is a cancer that almost always affects children under five years of age. It presents as a hard lump in the abdomen, often with anemia and weight loss. Surgical removal, followed by cancer chemotherapy is the only treatment.

In adults the most common malignant tumor is the *hypernephroma*. It usually begins on the periphery of the kidney and gradually grows into and replaces the body of the kidney. The usual presentation is blood in the urine. Often there is weight loss, fever, nausea, and vomiting and occasionally mild abdominal pain.

The diagnosis of hypernephroma is made by X-rays, ultrasound, and CAT scanning of the kidney. The treatment is surgical removal, followed by radiation therapy and/or chemotherapy to kill any remaining cancer cells. For more information about kidney cancer, call the Cancer Information Service, 1-800-4-CANCER.

Tumors of the Bladder

Bladder tumors, like tumors elsewhere, may be either benign or malignant. If they occur near the entry of the ureter into the bladder, they may obstruct the kidney, causing pain and swelling of the kidney *(hydronephrosis)*. If the tumor lies near the outlet to the urethra, it can cause difficulty urinating. The most common symptom, however, is painless bleeding into the urine (hematuria). Painful and frequent urination may also occur, with symptoms much like those that occur with inflammations of the bladder (see p. 328).

You should see your doctor whenever you develop urinary tract symptoms, especially if you notice blood in your urine. If a tumor is suspected, you will likely undergo X-ray diagnostic tests and cystoscopy, a procedure in which a thin tube is inserted into your bladder so that the bladder wall is directly examined internally. If indicated, a biopsy is then taken to determine the type of tumor.

Treatment. Bladder tumors may be destroyed by burning them out through a cystoscope, a process known as *fulguration*. If the tumor is malignant or extensive, part or all of the bladder may have to be removed. In the latter case, the ureters will be redirected to an opening in the abdominal wall and into a bag, or "external bladder" that must be emptied periodically. This is a relatively simple procedure that generally presents few problems.

Cross-section of the female reproductive organs

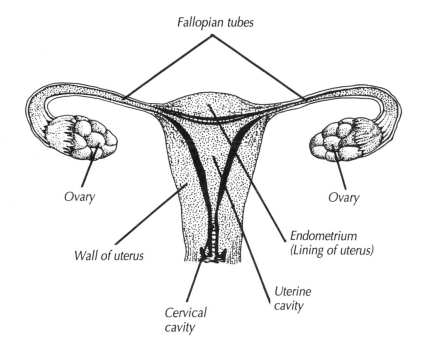

Fallopian tubes

Ovary

Ovary

Wall of uterus

Endometrium
(Lining of uterus)

Cervical
cavity

Uterine
cavity

Women's Medical Problems

We live in a time when women have unparalleled freedom, are better educated, have better health, and have greater health awareness than even a few years ago. For most women, the forces, both religious and social, that discouraged discussion of female sexuality, body development, and sexual body functions are now no greater than those for men. This is a welcome development because ignorance and reluctance to understand and discuss sexuality and sexually related medical problems have been responsible for untold woe. A healthy curiosity about all aspects of our bodies must be encouraged everywhere. As ignorance and misconception are overcome, so are shame, guilt, health neglect, disease, and disrupted lives avoided. Read on and teach your daughters well!

Disorders of Menstruation

The Normal Menstrual Cycle

The menstrual cycle begins with the first day of vaginal bleeding (day 1) and ends just before the next onset of bleeding. The average cycle length is 28 days however, relatively few women have a cycle exactly 28 days long. The normal range is from about 18 to 40 days. The interval between menstruations is most variable just after menstruation begins, the *menarche*, and just before menstruation ends, the *menopause*. Menarche usually occurs between the ages of 11 and 14 (generally earlier for overweight girls), whereas menopause usually occurs between ages 45 and 55 (average, 51). Once menstrual cycles have established regularity, the cycle seldom varies by more than 5 days. Bleeding usually lasts from 3 to 7 days. Normal blood loss varies from about 30 to 130 milliliters. Women taking birth control pills usually have less bleeding.

Menstrual blood may have an unpleasant odor, largely because of vaginal bacteria. Thus careful hygiene, with frequent changes of pads or tampons during menstruation, is important. There is no truth to the old myth that you should not bathe during menstruation. The mild constipation often accompanying menstruation is caused by the action of progesterone in slowing bowel activity. Add more fiber to your diet, and drink extra water at these times to prevent such constipation.

The menstrual cycle can be divided into three distinct phases. During the *preovulatory phase,* which begins with the first day of menstruation, the uterine lining is shed (menstruation) and then gradually begins to build up again. Follicle-stimulating hormone (FSH), secreted by the pituitary gland in the brain, begins to rise, stimulating one or more follicles in both ovaries to mature in preparation for ovulation. Later, luteinizing hormone (LH), also secreted by the pituitary, begins to rise, further maturing the ovarian follicle.

During the second, or *ovulatory phase,* LH and FSH surge, causing the egg(s) to be released from the mature follicle(s). Estrogen secretion also increases just before ovulation and progesterone levels in the blood begin to rise, preparing the uterus for implantation should the egg be fertilized by sperm. The temperature (measured just before rising in the morning) also increases about 0.6°F after ovulation.

The third, or *postovulatory phase,* is a relatively constant period, averaging about 14 days in the absence of pregnancy, that ends with the onset of a new menstrual cycle. During this phase, progesterone is secreted by the postovulatory follicle, called the corpus luteum, a period called the *luteal phase.* The uterine lining now reaches its maximum engorgement and the egg makes it way down the fallopian tube to be implanted in the uterine wall if fertilization occurs. If no fertilization takes place, the prepared uterine lining is shed, along with the unfertilized egg, during the ensuing menstruation.

Period of Fertility

Ovulation usually occurs about 14 days before the onset of the next menstrual period. However, sperm remain active for 5–7 days after intercourse. Consequently, the fertile period from the standpoint of intercourse extends on either side of the ovulatory period.

To determine with confidence the period during which you can become pregnant, the menstrual cycles must be fairly regular. To calculate this period, subtract 18 days from the length of the shortest of your previous 12 cycles and subtract 11 days from the longest. Thus, if your cycles vary between 26 and 29 days, you are likely to be fertile from day 8 (26 minus 18) through day 18 (29 minus 11) of each cycle.

Avoiding intercourse during this period in order to avoid pregnancy is known as the "rhythm method." Please understand that the rhythm method has a very high failure rate of 15–45% when relied upon as the sole method of contraception, which is why it is simply not a realistic method of contraception (p. 368).

Menstrual Irregularity and Absence of Periods *(Amenorrhea)*

As we have seen, a complex interaction exists between the brain, the pituitary gland and the ovaries to regulate the menstrual cycle. A failure at any level results in the absence of menstruation, called *amenorrhea*. Amenorrhea may be primary or secondary. Primary amenorrhea occurs when a woman entering adolescence fails to begin menstruating. Normally this is not suspected until after age 16. Secondary amenorrhea occurs when women who have begun menstruating regularly, subsequently fail to do so for 2 or 3 months. The most common cause of secondary amenorrhea is pregnancy, but there are many other causes as well.

Among these causes are intense physical activity (e.g., as in marathon runners) and excessive weight loss (*see* Eating Disorders, p. 318). Certain drugs used to treat breast cancer may also be responsible for amenorrhea, as can such disorders as thyroid and adrenal diseases. It is also normal not to menstruate for several weeks or months while nursing. You should consult your doctor if you are over 16 and have not menstruated, and whenever you go longer than two weeks without menstruating after having established a regular period cycle.

Remember that it is common to experience delayed menstruation for up to two months after stopping the use of contraceptive pills. Remember, too, that during amenorrhea, you may begin ovulating at any time. Therefore some form of contraception is advisable if you are sexually active during that time and wish to avoid pregnancy.

Infrequent Periods *(Oligomenorrhea)*

It is common to have infrequent or irregular periods soon after menarche and before menopause. Some women have infrequent periods throughout their menstrual life. Usually there is no medical significance attached to infrequent periods, although stress, intense exercise, overactive thyroid, obesity, and underweight may contribute to menstrual infrequency and irregularity. If you suspect that any of these factors may play a role in your infertility, consult your doctor.

Heavy Periods *(Menorrhagia)*

Bleeding for a prolonged time (e.g., longer than 7 days) or in excessive amounts (flooding or passing blood clots) are common menstrual problems. Heavy bleeding may occur as a result of hormonal irregularities that commonly accompany the onset of menopause, or it may be associated with uterine fibroids (*see* p. 351), endometriosis (*see* p. 352), pelvic infection (*see* p. 355), thyroid disease, or the presence of an intrauterine device (IUD). If you develop heavy periods after a period of regularity, reduce your level of activity. If bleeding does not lessen within 24 hours, consult your doctor.

Treatment. If your uterus is found to be normal, your doctor may prescribe a combination of estrogen and progesterone similar to birth control pills to control bleeding. If you use an IUD, your doctor will probably suggest a different contraceptive (*see* p. 368). In exceptional cases, when other measures have failed to correct or prevent anemia, a hysterectomy (surgical removal of the uterus) may be needed.

Remember, if you normally have heavy periods, you must increase your dietary iron to avoid anemia. Such foods as red meats, peas, beans, nuts, dried fruits, green leafy vegetables, and enriched grain products are good sources of iron. Do not take iron supplements without the advice of your doctor; excessive iron intake can be harmful to your liver and other organs.

Bleeding Between Periods

Bleeding between periods is never normal, although most causes are relatively benign. Women who use an intrauterine device (IUD) as a contraceptive measure may notice both heavier menstrual flow and "spotting" between periods. Usually this is tolerable because of the convenience of this form of contraception. However, if you also experience cramping, you should consult with your doctor about changing to another form of contraception (*see* p. 368).

Oral and implanted contraceptives may also be associated with bleeding between periods, especially just after their use is initiated. Many women will begin bleeding after skipping even a single pill. Continuing the regular pill schedule usually ends this problem. Remember, if you have forgotten to take pills longer than recommended as safe by the manufacturer, you must take additional contraceptive measures until you finish the packet. If spotting persists ask your doctor about the advisability of using a contraceptive preparation containing somewhat higher amounts of progesterone.

A variety of other causes may be responsible for vaginal bleeding, including cervical or uterine polyps, vaginal or cervical infections, and cervical or vaginal cancer. Each may also be associated with bleeding after intercourse. Consult your doctor since each of these has potentially serious consequences.

Menstrual Cramps *(Dysmenorrhea)*

There are two kinds of painful menses, known as primary and secondary dysmenorrhea. It is important to distinguish between them because the treatments for the two types are entirely different.

Primary dysmenorrhea is the most common form and is experienced at some times and degree by most women. This type usually starts within 3 years of the onset of menstruation and lasts 1 or 2 days each month. With increasing age and with the birth of children, these cramps may lessen, although they can last until menopause.

Secondary dysmenorrhea is the painful menses caused by another pelvic disease, such as pelvic infections, uterine fibroids, or endometriosis. This type usually begins later in life, increases in severity with time, is often associated with painful intercourse and is relieved when the pelvic condition is treated.

Primary dysmenorrhea is the result of the normal production of prostaglandins—chemical substances produced by the endometrium and released when it breaks up and is sloughed off at the end of the menstrual cycle. The prostaglandins make the uterus contract more strongly. In some cases, contractions can even cut off the uterine blood supply, temporarily depriving the uterine muscle of oxygen and thus causing pain.

The pain is usually experienced as cramping lower abdominal or pelvic pain. At times the pain may be constant, dull, low back pain, with or without radiation to the legs. The pain usually occurs with, or just prior to, menstruation, peaking in about 24 hours and lasting 1–3 days. Headache, constipation, nausea, vomiting, diarrhea, and urinary frequency may also accompany the cramps.

Treatment. The remedy that most women find effective is a drug that prevents the production of prostaglandins, namely one of the nonsteroidal anti-inflammatory drugs (NSAIDs), such as ibuprofen (Nuprin, Advil, Motrin). Naproxen (Naprosyn) and mefenamic acid (Ponstel) are prescription drugs that are approved to treat menstrual cramps. The recommended dose of ibuprofen is 200-400 mg every 4–6 hours. You should begin these drugs a day or so before you anticipate cramping in order to avoid pain altogether.

Aspirin—long the standard over-the-counter treatment for cramps—also inhibits prostaglandins, but appears to be less effective

PREMENSTRUAL SYNDROME

PMS is very common. The American College of Obstetrics and Gynecology estimates that 20–40% of all women suffer some symptoms of PMS, which it defines as "a recurring cycle of symptoms that are so severe as to affect lifestyle or work." The premenstrual syndrome (PMS) is a problem associated with the menstrual cycle that occurs in the last 7–10 days of the cycle (called the luteal phase), during which the ovary forms the *corpus luteum*.

The variety of symptoms ranges from the merely annoying to the downright disabling and appears to be related to the fluctuation of estrogen and progesterone produced during the menstual cycle. These symptoms can be grouped into four combinations:

1. Breast tenderness, swelling, weight gain, and bloating.
2. Emotional changes including depression, forgetfulness, crying, insomnia, and confusion.
3. Headaches, food cravings (especially sweets), increased appetite, fatigue, and dizziness.
4. Anxiety, nervous tension, mood swings, and irritability.

This list of symptoms is formidable and unfortunately they may vary or worsen with time. But almost no women ever experience all of them.

Treatment. No treatment regimen works for all women; often enough a treatment that works well on one occasion, fails completely on others. The most frequently prescribed remedy is a diuretic (e.g., hydrochlorothiazide, 50–100 milligrams daily) to control the water-retention effects of your own estrogens. Reducing your dietary salt intake and increasing your water intake (since water is itself a diuretic) are simple measures that may help.

Useful dietary changes include increasing your protein intake and decreasing your consumption of sugars and carbohydrates. Vitamin B_6 supplements may also be helpful. Get plenty of rest and exercise to help reduce tension. Keep a diary to document the onset and duration of your symptoms, along with those measures taken that seem to bring you relief. This will help your doctor individualize your treatment according to the type and severity of your symptoms.

Hormones may be needed if more conservative measures fail to help. Such treatments may include progesterone suppositories,

> injectable progesterone, or birth control pills. Recent studies have suggested that the drug naloxone may effectively reduce PMS symptoms in most cases. Other drugs that may be effective are alprazolam (Xanax) and fluoxetine (Prozac). Ask your doctor whether these may be useful for you.

than ibuprofen. Other over-the-counter preparations used to treat cramps are Midol and Pamprin, both of which contain a mixture of ingredients: an analgesic, a mild diuretic, and an antihistamine. They are worth trying if NSAIDs are ineffective for you.

Oral contraceptives are also effective in alleviating severe menstrual cramps resistant to other forms of treatment. Contraceptive pills disrupt the normal hormonal changes of the menstrual cycle, resulting in a thinner endometrium and a diminished production of prostaglandins. Vigorous exercise may also be of some benefit. It is thought that exercising raises the levels of beta endorphins, chemicals in the brain associated with pain relief.

Pads vs Tampons and Toxic Shock Syndrome

Though we don't read much about toxic shock syndrome any more, it has not gone away. Approximately 35 cases occur each month in the United States. Symptoms include high fever, nausea, vomiting, diarrhea, fainting, and a sunburn-like rash. The cause is a bacterial production of toxins that occurs most often in the particular vaginal environment created by highly absorbent tampons. If you develop any of the above symptoms while using tampons, discontinue their use at once and see your doctor.

Toxic shock syndrome can largely be avoided if pads are used, since they do not alter the vaginal secretions. However, most women prefer insertable tampons because of their greater comfort and convenience. Currently the incidence of toxic shock syndrome is about 1 in 10,000 menstruating women. Of these 2–3% are fatal. Thus the fatality is 2–3 per million menstruating women, not a high number, but infinitely high if you are the victim.

The safety of tampons can be greatly increased by proper selection and use. Tampons absorb between 4 and 16 milliliters of blood. You should select a low-absorbency tampon, such as Playtex slender-regular or regular, or Tampax junior, slender-regular or original-regular. Tampons should be changed every 4–6 hours, and ideally you should alternate tampons with pads. Tampons should never be worn overnight. Whether to use an applicator to insert tampons or not is a matter of personal preference. Avoid tampons that contain deodorants, since they don't prevent odors and may well cause an allergic rash. After childbirth, or surgery involving the vagina, uterus, or cervix, you should use pads rather than tampons until healing is complete.

Menopause

Menopause marks the ending of menstrual periods. For most women this is a gradual process caused by declining estrogen production and often accompanied by irregular and sometimes heavy periods. The age of onset for menopause normally varies between 40 and 60. By age 48, half of American women will have stopped menstruating, and by age 52, 85% will have stopped.

Menopause is a normal physiologic event in women's lives and may be associated with no other symptoms than a gradual cessation of menstruation. For the majority of women, however, menopause carries a price and for about 15% of women, symptoms are severe enough to seek medical relief. Such symptoms include heavy periods, headaches, backaches, fatigue, dryness of the vagina, painful intercourse, and hot flashes.

The *hot flash* is the classic menopausal symptom. It can come upon you, without warning, with the sensation of upper body heat, flushing, and sweating often profuse enough to soak the clothing next to your skin. Although many women find hot flashes embarrassing when they occur in social situations, more than likely no one else will notice; and if they do they will understand that this is a perfectly natural phenomenon, especially if you yourself make light of the matter.

Hot flashes can be better tolerated if you dress for them. Wear cotton and natural fibers for their greater absorbency and cooling properties. Wear layers of clothing that can be easily removed or added to as the situation demands. Colored fabrics show the telltale moisture more than whites and plain fabrics more than patterns. Since night sweats also occur, wear cotton nightwear and use cotton sheets as well as lightweight thermal blankets.

Reduced estrogen levels in your blood also cause the vagina to thin and become dry. This may lead to itching, occasional bleeding, and discomfort during intercourse (dyspareunia), problems that can be combatted with a vaginal lubricant. If over-the-counter preparations are unsatisfactory, your doctor can prescribe an estrogen cream, or a hormone replacement, that will reverse the thinning process.

Hormone Replacement Therapy

In hormone replacement therapy (HRT) a combination of estrogens and progesterone is prescribed which stops hot flashes and other menopausal symptoms, reduces the risk of cancer, and combats the inevitable bone loss *(osteoporosis)* that occurs after menopause. Osteoporosis is by far the most important consequence of menopausally reduced estrogen. Bone mass declines by about 1% per year after menopause, leading to fractures of the spine, hips, and wrist, often as a result of negligible trauma. Osteoporosis is an especially common problem for women who are slender, Caucasian, engage in little physical activity, smoke cigarets, or take corticosteroid medications. Remember that HRT must be combined with a high calcium intake (1000 mg/day) to reduce the likelihood of osteoporosis. *See* p. 405 for a more complete discussion of the nature and treatment of osteoporosis.

Though there are many advantages to HRT, there are also some drawbacks, the most important of which is they may restart your menstrual cycles. Thus women with mild menopausal symptoms and a normal bone mass (see your doctor about measuring this important factor) may elect not to begin HRT. Others for whom HRT may not be advisable are those who have had breast cancer, undiagnosed vaginal bleeding, or blood clots in the legs, as well as those with diabetes, epilepsy, and certain kinds of heart and liver diseases. For most other women, HRT should be seriously considered. With regard to the old bugaboo about estrogen replacement increasing the risk of breast cancer, most evidence indicates that modern formulations of low-dose estrogen, combined with small amounts of progesterone, do not increase your risk of breast cancer, or increase it only negligibly.

With regard to fertility during menopause, do not forget that, when pregnancy is unwanted, *you must still take contraceptive measures.* The possible period of fertility depends on your age at the time of your last period. If you are under 50, you should continue contraceptive measures for 2 years after your last period. If you are over 50, protection should continue for 1 year after your last period.

Remember that for most women, menopause marks the beginning of a period of new freedom, not the end of youth and vigor. There is no reason why your sexual relations with a loving partner should not continue indefinitely.

For more information about menopause write for NIH Publication No. 83.2461 from the National Institute on Aging, Information Center, PO Box 8057, Gaithersburg, MD 20898. It is available free!

To subscribe to the quarterly journal, *Midlife Wellness*, which deals with all aspects of menopause and midlife health concerns, write to: Center for Climacteric Studies, University of Florida, 901 NW 8th Avenue, Suite B1, Gainesville, FL 32601; 1-904-392-3184. Another newsletter, *Hot Flashes: Newsletter for Midlife and Older Women*, can be obtained from: The School of Allied Health Professionals, SUNY at Stony Brook, NY 11794.

Vagina and Vulva
Vaginal Hygiene

The vulva is the area around the entrance to the vagina and consists of the labia and a number of lubricating glands. The vagina is the internal pouch that separates the vulva from the cervix. The vagina is rich in fluid-producing glands that may, under certain circumstances, create ideal conditions for infection.

Manufacturers of "feminine hygiene" products would have you spend a lot of money on their preparations because it is the "nice" thing to do. But in reality, gentle washing of the vulva with soap and warm water during a shower or bath is usually all that is required to achieve cleanliness and avoid unwanted odor. Wear loose, absorbent clothing and cotton underpants. Douching is no longer recommended as a routine because it does not necessarily promote better hygiene and because of the possibility of introducing bacteria into the uterus and bladder. In fact, women who douche regularly are more likely to have pelvic inflammatory disease (*see* p. 355) and tubal pregnancies than women who do not douche.

Feminine sprays are also not usually recommended because of their role in creating local inflammation (*vulvitis*) caused by skin sensitivity to their ingredients. Odors, when present, most likely originate in the external genitals, not in the vagina. Such odors are best eliminated (and prevented) by your use of gentle (and inexpensive) soap and water, rather than high-priced douches. If you suspect an infection, don't douche before seeing your doctor; it will make the task of determining the cause of infection more difficult if one is present.

If you elect to douche, use a very low-pressure warm water or a vinegar/water solution (1 tablespoon per quart of water). Never force water into your vagina under pressure. Avoid commercial douche preparations. To avoid odors during menstruation, change tampons and pads every 4 hours. Sprays and perfumed tampons do nothing to prevent odors, and may cause sensitivity rashes.

Vaginal Infection *(Vaginitis)*

Several bacteria, yeasts, and other organisms can invade the vagina, producing vaginitis, or vulvovaginitis if the vulva is also infected. The most common of these are the yeast, *Candida albicans*, the protozoan, *Trichomonas vaginalis*, and the bacterium, *Gardnerella vaginalis*. Infections may result when the normal bacteria inhabiting the vagina are killed off, leading to an overgrowth of other organisms that cause infections. Such overgrowths occur when you are taking antibiotics for another infection, e.g., a strep throat, and are one good reason not to take antibiotics unless absolutely needed. Certain feminine hygiene sprays may also kill your normal bacteria, causing an overgrowth infection. Poor hygiene, as well as tight underclothes of synthetic fabrics that retain moisture, may predispose to infections.

The symptoms of such infections include itching and vaginal discharge. The discharge of *Trichomonas* infections may be greenish-yellow in color with an unpleasant odor. Occasionally vaginal bleeding and soreness during sexual intercourse may develop.

Treatment. You must see your doctor, who will take cultures to identify the causative organism. Antibiotics will generally be prescribed, either oral or in the form of vaginal suppositories or cream. If you have an infection that is usually transmitted sexually, e.g. trichomonas, chlamydia, and gonorrheal infections, your doctor will also advise treating your sexual partner to prevent reinfection (*see* Sexually Transmitted Diseases, p. 389). Douching is not usually advised because of the possibility of forcing the infection into your uterus or bladder. Discontinue the use of tampons during treatment. Avoid sexual intercourse until your treatment has been completed and take all prescribed medications for the full recommended course.

The itching associated with your vaginitis is caused by inflammation of the vulva; which is why these infections are known as vulvovaginitis. For itching, cleanse your vulva gently with soap and warm water, following the directions given below.

Itching of the Vulva *(Pruritus vulvae)*

As mentioned above, itching about the labia may be caused by infections. However there are several other causes of itching, including such medical conditions as diabetes, skin diseases, allergies, ringworm, pubic lice, as well as irritations attributable to contraceptive devices, contraceptive creams, clothing, sprays, and dyes. Itching associated with any of these conditions or irritations is not usually accompanied by excessive vaginal discharge.

Treatment. Wash the vulva gently with soap and warm water daily and dry carefully without rubbing the sensitive area. Wear your loosest cotton underwear instead of the synthetics that tend to hold moisture. Avoid talcum powder, which is irritating. Do not douche and avoid feminine hygiene sprays, which may only make itching worse. If itching does not subside within a few days, consult your doctor.

Atrophic Vulvar Dystrophy

Atrophic means shrunken or malnourished, and *dystrophy* is a kind of degeneration of tissues. Vulvar dystrophy usually occurs in women who are past menopause, when estrogen production ceases to stimulate growth and replacement of vulvar tissues. The symptoms include dry, itchy, reddened areas in the vulva that may become "papery" and shiny and the clitoris may shrink. In some cases the area may become thickened and white, a condition known as *leukoplakia*.

Diagnosis and treatment. For uncomplicated vulvar dystrophy, your doctor may prescribe a cortisone cream which is generally all that is necessary to relieve your symptoms. If leukoplakia has developed, your doctor will most likely recommend a biopsy, because its presence indicates an increased risk of vulvar cancer. While not usually a serious condition, atrophic vulvar dystrophy can give rise to cancer and periodic examinations are essential.

Sebaceous Cysts

The sebaceous glands are small glands associated with hair follicles that produce an oily substance that keeps the skin smooth and supple. If the opening of a sebaceous gland becomes obstructed, it can develop into a cyst that forms a soft, smooth lump in the skin, sometimes with a small, dark dot in the center. Sebaceous cysts can occur anywhere, including the vulva. They are quite harmless, unless they become infected, whereupon they become reddened and tender and may rupture and drain.

Treatment. If a sebaceous cyst becomes infected, your doctor will most likely prescribe an antibiotic. Cleansing the area with soap and warm water will relieve local soreness. Keep the area dry by wearing soft, cotton underpants. If a cyst enlarges to the point of being bothersome, it can be surgically removed under local anesthesia.

Vulvar Warts

Warts on or about the labia are relatively common. They are caused by a virus and are usually the same as those that occur on the hands and the rest of the body (*see* p. 453). In fact they may spread to the vulva by contact with the hands, or from a sexual partner.

Treatment. See your doctor, who will differentiate common warts (caused by the Herpes virus) from genital warts (caused by the human papilloma virus) that are sexually transmitted (*see* p. 395). Ordinarily common warts can be treated by application of a solution of salicylic acid or similar topical preparation. Cases resistant to medications may be treated with a laser beam or by *cryosurgery* (freezing with liquid nitrogen). Warts that are neglected have a potential for becoming malignant.

Bladder and Urethra

Bladder Infections *(Cystitis)*

In women bladder infections, called cystitis, are usually caused by bacteria that travel up the short urethra from the vagina into the bladder. The most common symptoms are pain or burning on urination and a frequent urge to empty your bladder. Occasionally the urine contains streaks of blood and may have a strong smell. Cystitis is common after intercourse during which mechanical forces push bacteria up into the bladder.

Treatment. Increase your intake of fluids. If symptoms persist more than a day or two, see your doctor, who may prescribe an antibiotic and an analgesic. To avoid cystitis, always wipe from front to back, away from the vagina, after a bowel movement. Remember to empty your bladder after intercourse to flush out bacteria that may have been forced into the bladder. Bladder infections that are not treated may lead to kidney infections.

Irritable Bladder *(Urge Incontinence)*

Some people experience a sudden overwhelming urge to urinate without having other symptoms of cystitis (*see above*). This may occur at night or during the day when you can't get to the bathroom soon enough; thus the so-called urge incontinence.

Treatment. If urge incontinence becomes more than an occasional event, you should see your doctor to make certain you do not have an infection or some correctable condition, such as prolapse of the uterus (*see* p. 354). If no obvious problem is found, your doctor may advise you to try holding your water as long as possible each time urgency occurs in order to strengthen your bladder muscles. In many cases this exercise alone can help you overcome this distressing problem.

Stress Incontinence

As women age, the muscles that form the floor of the pelvis become more relaxed and weakened. These muscles help support the bladder and close off the junction (*sphincter*) between the bladder and the urethra. Weakening of the sphincter leads to stress incontinence, i.e., involuntary loss of urine while straining, lifting, laughing, sneezing, and so on. Though stress incontinence occurs in men also, it is much more common in women.

Treatment. Often stress incontinence can be relieved by exercises designed to strengthen the pelvic-floor muscles. One such exercise consists of tensing your pelvic muscles in the same effort you would make to cut off your urine stream. By this exercise you strengthen your pelvic floor muscles, often completely correcting stress incontinence. Obesity aggravates stress incontinence, so you are encouraged to lose excess weight. A number of drugs can be prescribed for incontinence. However, these drugs often produce such side effects as dryness of the eyes and mouth, as well as retention of urine. Their use must be carefully monitored by your doctor.

If these measures fail to correct the problem, you should seek the advice of a urologist, who may recommend a surgical operation to tighten the pelvic-floor muscles. A very old remedy, and one still recommended for some, is the use of a pessary, a device worn inside the vagina to support the bladder. If a pessary is selected, scrupulous cleanliness is essential to avoid developing vaginitis (*see* p. 347).

Many women use sanitary napkins to absorb overflow urine. However, these are often irritating and tend to smell unless changed frequently. Usually there are better and less expensive alternatives that a urologist can suggest.

For more information about coping with incontinence, write to: The Simon Foundation, PO Box 815, Willamette, IL 60091; 1-800-23-SIMON, or to: Help for Incontinent People, PO Box 544, Union, SC 29379. Send a self-addressed stamped envelope for their newsletter.

Disorders of the Ovaries, Uterus, and Cervix

Disorders of the ovaries, uterus, and cervix are primarily structural problems or infections. Menstrual disorders are discussed on p. 339.

Ovarian Cysts

Cysts of the ovaries are fluid-filled sacs that in some cases may become quite large. Usually they cause no symptoms. If they become large enough, they may be felt as a lower abdominal swelling. In some cases they cause pelvic pain, especially during intercourse. They can also interfere with normal ovarian function.

FIBROIDS OF THE UTERUS

Fibroids are nonmalignant fibrous tumors that grow in the muscular wall of the uterus or project from a stalk into the uterine cavity. They are very common; about 20–30% of all women develop fibroids. Their growth rate is highly variable; sometimes they reach the size of a football within a year or two. However, in most women they grow slowly, remain small, and remain symptomless. Their most common symptom is excessive menstrual bleeding. Furthermore, fibroids grow primarily under the influence of estrogen and often shrink or disappear after menopause when estrogen production diminishes. If the tumors become large enough, abdominal swelling and even interference with pregnancy can result.

Treatment. If fibroids are small and result in excessive menstrual bleeding, they are frequently treated by a procedure known as dilatation and curettage (D&C). This is a minor operation, usually performed under general anesthesia, in which the cervical canal is widened with a dilator and the lining of the uterus is then scraped with a device known as a curette. During the process the fibroids are scraped away. If the fibroids are large, it may be necessary to remove the uterus entirely *(hysterectomy)*.

Treatment. Usually no treatment is necessary. If cysts cause discomfort, they may be drained by laparoscopy (a tube inserted into the abdomen), or surgically removed, depending upon your gynecologist's judgment. Removal does not usually lead to infertility.

Cancer of the Ovary

Cancer of the ovary is fortunately quite rare and most often develops after menopause. Because the ovaries lie within the abdomen, however, the cancer may be advanced before producing any symp-

---

ENDOMETRIOSIS

The endometrium is the normal lining of the uterus. When this tissue is found growing outside the uterus, the condition is known as endometriosis. The most common abnormal sites are within the abdomen and vagina, in the fallopian tubes, and in the ovaries or muscular walls of the uterus. It is commonly thought that endometriosis most often seeds into the abdomen by backflow of menstrual tissue through the fallopian tubes during menses. Since this tissue behaves like normal endometrium, it is under the influence of the pituitary and ovarian hormones that regulate the growth and shedding of the endometrium. Because the tissue has no means of escape, it swells, forming blister-like lesions wherever it happens to have implanted after seeding.

The most common symptom, if there are any at all, is pain, which is usually worse after menstruation. In some cases sexual intercourse may also be painful. Infertility is commonly associated with endometriosis. The symptoms usually cease with menopause. The diagnosis is usually made by laparoscopy.

Treatment. The treatment is highly individual, depending upon severity. Sometimes birth control pills to suppress the menstrual cycle can be given continuously for a period of time during which the body may rid itself of the abnormal tissue. In severe cases, large doses of synthetic hormones may be required to medically suppress ovarian function, although these tend to have many unpleasant side effects. In rare cases, hysterectomy and removal of the abdominal implants may be the only means of alleviating symptoms.

toms. These symptoms commonly include swelling of the abdomen, often due to the accumulation of fluid called *ascites*. Lower abdominal pain and unexplained weight loss are also symptoms that should prompt you to see your doctor.

Diagnosis. Early diagnosis—when the cancer is more easily cured—is most likely to be made by your doctor during a regular pelvic examination. X-rays and ultrasound are valuable procedures to determine the size and extent of the cancer. A tissue diagnosis is usually made by means of laparoscopy (passing a hollow tube through a small incision in the abdomen) or by laparotomy, in which a larger incision is made in the abdomen to reach the ovaries. If a biopsy is positive, surgical removal of the ovary and adjoining tissue is performed in the same operation.

Treatment. Usually both ovaries, the fallopian tubes, and uterus are removed to make certain that all of the tumor has been removed. After surgery, adjuvant chemotherapy with anticancer drugs or radiation is given to treat any cancer that may remain in you.

Risk Factors. Ovarian cancer is somewhat more likely to occur in woman who have experienced difficulty in conceiving and in women who have never been pregnant. There may also be some connection between ovarian cancer and breast cancer since women who have had ovarian cancer are four times more likely to develop breast cancer than women without ovarian cancer.

However, by far the most important risk factor for ovarian cancer is a family history of that cancer, which is thought to be inherited in an *autosomal dominant* manner. Sisters and daughters in ovarian cancer-prone families having two or more affected first-degree relatives (mother, sister, daughter, who share half their genes) may have up to a 50% chance of developing ovarian cancer. This compares with a 1 in 70 chance for women without such a family history of ovarian cancer. The risk of developing ovarian cancer with one first-degree and one second-degree relative (grandmother or aunt) or two or more second-degree relatives (who share one-quarter of their genes) is less than 50%.

Such high risks of developing a cancer that is difficult to detect in its early stages, and for which only a few good screening tests exist, may require extraordinary preventative measures. Many cancer experts recommend prophylactic removal of the ovaries (*oophorectomy*) in these rare cases. Early genetic counseling is also needed to clearly understand the risks of passing the cancer gene to a daughter. If there is a family history of ovarian cancer and you find prophylactic oophorectomy unsettling, semiannual pelvic and abdominal examinations are recommended, along with periodic Doppler ultrasound imaging of the ovarian blood supply.

For further information about cancer therapy, *see* p. 9.

Prolapse of the Uterus

Prolapse of the uterus is a condition of older women, usually those who have had several children. Prolapse is a downward displacement of the uterus into the vagina caused by weakening of the muscles and ligaments that form the pelvic floor.

The symptoms of prolapse are a sensation of heaviness and discomfort in the pelvis, along with back pain when lifting or straining. A noticeable bulge may be felt in the vagina. In very severe cases the uterus may actually protrude out of the vagina.

Stress incontinence is also common with prolapse (*see* p. 350).

Treatment. You can often correct uterine prolapse by yourself through exercise and diet. Muscle strengthening exercises consist of tensing your pelvic floor muscles several times each day. This is done by contracting the muscles in the same way that you would cut off the flow of urine. The same muscles that constrict the urethra support the uterus. If you are overweight, ask your doctor for a diet appropriate for you. Increase your dietary fiber in order to avoid constipation; straining at stools makes prolapse worse. So does a chronic cough and other maneuvers that increase abdominal pressure, e.g., lifting.

If these simple measures fail, your doctor may recommend a surgical procedure to correct the prolapse, or may recommend that you be fitted with a pessary, a device rather like a large sewing thread spool inserted into the vagina to support the uterus.

Retroversion of the Uterus

Normally the uterus lies in the posterior part of the pelvis with the upper pole tilted forward. In about one woman in five, however, the uterus is tilted backward, or retroverted. Usually this causes no symptoms. Nevertheless in some women it may give rise to backaches, painful menstruation, and painful intercourse. The diagnosis is made by simple pelvic examination.

Treatment. If significant symptoms are associated with retroversion of the uterus, your doctor may recommend an operation called ventrosuspension, in which the uterus is moved to a more forward position.

Pelvic Infections *(Salpingitis, Pelvic Inflammatory Disease)*

Bacteria enter the uterus through the cervix and then into the abdomen through the fallopian tubes. Women often suffer infections following sexual intercourse, childbirth, or abortion, or they may be associated with the presence of an intrauterine device, though in many cases there is no recognizable cause.

These infections may be either acute or chronic. Acute infections often cause severe lower abdominal pain, tenderness, and fever. (Gonococcus and chlamydia are the commonest bacteria to cause these acute infections. In chronic infections the pain is more nagging and often there is no fever. Either type of infection may be associated with excessive vaginal discharge, sometimes foul-smelling, irregular menstruation, back pain, and painful intercourse.

Treatment. The occurrence of any of the above symptoms should prompt you to see your doctor at once. Failure to treat pelvic infections with appropriate antibiotics can lead to peritonitis, an infection of the entire abdominal cavity, which is life threatening. Bed rest and the avoidance of sexual intercourse are also recommended. If the causative bacteria has been transmitted sexually, your partner will also require treatment.

Cancer of the Cervix

Cancer of the cervix accounts for about 6% of all cancers in women and occurs most commonly in the age range 40–60. Risk factors for cervical cancer include:

- Having sexual intercourse before age 18
- Having had many sex partners

The venereal transmission of human papilloma virus and herpesvirus type 2 have also been implicated as important in causing cervical cancer.

Women who undertake estrogen replacement therapy after menopause (*see* p. 345) and women who have had no children are at *lower* risk of developing cervical cancer.

Symptoms. The most common symptom of cervical cancer is a bloody vaginal discharge, which may be heavy and have an unpleasant odor; bleeding or spotting between periods, after intercourse, or after menopause may also be signs of cervical cancer.

SCREENING FOR CERVICAL CANCER

A program of regular examinations and Pap smears is very successful in detecting either cervical dysplasia (a type of precancer) before it develops into cervical cancer, or in detecting cancer itself at an early stage, while there is still a good likelihood of cure. (*See* p. 16 for the current recommendations for Pap smears.) Between 1950 and 1970, such screening programs led to a 50% decline in the incidence and mortality rates of cervical cancer. Both rates have continued to decline since 1970.

Diagnosis. When cancer of the cervix is suspected, a Pap smear will be made of cells scraped from your cervix and examined under a microscope. If the Pap smear is abnormal, a biopsy, and possibly a D&C, will be performed to determine whether cancer has spread into your uterus.

Treatment. As with most cancers, the treatment depends upon the stage (extent) of your cancer at the time of its diagnosis. Usually the cervix is removed, and if the cancer is advanced, the rest of the uterus, ovaries, and fallopian tubes will be removed. Your decision to treat with postoperative radiation therapy also depends upon the stage of disease. Chemotherapy is usually reserved for cancers that have spread to distant organs.

Cancer of the Uterus *(Endometrial Cancer)*

Cancer of the uterus starts in the endometrium and spreads to the walls of the uterus, fallopian tubes, ovaries, bladder, and rectum, and by the lymphatic system to distant organs. This is a slow growing cancer and, if detected early, is usually curable. Cancer of the uterus is the second most common genital cancer in women after cancer of the cervix. It is predominantly a cancer of older women, usually occurring in the age range 55–70.

Though the cause of cancer of the uterus is not known, there are certain identifiable risk factors. These include:

- Obesity
- Diabetes
- Infertility
- Late menopause
- Any condition that increases blood estrogen levels, including hormone medications containing *only* estrogen. Almost all modern

---

SCREENING FOR UTERINE CANCER

Pap smears do not adequately screen for the presence of uterine cancer. And most doctors do not recommend routine D&Cs to detect asymptomatic uterine cancer. This is a traumatic and expensive procedure and the detection rate is low. However, some doctors do recommend screening D&Cs for women who are at high risk of developing uterine cancer. If you are in doubt, ask your doctor's recommendations.

---

birth control pills contain a combination of estrogen and progesterone that actually *decreases* the incidence of cancer of the uterus. For this reason the incidence of cancer of the uterus in the United States is declining.

Symptoms. Abnormal vaginal bleeding after menopause is the most common symptom. A bloody discharge does not always indicate the presence of cancer, but it does demand that further tests be undertaken to rule out the possibility of cancer.

Diagnosis. When cancer of the uterus is suspected, your doctor will most likely recommend a D&C in which a portion of the endometrium is scraped out and examined for the presence of cancerous cells. If cancer is found, additional X-ray procedures will be ordered to determine the extent of the cancer (the stage).

Treatment. When cancer of the uterus is confirmed, the uterus is usually removed, along with your ovaries and fallopian tubes. In some cases radiation or chemotherapy are also recommended. For more information on cancer care and cancer resources, *see* p. 9.

Other Cervical Lesions

The Pap smear is also useful in differentiating two other cervical conditions from cervical cancer, i.e., *cervical erosion* and *cervical dysplasia*. Cervical erosion is a benign condition in which the inner lining (epithelium) of the cervix extends down onto the vaginal portion of the cervix. Since this lining is more vascular than normal cervical epithelium, bleeding may occur following intercourse. The treatment of cervical erosion is simple chemical or electrocauterization to remove the abnormal epithelium.

Cervical dysplasia is a potentially cancerous change in the cervical epithelium that is readily detected by microscopic examination. The areas of dysplasia are removed by laser beam treatment or by simple surgery.

Cervical polyps are benign grape-like growths on the cervix that may have all of the symptoms of cervical cancer—heavy discharge and bleeding after intercourse and after menopause. The diagnosis is easily made by pelvic examination and Pap smear. Removal is simple and recurrence is unlikely.

Breast Disorders

Lumps in the Breast

For most women, the first reaction to finding a lump in her breast is likely to be, "Oh, no! I have cancer." For some the response is anxiety and fear of seeking medical attention lest the doctor confirm the worst. So let us emphasize at the outset that most (more than four out of five) breast lumps are not cancerous. There are five common kinds of benign breast lumps: lipomas, fat necrosis, infections, fibroadenomas, and cystic disease.

Lipomas

These are soft, painless, movable, fatty growths that commonly develop in the breasts and elsewhere in older women. They grow slowly and have no consequence, unless they become large enough to cause concern cosmetically.

Fat Necrosis

These lumps commonly form in older women and women with large breasts, most often in response to a bruise or some trauma to the breast. The injury causes the fatty tissue of the breast to form painless round lumps that usually disappear after a time.

Fibroadenomas

These are small, firm, rubbery, movable lumps that usually form in young women and are more common among black women. They can most reliably be distinguished from cancer by mammography, a type of breast X-ray. They are most often treated by surgical removal and do not recur.

Breast Infections

It is not uncommon for bacteria to enter your nipple and form small abscesses in the milk ducts beneath the nipple. Usually these are painful, tender, and sometimes reddened. The lymph nodes under the arm on the same side may become swollen and tender as a result of

---

FIBROCYSTIC DISEASE

This is the most common disease of the female breast in middle-aged women. Fibrocystic disease is characterized by the development of fluid-filled cysts arising out of the milk ducts. Fibrocystic production appears to be stimulated by estrogen, since the condition commonly disappears with menopause. The cysts may enlarge and become tender just before menstruation and then subside after menstruation. Women with fibrocystic disease have a 2 to 5 times higher risk of developing breast cancer. Therefore regular breast examinations and routine mammography are especially important if you are one of these women.

Treatment. Usually no specific treatment is required. There is evidence to suggest that eliminating substances containing methylxanthine from your diet is helpful in reducing the severity of cystic disease. These include coffee, tea, colas, and chocolate. It may also be useful to take vitamin E in doses of 600–800 IU per day if fibrocystic disease is troublesome. Birth control pills also tend to reduce the severity of fibrocystic disease. Consult your doctor about these possibilities. Contrary to popular notions, aspirin does not appear to worsen fibrocystic disease.

---

infectious drainage. Breast infections also occur while women are nursing. The usual treatment for these infections is an antibiotic and a pain reliever. In rare instances an abscess must be surgically drained. To prevent nipple infections during nursing, keep your nipples clean and dry. Apply petrolatum on the nipples if they tend to crack.

A WORD OF CAUTION

The purpose of describing the benign breast conditions above was to explain the origin of most lumps in the breast. It was not meant to encourage you to try to make your own diagnosis. If you feel a new lump in your breast that does not go away after menstruating, see your doctor soon to obtain a professional opinion about the nature of the lump and what must be done about it.

Breast Cancer

Breast cancer is the most common malignancy among women, and accounts for a greater number of deaths than any other single form of cancer in women. It occurs in about 1 in 9 white women and about 1

BREAST CANCER RISK FACTORS

Risk factors that tend to increase the likelihood of developing breast cancer include:

1. A close relative with breast cancer (mother, grandmother, sister)
2. Early age of menarche
3. Advancing age
3. Obesity, especially during adolescence
4. Late pregnancy or childlessness

---

in 14 black women in the United States. The cancer is rare before age 30, but the incidence rises rapidly after menopause.

Some recent studies suggest that alcohol consumption may also increase such risk, although the increase appears to be slight.

There are several different types of breast cancer, but they all begin as lumps, local hardness, or changes in the contour of the breasts that have been detailed above. When any of these changes is noticed, see your doctor at once.

After examining your breasts, your doctor will order a mammogram to help determine what type of mass is present. In some cases, your doctor will recommend aspiration of the lump, using a needle to withdraw fluid or a small amount of tissue. If the lump appears to be a simple cyst, often it will be observed and no further treatment undertaken if the lump does not reappear.

Often it will be recommended that the lump be biopsied, since this is the only sure way to know whether or not cancer cells are present. At this point an important choice must be made. You must decide whether, if cancer is found, you want the surgeon to go ahead and remove the cancer, a so-called *one-step* procedure. Or you may decide just to have the biopsy, and, if necessary, undergo definitive surgery a week or so later, a *two-step* procedure. There is no known disadvantage to the short delay of the two-step procedure, and this may give you an opportunity to review your options, or possibly even to have a second opinion about the type of surgery recommended for you (*see* pp. 4 and 9 for information about second opinions and getting the best cancer care). Many surgeons prefer the two-step procedure, because it provides an opportunity to undertake additional tests to help determine the extent of the disease, as well as whether or not the tumor is likely

---

STAGES OF BREAST CANCER

- Stage I means that the tumor is 2 centimeters (about 1 inch) or less in diameter, and has not spread outside the breast.
- Stage II breast cancer is from 2 to 5 cm in diameter, and/or has spread to the lymph nodes under the arm.
- Stage III cancer is larger than 5 cm, has spread to the lymph nodes under the arm to a greater extent and/or has spread to other lymph nodes or other tissues near the breast.
- Stage IV cancer has spread (metastasized) to other organs of the body, most often to the lungs, bones, liver, or brain.

---

to respond to certain types of chemotherapy. Remember that four out of five breast lumps are not cancer.

Staging of Breast Cancer

There are several factors that determine the specific therapy most appropriate for you. These include your medical history, age, general health, and the type and extent of the cancer. The extent of the cancer is known as its stage. In breast cancer, the staging system used is outlined in the box above.

Carcinoma *in situ* is very early breast cancer. Cancer is present only in the immediate area of the lump.

Treatment Options. The four standard ways of treating breast cancer are surgery, radiation therapy, chemotherapy, and hormone therapy. The type of therapy will largely depend on your health and the stage of disease.

Surgery is the most common treatment for breast cancer. Again, there are several types of surgery that can be performed. From least to most extensive, the types of surgery are given in the box on the following page.

CHEMOTHERAPY AND HORMONAL THERAPY

Chemotherapy, using cytotoxic drugs, is often given during surgery to destroy any cancer cells that may get into the bloodstream during the operation. These drugs are also useful in prolonging life in patients with Stage III and IV disease, and with recurrent breast cancer (about 20% of cases).

In women whose cancer cells contain special estrogen receptors, the anti-estrogen drug, tamoxifen, may be useful in stopping or slowing tumor growth because these tumors appear to depend on a supply of estrogen to maintain their cancer growth.

TYPES OF BREAST CANCER SURGERY

- *Partial or segmental mastectomy*, also called *lumpectomy*, in which only a portion of the breast is removed, including the cancer and a surrounding margin of healthy breast tissue. Most surgeons also remove some of the lymph nodes in the armpit, and usually follow up with radiotherapy. This procedure is commonly recommended for carcinoma *in situ*. In some cases radiation implants may also be used as supplemental therapy.
- *Total simple mastectomy*, which means complete removal of the breast. Some of the lymph nodes may also be removed.
- *Modified radical mastectomy*, which involves removal of the breast, the underarm lymph nodes, and the lining of the chest muscles. It is the most common operation for Stage I and II breast cancer.
- *Radical mastectomy* removes the breast, lymph nodes, and the chest muscles. This procedure, which used to be common, is now used only occasionally because it is disfiguring, there is often residual swelling (edema) of the arm, and less extensivel operations give just as good results.

Several recent studies have shown that women with relatively early breast cancer—those with a low risk of recurrence—have a better chance of surviving when chemotherapy or hormonal therapy is combined with the standard surgery and radiotherapy programs. These treatment programs are known as *adjuvant* chemotherapy and have dramatically altered medical thinking about breast cancer. Adjuvant chemotherapy increases the number of complications breast cancer patients will experience, but the additional lives saved or lengthened appear to warrant the added therapy.

REHABILITATION

Breast cancer surgery is often quite traumatic, interrupting nerves, lymph nodes, and general vitality. Good nutrition and adequate exercise after surgery are essential for your speedy recovery. The Cancer Information Service at 1-800-4-CANCER can send you several publications on diet and nutrition during cancer treatment, control of pain, recovery from surgery, and coping with radiation and chemotherapy.

The American Cancer Society's Reach to Recovery program is also very useful to breast cancer patients. It is staffed by volunteers who themselves have had breast surgery and can help with exercises and assist in obtaining prosthetic breast forms and clothing adjustments.

Finally, a word of caution about continued breast cancer surveillance. Of women who develop cancer in one breast, about 15% will develop cancer in the opposite breast some time later. This means that a program of breast self-examination (*see* p. 365), mammography, and periodic examinations by your doctor are important.

BREAST PROSTHESES AND IMPLANTS

To overcome the disfigurement of mastectomy, you may choose to wear a breast form (prosthesis) that comes in a wide variety of types and materials. These prostheses are sold in surgical supply stores, in lingerie and corset shops, and in the underwear sections of large department stores. It is important to shop around for one you find comfortable, is convenient to wear, and makes you look your best.

In the past 20 years, more than two million women have elected to have breast implants for reconstruction after breast surgery and, rather more often, for augmentation of breast size. By far the most popular has been the silicone gel implant, which consists of a silicone rubber pouch filled with silicone gel. A smaller number of saline-filled devices has been implanted, though they are considered less "natural."

In recent years several reports have questioned the safety of silicone gel-filled implants, and in April, 1992, the US Food and Drug Administration restricted their availability until more information is gained. The safety questions concern the body's various reactions to silicone. All implants tend to "bleed" small amounts of silicone from the implant, and in a certain number of women the implant ruptures, releasing large amounts of silicone gel into surrounding tissues. The following problems have been known to occur:

1. A certain number of women develop *capsular contracture*, a shrinking of scar tissue around the implant that can cause painful hardening of the breasts.
2. Some women develop an immune-related disorder of connective tissue, akin to scleroderma, rheumatoid arthritis, and lupus.
3. In some women the implant has hidden the development (probably unrelated to the implant itself) of a second breast cancer by interfering with the ability to interpret mammograms.
4. There have been some concerns about implants causing cancer. This question has been associated most frequently with a particular polyurethane-coated implant which was withdrawn from the market in April, 1991.
5. Finally, there is the question of failure rate. Breast implants of any

type can rupture, and when they do, it is advised that the implant be removed. The failure rate is not really known; manufacturers report rupture rates between 0.2 and 1.1%.

At this time silicone gel-filled implants are available for reconstruction after breast cancer surgery to any woman who needs and wants them, provided they enter a protocol (a study monitored by the FDA) designed to answer the above enumerated safety questions.

Saline-filled implants are still available without restriction for both augmentation and reconstruction. Although the safety of these implants have not been proven, a rupture only releases saline, which is not harmful to the body. However, like silicone gel-filled devices, saline implants are encased in a silicone rubber envelope that may not be entirely risk-free.

The silicone gel-filled implants are available to women for the purpose of breast augmentation only under limited circumstances and only to numbers sufficient to answer questions of safety. Safety is of greater concern for younger women with normal breast tissue because of the potentially longer exposure to silicone and the need for continued breast cancer surveillance by mammography.

For more information about breast implants, write or call:

FDA, Breast Implant Information, HFE-88, 5600 Fishers Lane, Rockville, MD 20857, or call 1-302-443-3170.

The National Cancer Institute provides brochures, treatment information, and local resources: 1-800-4-CANCER.

Y-Me, a breast cancer support group that provides information and counselling. Write: 18220 Harwood Ave, Homewood, IL 60430, or call 1-800-221-2141.

Command Trust Network, Inc., an advocacy organization for support and information about breast implants and breast implant surgery. Send $1 and a self-addressed, stamped envelope to P.O. Box 17082, Covington, KY 41017.

If You Have An Implant ...

Most women with breast implants do not experience serious problems. And, it should be emphasized, that *if you are not having problems, there is no need to have your implant removed.* Although the possibility cannot be ruled out, there is currently no evidence that silicone gel-filled implants increase the risk of cancer. This applies equally to the 10% of women who have had the polyurethane covered implants.

BREAST SELF-EXAMINATION

Women's breasts change throughout their lives. Factors such as pregnancy, birth control, the menstrual cycle, and especially age all effect the size and consistency of the breasts. You must develop a clear understanding of how your breasts should look and feel. Because more than 90% of breast cancers are discovered by women themselves, the breast self-examination plays a vital role in cancer surveillance.

Get in the habit of examining your breasts each month. All women over 20 years of age should undertake this regular examination. It is important to examine them at the same time after your last menstrual period, since your breasts change with the menstrual cycle. A good time is about a week after your menstrual period since breast swelling is at a minimum at this time.

1. Begin with a visual inspection. Stand before a mirror and inspect both breasts for any unusual appearance, such as discharge from the nipples, redness, scaling, puckering, or dimpling of the skin. Remember that the breasts are normally somewhat asymmetrical.
2. Clasp your hands behind your head and press your hands forward. Notice any change in the shape or contour of your breasts.
3. Next, place your hands firmly on your hips and bow slightly forward toward the mirror.
4. Next, examine the texture of each breast. Many women prefer to do this in the shower, letting fingers glide over soapy skin to better feel the tissues beneath. Raise your left arm. Use three or four finger of your right hand to explore your left breast firmly and thoroughly. Beginning at the outer edge, press down on your breast, moving your fingers in small circles all over the breast. Gradually work toward the nipple. Pay special attention to the area between the breast and the armpit, including the armpit itself. Feel for any unusual lumps beneath the skin. Repeat this step examining your right breast.
5. Gently squeeze each nipple and look for a discharge.
6. Now lie down with a pillow beneath your shoulder. Raise first your left arm over your head and repeat step 4. Lying down allows you to palpate the lower part of your breasts more easily.

Get to know how each breast feels. Remember that it is normal for your breast tissue to feel somewhat lumpy and uneven; it is changes in that familiar texture that you must notice. Look for any differences since the last month. Note especially any thickening or hardening of pea-sized lumps. For an illustrated brochure on breast self-examination, write for NIH Publication No. 85.2000 to: National Cancer Institute, 9000 Rockville Pike, Bethesda MD 20892.

However, you should be aware of the potential for a problem. Here is what you should do:

- If you experience any breast discomfort, change in the size or shape of your breast, or any symptoms you think may be related to your implants, see your doctor at once. A ruptured implant should be removed.
- You should have periodic (at least yearly) checkups by your doctor and you should do monthly breast exams (*see* previous page).
- You should have screening mammography at the same intervals recommended for all women in your age group (*see below*).
- If you develop symptoms associated with an immune-related or connective tissue disorder, see your doctor at once. These symptoms include:

  1. Joint pain and swelling
  2. Skin tightness, redness or swelling
  3. Swollen glands or lymph nodes
  4. Unusual and unexplained fatigue
  5. Swollen hands and feet
  6. Unexpected hair loss

Naturally, all of these symptoms can occur with non-immune disorders and your doctor will conduct a proper diagnostic workup.

To Report a Problem

To report a problem with an implant, write to The Problem Reporting Program, 12601 Twinbrook Parkway, Rockville, MD 20852. A copy of your report will be forwarded to the manufacturer and to the FDA. Include the following information, if known:

- Product brand name and manufacturer.
- Style, size, and lot number.
- Dates of all implant surgeries.
- Age at time of first implant.
- Whether the procedure was for augmentation or reconstruction.
- Nature of problem and date of onset.
- Name and address of surgeon and the facility where surgery was performed.
- Your name, address, and telephone number.

THE VALUE OF ROUTINE MAMMOGRAPHY

Mammography is a special X-ray technique that uses low-energy X-rays to clearly visualize the soft tissues of the breast. Newer equipment delivers a very low radiation dose to the breasts and entails a negligible risk from the radiation itself. Mammography is much more accurate than either ultrasound or thermography in detecting breast lesions. Be sure to ask your doctor whether the mammography equipment used in your studies was especially designed for mammography.

The procedure should not be painful; if it is, tell the technicians so they are more sensitive and careful with their technique. Breast lesions can be detected by mammography that are only half the size you are likely to detect by your own breast evaluation , even if you are very skilled in self-examination.

How Often Do You Need a Mammogram?

The American Cancer Society (ACS) recommends a baseline mammogram for all women between the ages of 35 and 40 and even earlier for women with known risk factors, such as a family history of breast cancer. This baseline mammogram can then be compared to all subsequent mammograms to aid in cancer detection.

For women 40–49 years of age, the ACS recommends mammograms every other year. After age 50 every woman should have an annual mammogram. The great value of routine mammography is that it allows earlier detection of breast cancer—when there is a greater chance of cure and when less disfiguring surgery will be needed to control the cancer. These recommendations will change as new information is gained. Consult your doctor.

Other Resources

For more information, contact the Cancer Information Service, 1-800-4-CANCER (in Alaska, 1-800-638-6070; in Hawaii, 524-1234) to receive free brochures providing information on all aspects of breast cancer and its treatment. The American Cancer Society, 90 Park Avenue, New York, NY 10016; 1-212-599-3600 is a national voluntary organization that offers a wide range of services to cancer patients and their families. See your telephone directory for their local chapter. Most YWCA offices sponsor an Encore program that offers exercise and group discussions for women who have had breast cancer.

For brochures with the latest information on breast cancer, write: Woman's Breast Cancer Advisory Committee, Box 224, Kensington, MD 20895.

For more information about breast surgery, call the Cancer Information Service, 1-800-4-CANCER and ask for the pamphlet: *Mastectomy: A Treatment for Breast Cancer.*

Contraceptive Measures for Women

Paradoxically the contraception options for women in the United States have decreased with time as more and more intrauterine devices (IUDS) have been withdrawn from the market because of complications and lawsuits. The most publicized example is the Dalkon Shield, which caused pelvic infections in many users. European women enjoy more options, including drugs that stop ovulation for as long as 5 years, and the "morning after" pill that interferes with implantation of a fertilized egg into the uterus. Still, women in the US have access to a number of effective contraceptive measures.

Birth-Control Pills

Most oral contraceptives contain small amounts of estrogen and progesterone, the female hormones that regulate the uterine cycle and ovulation. "Birth-control pills" (BCPs) are about 98% effective in preventing pregnancy, the highest success rate of any method after sterilization. The other advantages of BCPs are lighter, more regular, and cramp-free menstrual periods; protection against cancer of the uterus and ovaries; and decreased risks of benign breast disease, ovarian cysts, and pelvic inflammatory disease.

BCPs are usually the most effective and well-accepted form of contraception among young women. Supervision and annual examinations by a doctor are essential for their effective use and the avoidance of complications. Complications of BCPs include side effects similar to early pregnancy, such as nausea, breast tenderness, and fluid retention. Usually these side effects disappear after about three months of use. Increased blood pressure and mental depression occur rarely; your doctor can usually control these side effects by reducing the dose of estrogen. Women who develop breakthrough bleeding are usually managed by *increasing* the dose of estrogen.

Such side effects as weight gain, acne, and nervousness may be corrected by altering the dose of progesterone in the combination.

Be certain to consult your doctor about the correct timing for restarting BCPs after pregnancy or a miscarriage and their proper use during breast feeding.

BCPs and Breast Cancer

It has now been almost 30 years since birth control pills were introduced in the United States—long enough for their safety to be established and their side-effects known. Very early on it was postulated

WHO SHOULD NOT TAKE BCPs?

It is estimated that since their introduction, more than 80 million women have used BCPs. Among women who are currently in their childbearing years, almost half have used BCPs at some time or another. Taking all of these women into account, BCPs have demonstrated an extraordinary safety record. Nevertheless, there are certain women who are at greater risk of various complications from BCPs than others:

- Women who smoke. Smoking definitely increases the risk of high blood pressure, heart attacks, blood clots, and strokes in women who use BCPs.
- Women with blood clotting disorders, high blood pressure, or heart disease should not take BCPs without the advice and close supervision of their doctors.
- Women who are or may be pregnant.
- Women with liver disease or diabetes
- Women with known or suspected breast cancer.
- Women who take certain drugs, such as barbiturates, sulfonamides, cyclophosphamide, and rifampin which may act to make BCPs less effective. Be sure to tell your doctor what medications you are taking when discussing oral contraceptives.

that the estrogen in birth control pills might cause, or at least stimulate, the development of breast cancer. However, several large studies found no relationship between BCPs and breast cancer in women, even though its incidence among women in the United States has been steadily increasing.

Recently, a few isolated studies have again brought up the question of a link between breast cancer and BCPs, although the findings were in some cases contradictory and an expert panel of the Food and Drug Administration has not found the current evidence sufficient to change package recommendations of any of the contraceptive combinations. Furthermore, the panel urged that the data concerning breast cancer be viewed in perspective:

- There is ample evidence that BCPs actually *prevent* endometrial and ovarian cancer and these effects alone would cancel out the slight increases in breast cancer reported by the recent studies.

- With the decreased marketing of other contraceptive devices, such as IUDs, and given the lesser effectiveness of "barrier techniques" such as condoms and diaphragms, BCPs offer one of the few truly effective means of contraception. This is especially important in view of the fact that the risk of dying from a pregnancy complication is 8 in 10,000, much higher than a young women's potentially increased risk of breast cancer or other BCP-related complication.
- Other conditions, such as irregular menstrual bleeding, endometriosis, and benign breast disease are all favorably affected by BCPs.

Contraceptive Implants

The newest method of delivering contraceptive hormones is by implanting small rubber tubes containing the hormone beneath the skin, where a near-constant amount is then released into the blood stream each day. The first of these to be developed is Norplant, which consists of six small silastic tubes inserted beneath the skin on the inner side of the arm just above the elbow. The surgical insertion is simple, relatively painless, and requires only about 15 minutes. The tubes contain enough hormone to last about five years, at which time they can be removed as simply as they were inserted. The great advantages this contraceptive method affords are the convenience of not having to take daily pills and the long period of its effectiveness. The failure rate of such implants is about the same as that for birth control pills—about 1% per year. Should you desire to become pregnant, the implants can be removed and normal ovarian cycling begins almost at once.

What are the drawbacks of implants? Essentially, they are the same side effects associated with oral contraceptives *(see above)*. Of these, the most common are spotting and irregular menstrual periods.

Intrauterine Devices (IUDs)

These are small pieces of plastic or copper inserted into the uterus; they act to prevent fertilization of the ovum by the sperm. One brand, Progestasert, depends on the release of small amounts of the hormone progesterone as the contraceptive action. The presence of progesterone makes the uterine lining unfavorable for implantation of the ovum. IUDs must be inserted by a doctor and can be left in place for a year or longer. They are about 95% effective in preventing pregnancy, and there is not much difference in effectiveness between different brands.

The most common complications include cramping and bleeding, which occur in about 15% of users during the first year and 7% during the second year. IUDs may in rare cases contribute to pelvic infections and ectopic pregnancy, i.e., the development of a fetus outside the uterus, which necessitates surgical removal. Perforation of the uterus is another very rare complication.

Automatic expulsion of the IUD occurs in 20–30% of users during the first year and 10–15% during the second year. Your doctor will show you how to regularly check for correct IUD placement.

IUDs are generally recommended for women who are over 25, have had at least one child, and have no history of pelvic inflammatory disease or ectopic (fallopian tube) pregnancy. IUDs are not recommended for women who have *multiple* sex partners because they do not protect against sexually transmitted diseases as well as barrier methods do, and the presence of an IUD increases the risk of pelvic inflammatory disease in such circumstances.

Diaphragms

A diaphragm is a dome-shaped rubber cap that fits over the cervix and acts as a barrier to sperm entering the uterus. Used in conjunction with a spermicidal preparation, diaphragms are 80–95% effective in preventing pregnancy. They must be fitted by your doctor, who will also instruct you in proper insertion, removal, and care. The diaphragm should be inserted prior to coitus and left in place for 8 hours afterward. Additional spermicide should be added prior to each act of intercourse to improve effectiveness. Do not douche after intercourse; this will only reduce the effectiveness of the spermicide.

Cervical Cap

The cervical cap is similar to a diaphragm, only smaller and less fragile. It comes in several sizes and must be fitted initially by your doctor, since it is generally more difficult to insert than a diaphragm. Once inserted, it may be left in place for up to 48 hours; longer wear will result in an unpleasant odor. When used with a spermicide, the effectiveness is similar to that of a diaphragm. The cervical cap is recommended only for women with a normal Pap smear, and this test must be repeated after three months use.

Vaginal Spermicides

Available as foams, creams, jellies, suppositories, and sponges, these over-the-counter preparations contain an agent, usually nonoxynol-9, that kills or immobilizes sperm on contact. These preparations must be placed into the vagina before each intercourse, and for maximum effectiveness, no longer than an hour before each occasion. Thus effective use requires a cool attitude, one that is not flustered or distracted in times of passion. Possibly for this reason, the effectiveness of vaginal spermicides (70–80% when used alone) increases with age (and experience). The contraceptive sponge has the advantage that it can be inserted as long as 24 hours prior to intercourse and consequently may interfere less with one's sense of spontaneity. The sponge must be left in place for six hours after the last occasion of intercourse. Despite some publicity to the contrary, use of spermicides does not increase the risk of birth defects in those pregnancies that occur in spite of the spermicide.

Sterilization

For women, sterilization is slightly more complex than vasectomy is for men. Usually an abdominal incision is made and the fallopian tubes are tied (tubal ligation) or cauterized with an electric current. Though general anesthesia is usually recommended, hospitalization is seldom required. Nor does tubal ligation after delivery prolong hospitalization. Often the sterilization procedure can be accomplished through a laparoscope inserted into the abdomen. In women with severe menstrual problems or with uterine tumors, a vaginal hysterectomy is often the recommended sterilization procedure.

Reversal of tubal ligation is about 75% effective, should you later desire to become pregnant. For more information about sterilization and its reversal, send a stamped, self-addressed business-size envelope to: Association for Voluntary Surgical Contraception, 122 E. 43rd St., New York, NY 10168.

Condoms for Women

Recently, the US Food and Drug Administration has approved a condom designed to be inserted into the vagina by the woman herself. These new condoms provide not only protection against unwanted fertilization, but a barrier against sexually transmitted disease as well. At this time it is too early to advise how successful these new condoms will be in preventing either pregnancy or disease, or how well they will be accepted by women and their partners. But the development is a step toward providing women with greater control and freedom, which is most certainly a step in the right direction.

The male reproductive organs

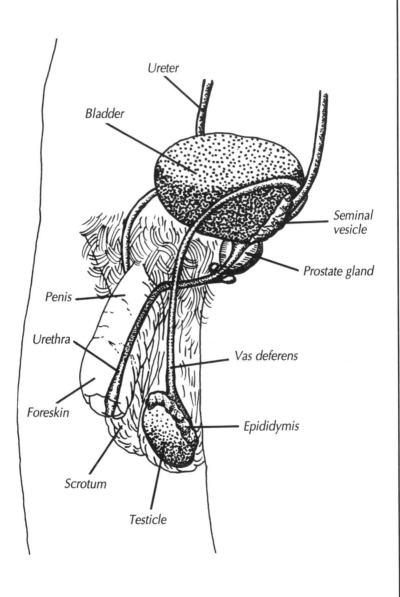

Ureter

Bladder

Seminal vesicle

Prostate gland

Penis

Urethra

Vas deferens

Foreskin

Epididymis

Scrotum

Testicle

Men's Medical Problems

The Testicles and Scrotum

The testicles are the two male glands that produce sperm and the hormones responsible for male sexual characteristics. Their relationship to the penis, bladder, and prostate gland are shown in the figure on the opposite page. The principal medical problems of the testicles and scrotum are inflammation and the unwanted presence of various masses that need to be distinguished.

Epididymitis

Epididymitis is an inflammation of the epididymis, the worm-like appendage at the back of the testicle that serves as the organ's sperm collecting system and can be felt as a cord running upward into the groin. Infections of the epididymis occur when bacteria descend into it from the urethra through the vas deferens. In fact, epididymitis is usually a complication of urethritis (*see* p. 391) or prostatitis (*see* p. 379). Often the testicles will be inflamed as well *(orchitis)*.

The hallmark of epididymitis is a warm, sausage-like swelling at the back of the testicle that is exquisitely painful and tender to touch. *Fever, nausea, and vomiting provide ample indication that you need to see your doctor at once.*

Treatment. Symptomatic treatment consists of bed rest, elevation of the testicles using a scrotal support, and ice packs. Appropriate antibiotics are selected for the particular bacteria responsible. The most common bacteria that cause epididymitis are those that cause gonorrhea and chlamydia, both sexually transmitted (*see* p. 389). Therefore your sexual partner may also need to be treated with antibiotics to prevent reinfection. In the rare cases in which an abscess develops, surgical drainage is required.

Torsion of the Testicle

Torsion of the testicle is a condition that often must be distinguished from epididymitis. It occurs when the testicle twists within the scrotum because the back of the testicle is not firmly attached to the scrotum, in a way that cuts off its own blood supply.

375

The swelling, pain, and tenderness of the involved testicle often make torsion so difficult to distinguish from epididymitis that the distinction can often only be made by radiographic tests that determine how much blood is flowing to the testicle.

Treatment. Surgery within a few hours of onset of pain is the only measure that will save the testicle. After untwisting the spermatic cord, the testicle is then fixed in place to prevent a recurrence. If surgery is not undertaken promptly, the testicle will atyrophy. However, loss of function in one testicle usually does not mean sterility, since enlargement of the opposite testicle produces sufficient sperm to ensure fertility.

Injury to the Testicle

Because of their exposure, the testicles are sometimes injured, resulting in pain severe enough to double you over. Being kicked in the groin, often in the context of sports, is probably the most common cause of testicular injury.

Treatment. Usually no treatment is necessary. However, *if pain persists and swelling of a testicle results, see your doctor at once.* Surgical removal of a blood clot (hematoma) may be the only procedure that will save the testicle. In some cases after injury, a painless accumulation of blood within the scrotum develops slowly over time. This is known as a *hematocele*, and is similar to a *hydrocele (see below)*, except that light from a flashlight will not shine through a hematocele. If the hematocele does not disappear by itself, it may have to be removed surgically to prevent infertility.

Hydrocele

Hydrocele is a swelling caused by fluid accumulating inside the scrotum. The hydrocele usually develops on one side and may become large enough to cause discomfort. You can distinguish a hydrocele from a hematocele *(see above)* by the fact that light from a small flashlight shines through the hydrocele. The treatment is surgical removal if the mass causes discomfort. Fluid can also be drained by needle aspiration, however, the fluid usually reaccumulates and there is also a danger of inducing infection.

Varicocele

Varicocele is an accumulation of dilated veins that more often occurs in the left scrotum and has often been described as feeling to the touch like a "bag of worms." The swollen veins disappear when you lie down, as a result of normal postural drainage. The condition is harmless, although their presence may reduce fertility. They are best tolerated by wearing tight-fitting underwear. If they cause discomfort, or you are worried about possible infertility (they do not in any way affect male potency), see your doctor, who may advise surgical removal of the veins.

In some men with fluid in the abdomen (ascites), a portion of the fluid may leak into the scrotum, causing swelling on both sides. The treatment is the use of a scrotal suspensory, much like a jock strap. In severe cases, surgery may be recommended to close communication between the abdomen and the scrotum.

Cysts of the Epididymis

Small cysts may develop in the sperm collecting tubules within the epididymis. They are common in men over the age of 40, appearing as minor, painless swellings in the upper rear part of one or both testicles. They are quite harmless unless they become large enough to cause discomfort. In such cases they may require surgical removal. If you are uncertain whether a lump is actually a part of the testicle, see your doctor.

Blood in the Semen

The appearance of blood in the ejaculated semen is known as *hemospermia*. It is relatively common, is painless, and there is almost always no need for alarm. The usual cause is the rupture of a small vein in the upper part of the urethra during erection. Usually the semen contains only reddish or brownish streaks of blood, although in rare cases blood may appear in the semen for several days. No treatment is necessary. If, however, you notice blood in your urine, see your doctor, because this may signify a serious bladder or kidney problem.

Undescended Testicle

During fetal development the testicles descend from near the kidneys, through the inguinal canal, and into the scrotum. In a small number of boys, one or both testicles fail to descend completely. Such boys must be examined periodically, and if the testicle(s) has/have not descended by age two, a surgical procedure known as orchiopexy to secure the testicle in the scrotum is usually recommended. Delay of surgery beyond age five may lead eventually to compromised sperm formation. In some cases injections of a hormone may induce descent. If an undescended testicle is not detected until after puberty, surgical removal is recommended because of the increased probability that such a testicle will develop cancer.

Mobile testicles that retract into the abdomen when the scrotum contracts are common and require no treatment, although the likelihood of an inguinal hernia is increased for such boys.

Inguinal Hernia

Incomplete closure or tissue weakness may result in enlarging the inguinal canal in the floor of the abdomen through which the spermatic cord passes. If this opening is wide enough, the intestines may slip through and into the scrotum. When a *femoral hernia* exists, the opening is to the side of the inguinal canal and the intestines may protrude into the upper thigh.

Treatment. Both types of hernia should be closed surgically because of the danger that the blood supply to the segment of intestine that passes through the hernia may be cut off. Such an interruption of blood supply is known as *strangulation* of the hernia.

Cancer of the Testicle

Unlike most cancers in men, testicular cancer primarily affects young men between the ages of 15 and 35. Fortunately, it is a disease with a high rate of cure when found early. Undescended testicles (*see above*) develop cancer much more often than normally descended testicles. A family history of testicular cancer or having had mumps orchitis are additional risk factors.

The earliest sign of testicular cancer is a small painless lump in the body of the testicle that grows slowly. Usually it will not be recognized unless you develop the habit of examining your testicles periodically (*see below*). *If you find a testicular mass, see your doctor at once.*

Treatment. Several diagnostic tests are available to determine the type of a testicular tumor and the extent of its development. The initial treatment is removal of the involved testicle. Depending on the cancer's stage of development, radiation therapy or chemotherapy may also be recommended. With early detection, modern treatment results in cure in 80–90% of cases. In most cases the uninvolved testicle is spared, preserving fertility and potency.

For more information, call the Cancer Information Service of the National Cancer Institute: 1-800-422-6237.

SELF EXAMINATION OF THE TESTICLES

The key to early detection of testicular cancer is a simple, two-minute self examination every month beginning right after puberty. The best time is after a warm bath or shower, when the scrotum is relaxed. Roll each testicle gently between your thumb and index finger of both hands. If you find a hard lump in one of your testicles, see your doctor as soon as possible.

Parents should explain the importance of self examination to their sons, because most school health programs omit such training. If you are reluctant to approach this subject, ask your doctor to teach your sons how to examine themselves.

Disorders of the Prostate Gland

The prostate gland is a small organ that surrounds the urethra as it leaves the bladder. The chief function of the prostate is to add essential fluid to ejaculated sperm. The principal problems arising in the prostate are enlargement, inflammation, and tumors.

Inflammation of the Prostate *(Prostatitis)*

Prostatitis, an infection of the prostate, often accompanies urethritis (*see* p. 382). Acute infections are characterized by chills, fever, the frequent urge to void small amounts of urine, pain and burning on urination, and dull pain in the low back or testicles, often radiating down the backs of the legs.

Treatment. A full course of antibiotics is prescribed, along with bed rest, analgesics, and increased fluid intake to wash out the urinary tract and prevent bacteria from entering the bladder. It is important to follow your doctor's instructions carefully to prevent the infection from developing into chronic prostatitis.

Nonbacterial Prostatitis

Even more common, particularly in older men, is a type of chronic prostatitis in which no disease-causing bacteria can be found (*nonbacterial prostatitis*). The cause is unknown and antibiotics do not relieve the symptoms, usually dull pain in the genitals, or anus, sometimes radiating down the backs of the legs. Periodic prostatic massage by your doctor may bring temporary relief. Also try acidifying your urine by taking 1000 milligrams of Vitamin C orally each day. An alkaline urine tends to precipitate deposits of prostatic secretions, which may then become a source of irritation.

Enlarged Prostate *(Benign Prostatic Hypertrophy)*

Enlargement of the prostate gland *(prostatic hypertrophy)* is very common; approximately half of all men in the United States over the age of 50, and 80% of men over 60 suffer from it. The cause is unknown. The result in many men is a gradual obstruction of the urethra, which reduces the force of the urine stream, particularly first thing in the morning. Certain drugs, such as antihistamines, decongestants, and others, significantly worsen the obstruction. Pain is seldom encountered, but as a consequence of being incapable of emptying the bladder, frequent and urgent urination is common. Some men find they are incapable of holding their urine because of overflow incontinence. With urinary stagnation, bladder and kidney infections may result. There is also a danger of sudden, acute obstruction in which urine cannot be voided at all—this is a medical emergency.

Treatment. In at least one out of three cases of mild prostatic enlargement, symptoms disappear without treatment. However, if symptoms persist, your doctor may recommend surgical removal of some of the prostatic tissue. The preferred method is known as a transurethral resection of the prostate (TURP), in which the tissue is removed by a surgical instrument introduced through the urethra, thus sparing an incision. In other cases, especially with very large prostates, removal must be accomplished through an abdominal incision.

The results of prostatic surgery are usually quite satisfactory. However, overall success depends greatly on the skill of the surgeon in preventing such complications as incontinence, impotence, and infections. Shop around for the best surgeon you can find (*see* p. 1). One common change after prostatectomy is retrograde ejaculation, in which sperm is diverted into the bladder and later washed out during urination. This is of no concern unless a pregnancy is desired.

Recent advances in the drug treatment of BPH are encouraging. One new drug, finasteride (Proscar), inhibits the conversion of testosterone to dihydrotestosterone, a hormone that promotes growth of prostate tissue. In some patients finasteride slowly shrinks the prostate sufficiently to reduce obstruction and increases the urine stream to a satisfactory degree. Several months of therapy may be required

---

CANCER OF THE PROSTATE

Cancer of the prostate is now the third most common cancer in men over 55 years of age, after lung cancer and colon cancer. It has been estimated that, by age 80, virtually every male has microscopic prostatic cancer, although many fail to spread and thus cause no symptoms. Interestingly, there appears to be no relationship between benign prostatic hypertrophy and the development of prostatic cancer.

Many men have no symptoms at all when prostate cancer is first detected by physical examination, or at the time of surgery for prostatic enlargement. This is why it is important for men over 50 to have a rectal examination annually. If the tumor becomes large, urinary obstruction causes the symptoms for prostatic enlargement described above. If the cancer spreads to bone, bone pain and weight loss may be the first symptoms.

Recent studies suggest that measuring serum prostate specific antigen (PSA) may increase early detection of prostate cancer by 30%. Ask your doctor if this test may be appropriate for you.

Treatment. If the cancer is localized, either surgical removal of the prostate or radiation therapy will most likely be recommended. For more advanced disease, hormone therapy significantly retards progression of the cancer, which depends on testosterone for active growth. Previously this was accomplished by castration or by administering estrogens. More recently a drug known as *leuprolide* (Lupron) has been found to accomplish the same end without the undesirable cardiovascular side effects of estrogens. An antiandrogen, flutamine, also offers promise in hormone control of the cancer. An anticancer drug, Suramin, is currently under study.

For more information, call the Cancer Information Service of the National Cancer Institute: 1-800-422-6237.

---

to produce noticeable effects. Side effects include impotence and reduced libido in a small number of patients taking the drug.

A second drug, terazosin (Hytrin), is an antihypertensive drug that relaxes smooth muscle and may relieve prostatic obstruction immediately. In some individuals a combination of these drugs may be appropriate. Ask your doctor.

Disorders of the Penis

Inflammation *(Balanitis)*

Balanitis is an inflammation of the foreskin and the tip of the penis (the glans). There are many causes—infection, including genital herpes (*see* p. 394), chancroid (*see* p. 393), tinea cruris (*see* p. 449), and a variety of yeasts. Other causes include irritation by moist underwear, failure to remove smegma from beneath the foreskin, and allergic reactions to condoms or contraceptive creams.

Treatment. Most cases of balanitis disappear spontaneously if the cause is found and eliminated. Good hygiene is essential. If you are not circumcised, carefully retract the foreskin and wash gently with soap and water during showering and bathing to remove irritating smegma. If you have difficulty retracting your foreskin *(phimosis)*, consult your doctor about the advisability of having a circumcision. If redness, swelling, pain, and pus are present, see your doctor for antibiotic treatment.

To prevent irritation from perspiration, use a medicated talcum powder (e.g., Dr. Ammons' Powder) to dust your groin region and wear looser fitting cotton underwear and trousers during warm seasons. Change your underwear daily and after exercising.

Urethritis

Urethritis, inflammation of the urethra in men, is usually caused by one of the sexually transmitted diseases. The major symptoms include penile discharge, burning, and frequent urination. The most common causes are nonspecific urethritis (*see* p. 391) and gonorrhea, *see* p. 389).

Priapism

Priapism is a persistent, painful erection in the absence of sexual desire or excitation. Causes vary from pelvic blood clots to tumors, nerve dysfunction, and reaction to certain drugs. Often the cause is never found.

Treatment. Priapism is an emergency. Do not waste time—apply cold compresses and call your doctor, or go to an emergency room, at once. Failure to treat the condition promptly may result in permanent impotence. Treatment may involve spinal anesthesia, surgical decompression, and drugs to lower blood pressure.

Premature Ejaculation

Premature ejaculation is one of the most common sexual problems in men, particularly among younger men. The causes vary, and most often stem from anxiety—fear of unwanted pregnancy, of contracting a sexually transmitted disease, of not being considered manly, or even fear of the sheer sinfulness of the act. It should also be understood that most men can achieve orgasm within about two minutes of commencing intercourse, whereas women are seldom able to reach that point so quickly. Satisfactory intercourse, then, is almost always a matter of the man's learning to delay orgasm until harmonized with his partner.

Treatment. There are a number of techniques whereby a man can learn to forestall orgasm. Needless to say, they should be practiced with women who are sympathetic to the problem, so that good interpersonal communication is essential.

The "stop-and-start" technique involves stimulating the penis, either manually or through intercourse, until the approach of orgasm. Stimulation is stopped (even if withdrawal is necessary) for 20–30 seconds, and is then recommenced. This is repeated three or four times, after which the orgasm is allowed to take place. With repeated experience and with an understanding partner, the man will learn to prolong intercourse without interrupting the act.

Stimulation of the penis may also be stopped by the "squeeze" technique, whereby it is squeezed at the junction of the head and the shaft for 3–4 seconds. This interrupts orgasm and reduces the erection slightly. After a short while, intercourse may be resumed.

A variety of desensitizing preparations can be applied to the penis to retard orgasm. These are normally used in conjunction with a condom in order to prevent simultaneous desensitization of the partner. It is probably wise to experiment with such techniques before coupling.

For more information and for a list of sex counselors in your area, consult: American Association of Sex Educators, Counselors and Therapists, 435 N. Michigan Ave., Suite 1717, Chicago, IL 60611; 1-312-644-0828.

Impotence

Impotence in men is defined as an inability to attain or maintain an erection satisfactory for sexual intercourse. It used to be thought that

90% of such problems were psychological in origin, i.e., that impotence is caused by depression, anxiety, lack of confidence, or, in many cases, boredom with the sexual partner. It is now thought that only about half of all cases are psychological; the rest are caused by organic problems. As the male population ages, this percentage will no doubt become larger.

Organic Causes of Impotence

Physical factors responsible for impotence include several systemic diseases, including diabetes, syphilis, alcoholism, thyroid and pituitary diseases, and drug dependency. Any condition that reduces blood levels of the male hormone, testosterone, can lead to impotence. Vascular disorders contributing to impotence include aortic aneurysm and pelvic thrombosis. Neurologic disorders leading to it include multiple sclerosis and spinal cord lesions. Several drugs also affect potency; most common are high blood pressure medicines, sedatives, tranquilizers, and central nervous stimulants, such as amphetamines. Impotence is not common after transurethral prostatectomy (TURP), although retrograde ejaculation (ejaculation into the bladder) does occur. Neither is aging itself a cause of impotence, although ejaculatory force and sexual drive diminish, often not until quite late in life.

Treatment. Treatment of an underlying disease, especially if diabetes is the cause, may correct impotence. If a medication, such as a blood pressure drug, is responsible, a change in your medication often resolves the problem. For example, the drugs known as ACE inhibitors are less likely than most other antihypertensive drugs to interfere with sexual function. If impotence has been long-standing, however, counseling of both partners may be necessary because psychologic impediments to sex can develop over time. In rare cases, injections of testosterone may cure impotence.

Recently, the drug yohimbine, often found in folk remedies for various diseases, has been promoted as helpful in some cases of impotence. Yohimbine is not a sexual stimulant, but causes the smooth muscle in certain blood vessels to dilate. In the penis, yohimbine may act in such a way as to favor erection. Ask your doctor whether this may be a solution for you. Please avoid the untested preparations offered in some catalogs, such as those that contain rhinoceros tusk or an extract of whale testicles. There is absolutely no proof that substances of this sort work and their use necessarily involves the needless killing of endangered animals.

MALE INFERTILITY

About half of all cases of infertility are caused by problems of the male. In some cases, impotence, described above, is responsible, but more often the cause is low sperm count. The following are the more common causes of low sperm count:

- *Previous infections.* Mumps orchitis causes scarring of the testicles that may result in low sperm count. More common than this is previous venereal disease, especially gonorrhea, that causes scarring of the sperm ducts. Very little can be done to correct either of these problems, although in cases of a blocked vas deferens, microsurgery may restore fertility.
- *Drugs.* Prescription drugs, such as sulfasalazine (used in ulcerative colitis) and some steroids, may reduce sperm count. Marijuana can also have this effect.
- *Varicocele.* This problem has been described on p. 376. Surgical removal of the dilated veins often raises sperm count.
- *Heat.* Sperm production is sensitive to temperature. In some cases, tight-fitting clothing can raise testicular temperature sufficiently to reduce sperm count. Wearing boxer shorts and looser slacks may correct this problem.
- *Injury.* Previous trauma or radiation can cause irreversible testicular injury.
- *Hormone deficiency.* In rare cases decreased testosterone production can cause reduced sperm count. Occasionally this can be corrected by testosterone injections.

Neurogenic and vascular causes of impotence are frequently not treatable. In motivated individuals, semirigid and inflatable implants may be inserted surgically into the penis. Although these prosthetic devices do not restore orgasm, they are often satisfactory in providing pleasure to the partner.

In some cases so-called "external management systems" provide a satisfactory alternative to penis implants. For example, the use of a vacuum pump can cause engorgement of the penis sufficient for penetration. Placing a constricting band around the base of the penis prevents deflation. In many cases satisfactory orgasm can be achieved.

Men who can achieve an erection with certain women, but not others, or who can masturbate satisfactorily, usually have a psychological cause of impotence. Such problems can often be successfully treated by sex therapy. For example, Masters and Johnson have developed a three-stage method involving, successively nongenital pleasuring, genital pleasuring, and nondemanding intercourse that, with counselling of both partners, may overcome psychic inhibitions to sexual performance.

Occasionally men experience pain with intercourse. This may be caused by infections, or in rare instances, by sensitivity to a spermicidal preparation. Such problems generally require consultation with your doctor to resolve.

Male Breast Enlargement *(Male Gynecomastia)*

Breast enlargement in men is relatively common. Most adolescent boys go through a brief period during which the breast tissue just beneath the nipples swells slightly and may even become tender. As adolescence progresses and the newly increased hormone levels begin to balance, the enlargement goes away. If it does not, your doctor should be consulted to rule out the possibility of a testicular or pituitary tumor.

In older men enlargement of only one breast is an occasional problem. Usually this condition is temporary and will disappear. In any case, you should see your doctor to make certain that this enlargement is not caused by male breast cancer *(see below)*.

Enlargement of both breasts in men may be caused by severe liver disease and by certain drugs if taken for prolonged periods. Drugs that cause breast enlargement include digitalis, cimetidine (Tagamet), various tranquilizers, and drugs that lower high blood pressure.

The normal fat redistribution that occurs in most men after age 40 also causes accentuation of the breasts, especially among the sedentary. If you are sensitive to this normal change, consult a fitness specialist, but by no means is it likely to be gynecomastia.

Breast Cancer

Breast cancer in men is rare, and when it occurs, usually appears in men over 60 years of age. The tumor usually appears as a painless lump near the nipple. Any hardened breast lump or sore near the nipple should be examined by your doctor at once. *See* Treatment of Breast Cancer, p. 361.

Contraceptive Measures for Men

At this time there are only two contraceptive measures available for men—condoms and vasectomy.

Vasectomy

Vasectomy, or "tying the cords" is the surgical cutting and tying off of the spermatic ducts from each testicle. This is a simple, inexpensive operation that can be performed under local anesthesia in about 20 minutes and does not require hospitalization. Permanent sterilization results after about 15–20 ejaculations to empty residual sperm from the spermatic ducts. Remember that sterilization should not be assumed until semen analysis by your doctor demonstrates two sperm-free ejaculates; numerous children have been born of recently vasectomized fathers. Vasectomy has no effect on sexual desire or performance, unless it is to increase both by freeing the couple of the anxiety of unwanted pregnancy. For this reason, vasectomy may be encouraged whenever a couple decides that their family is complete.

Condoms

Condoms or prophylactic sheaths are about 90% effective in preventing pregnancy and may also be more effective in preventing such sexually transmitted diseases as herpes and AIDS than other contraceptive measures. The most effective condoms are those that contain a spermicidal lubricant, such as nonoxynol-9. The principal drawback of condoms is reduced sensitivity for the man, which lessens their acceptance. In rare instances, sensitivity to rubber causes a rash of the penis. This type of contact dermatitis, described more fully on p. 441, can be prevented by switching to a condom made of sheep gut (e.g., lambskin), which may also improve sensation for the man.

Prelubricated condoms are usually preferred. If you buy a nonlubricated latex condom, lubricate it with a water-based lubricant, such as K-Y Jelly, or saliva. *Do not use an oil-based product,* such as Vaseline, Intensive Care lotion, baby oil, Nivea hand cream, or other oily product, since oils can dissolve the rubber and cause the condom to break within minutes. When buying condoms, read the directions. Improper use understandably can have disastrous consequences.

Unprotected sex using such methods as coitus interruptus and periodic abstinence (the "rhythm method") cannot be treated as contraceptive measures because they are either useless or highly ineffective for most couples.

AIDS

ACQUIRED IMMUNODEFICIENCY SYNDROME

lymphogranuloma venereum

CHLAMYDIA

URETHRITIS

gonorrhea

TRICHOMONA

genital herpes

GRANULOMA INGUINALE

genital warts

chancroid

syphilis

Sexually Transmitted Diseases

Prevention and Cure

In our current national preoccupation with AIDS, we tend to forget about the other sexually transmitted diseases and how common they are. For example, it is estimated that 3 million persons in the United States and more than 250 million worldwide are infected with gonorrhea each year. The annual worldwide prevalence of syphilis is about 50 million, with 400,000 new cases each year in the United States. In short, these are among our most common communicable diseases.

Despite advances in diagnosis and treatment, sexually transmitted diseases are on the rise. The factors thought to be responsible for this are:

- More permissive attitudes toward sexual behavior
- Widespread use of contraceptive pills decreases the likelihood of pregnancy
- Increased numbers of sexual partners
- A highly mobile population
- More varied sexual practices, including orogenital and anogenital sex
- The evolution of antibiotic-resistant microorganisms

These, combined with an uneducated public that is often unwilling to seek treatment, create a fertile climate for the spread of disease.

Gonorrhea

One of the most common venereal diseases, gonorrhea is caused by the bacterium, *Neisseria gonorrhoeae*, which attacks the mucous membranes of the genital tract, anus, and mouth.

In men, the most common symptoms of acute gonorrhea are pain, burning, and urgency and frequency of urination, along with a yellowish discharge from the penis. These symptoms develop from 2 to 14 days following exposure.

In women, the symptoms are generally milder, consisting of burning and, occasionally, frequency of urination and a yellowish vaginal
discharge. The symptoms usually begin from 7 to 21 days after contact. Frequently, women who are not treated enter a "carrier" state in
which they are infectious to male partners, but entirely without symptoms. Such women are often surprised and *angry* when accused by a
recent sex partner of responsibility for an infection.

Complications of gonorrhea include infections of the prostate
or testicles in men, and acute abdominal pain and infection (pelvic
inflammatory disease) in women. Infertility is an occasional sequel
if the infection scars the Fallopian tubes. Other complications are
acute arthritis and a generalized illness that includes fever, prostration, and skin lesions. Infections of the throat and anus frequently result from orogenital and anogenital sexual activities with
an infected partner. These may cause an acute sore throat or rectal pain and discharge, or may be entirely without symptoms.
The diagnosis is made by the identification of *N. gonorrhoeae* microscopically or by culturing swabs.

Treatment. Nonresistant gonorrhea is relatively easily treated with
one of three treatment regimens:

1. Aqueous procaine penicillin (4.8 million units) is administered intra-
   muscularly (divided, and given at two sites) plus simultaneous oral
   probenecid given orally to prolong the effect of penicillin.
2. Ampicillin (3.5 grams) or amoxicillin (3 grams) are given orally
   with simultaneous probenecid.
3. Tetracycline (500 grams) is given orally 4 times daily for 5 days.

For suspected rectal infection, the intramuscular penicillin regimen
is preferred. For suspected pharyngeal infection, ampicillin should
be avoided. Men should not squeeze their penises in search of ure-
thral discharge, as this forces bacteria into the prostate and testes and
risks causing prostatitis and/or epididymitis. All sexual activity must
be avoided until cure is confirmed by your doctor.

One week following initial treatment, cultures should be taken to
confirm cure. If the disease continues, cultures should be tested for
antibiotic resistance, although most treatment "failures" are caused
by reinfection (often from the same partner from whom the first infection was contracted). In men, a continuing discharge may also be
caused by chlamydia infection *(see below)* that is not sensitive to penicillin and that was contracted simultaneously with the gonorrhea.

All recent sexual partners should be contacted and notified that they will require treatment as well. (Sex partners are treated whether or not they develop symptoms.) Approximately 3 months after treatment, a test for the presence of syphilis should be made by your doctor to identify any possible simultaneous infection that was not adequately treated by the therapy for gonorrhea.

Nonspecific Urethritis (NSU)

In many people with the symptoms of gonorrhea described above, but in whom *N. gonorrhoeae* cannot be found, the cause of the infection may be either *Chlamydia trachomatis* or *Ureaplasma urealyticum*. These infections have been called nonspecific urethritis (NSU) or nongonococcal urethritis (NGU) because the causative organism could not be identified. Now, special laboratory techniques can usually pinpoint these organisms, and they are thought to be the most common of all sexually transmitted diseases.

In men the sensation of burning during urination is usually more mild than in gonorrhea and the discharge from the penis may be clear or slightly yellow. Discharge is most easily found in the morning when the penis may be encrusted and the underwear stained. The symptoms usually appear 7–28 days after sexual contact.

In women the symptoms are also milder than those occurring in gonorrhea. In both women and men, throat and anal infections may develop after oral or anal sex with an infected partner.

Chlamydia infections are much more serious in women than in men because of their potential to cause *pelvic inflammatory disease*. If the organisms ascend into the Fallopian tubes or into the abdomen, an acute abdominal infection with pelvic pain and high fever may result. In a high percentage of these women, the tubes are scarred closed, resulting in infertility. There is also an increased chance of tubal pregnancy, in which the fetus begins to grow outside the uterus, leading to pain and possibly fatal hemorrhage. Women with chlamydial infections also transmit the infection to their newborn babies in about 60% of cases.

Treatment. Most infections are effectively treated with oral tetracycline or doxycycline for 7 days. It is important to continue your medication for the full prescribed period to prevent recurrence. During this time all sexual activity must be avoided. Again, a serologic test for syphilis should be obtained 3 months after treatment. Recent sexual contacts must be notified that they also require treatment.

Syphilis

Syphilis is caused by the spirochete *Treponema pallidum*. Syphilis has been called "the great imitator" because it can affect any organ of the body, mimicking numerous other diseases during its varying stages. The disease is particularly insidious now because its relatively low incidence (in the age of penicillin) makes it less likely to be considered by doctors and the public alike. In fact, the disease is increasing among the sexually active.

Primary Syphilis

The primary lesion in syphilis is the *chancre*, a small, painless sore that appears as a reddened ulcer with a hardened rim, located on the shaft of the penis, the vulva, lips, anus, vagina, or mouth, depending upon the focus of sexual contact. The primary lesions appear within 3–4 weeks of contact and usually heal within 4–8 weeks. Often local lymph nodes are enlarged, but not tender. Since chancres do not bleed and are painless, they are often ignored, thus permitting the onset of secondary syphilis.

Secondary Syphilis

Skin rashes follow the appearance of the chancre; often the chancre will just be healing as the rashes appear. The rashes, which *do not itch*, occur most often on the palms, soles, arms, trunk, and in the mouth. They are tan or copper-colored (in blacks they are pigmented), slightly raised, and rounded. The hair may fall out in patches, leaving "moth-eaten" round bald areas. During the secondary phase, which lasts 3–4 weeks, fever, muscle aches, joint pain, and neck stiffness are common. Nearly every organ in the body may be affected.

Latent Syphilis

Skin and lip lesions may reappear during the first two years after a syphilis infection, and these too are infectious. After two years, however, skin lesions do not generally reappear, and the disease ceases being infectious.

Late or Tertiary Syphilis

About one-third of untreated patients develop tertiary syphilis, often several years after the primary infection. Any organ in the body may be affected, but most commonly these are blood vessels and the brain. Brain damage is marked by dementia, weakness, an unsteady walk, hence its other name, *general paresis*. At this stage, the diagnosis may be difficult to make.

Diagnosis. Primary syphilis is diagnosed by microscopic detection of spirochetes from the chancre. In secondary and tertiary syphilis, there are several blood tests that identify the presence of *T. pallidum* reliably.

Treatment. The treatment for all stages of syphilis is penicillin. If you are allergic to penicillin, erythromycin can be substituted. Most patients with early syphilis develop what is known as a *Herxheimer reaction* within 6–12 hours after starting their course of antibiotics. Its symptoms include fever, headache, sweating, and muscle aches lasting about 24 hours. The cause of this reaction is massive destruction of the infecting spirochetes by the antibiotic.

Treated patients need to be watched closely by their doctors to make certain that cure has been complete. All recent sexual contacts must be notified that examination and treatment are required. *Sexual activity must be suspended until treatment is complete.* Patients with tertiary syphilis may need to be examined periodically for life.

Chancroid

Chancroid is caused by the bacteria *Hemophilus ducreyi*. The disease begins as small painful blisters that later become pus-filled ulcers on the genitals. The ulcers develop only 3–5 days after contact. Local groin nodes (buboes) become swollen, tender, and may even rupture and drain. The diagnosis is usually made from its characteristic appearance, though the organism can be cultured with difficulty.

Treatment. Several antibiotics are effective. *As with all sexually transmitted diseases, every sexual contact of the patient should be examined and treated.* Patients should be examined periodically for three months and retreated if necessary. It is essential to avoid sexual contact until cure is complete. A blood test for concurrent syphilis infection is a routine part of the treatment.

Lymphogranuloma Venereum

This is another disease caused by *Chlamydia trachomatis*, which is immunologically distinct from the bacterium that cause nonspecific urethritis and conjunctivitis. From 3 to 12 days after contact, a small, painless blister develops on the genitals. Local lymph nodes usually become swollen. Often this primary stage will go unnoticed. Months to years later the inguinal lymph nodes will swell, become tender, and fluctuant *buboes* appear. The overlying tissue may rupture, with drainage of blood and pus. The diagnosis is confirmed by special blood tests.

Treatment. The usual treatment is tetracycline for 10–14 days. All sexual contacts of the patient must be located and examined for possible treatment. Sexual activity must be abstained from until all evidence of infection clears.

Granuloma Inguinale

This disease is largely found in tropical and subtropical regions, and is caused by a bacterium, *C. granulomatis*. The initial lesions develop from 1 to 12 weeks after contact. They grow slowly and become elevated , irregular, velvety masses that appear on the penis, scrotum, groin, and thighs in males and the vulva and vagina, anus, or buttocks of women. The disease spreads by self inoculation. If untreated, the granulomas can form confluent masses about the entire genital region. Treatment is effective with several antibiotics. Sexual activity must cease and sexual contacts must be notified and examined for treatment.

Genital Herpes

Infection of the genital and anal regions with herpes simplex virus (HSV) is one of the most common causes of venereal disease in developed countries. Symptoms begin 4–7 days after sexual contact, first as a localized burning and tingling. Shortly thereafter small fluid-filled blisters form that rupture and ulcerate. The ulcers are painful and occur on the foreskin, glans, and shaft of the penis in men and the labia, clitoris, vagina, and cervix in women. In rectally exposed men and women, blisters may occur in the rectum and about the anus.

The blisters last 3–5 days, after which they crust over and disappear in about 10 days, with or without scarring. During the infection, the groin lymph nodes may be swollen and tender. Generalized symptoms of fever and malaise may accompany the infection. Upon clearing, the virus recedes to the regional nerve ganglia, from whence it may emerge at varying intervals to reinfect the skin. Episodes of recurrence may be triggered by high fever, illness, sunburn, or emotional stress. These recurrences recede in 7–9 days and are usually less severe than the primary episode.

Complications of HSV infections, both oral and genital, include meningitis and peripheral nerve involvement (including constipation, inability to urinate, and impotence in men). Infants, elderly adults, and people with immune compromise (those on long-term steroids, suffering AIDS, etc.) are particularly susceptible. Pregnant women with active genital herpes may require a cesarean section to prevent infections of their newborns with a variety of severe illnesses, and with mental retardation. Patients with atopic dermatitis (*see* p. 444) may develop a fatal form of HSV infection (*eczema herpeticum*).

Treatment. Currently there is no cure for genital herpes. Analgesics (aspirin, acetaminophen) are appropriate for the pain of herpes. Saline (1 teaspoon of salt per glass of water) compresses are soothing and help keep the blisters clean. Your doctor will prescribe acyclovir in topical or oral form. This drug is effective in reducing the severity of symptoms in primary and secondary infections, and when used prophylactically, reduces the rate of recurrence. However, the drug, even when used early in primary infections, does not prevent recurrent disease.

Vitamin and mineral treatments, dye treatments, light therapy, and special diets are all ineffective in treating HSV infections.

It should be borne in mind that oral herpes can be transmitted to the genitalia, resulting in genital herpes (*see* p. 267 for a discussion of cold sores caused by HSV). Therefore orogenital contact should be strictly avoided during active oral infections. During active genital infections, sex should be protected with condoms.

Genital Warts *(Condylomata Acuminata; Venereal Warts)*

Genital warts are caused by the human papilloma virus and are most often transmitted by sexual contact. They develop in 1–6 months after contact as soft , moist, pink swellings that grow rapidly, developing a stalk that makes them look like tiny cauliflowers. They occur on the penis in men and on the vulva, vaginal wall, and cervix in women. They may develop around the buttocks and anus in both men and women who have had anal sex.

Treatment. Warts must be treated by a doctor experienced in dealing with them. They may be treated by topical podophyllin, electrocauterization, laser therapy, cryotherapy with liquid nitrogen, or by surgical removal. No form of therapy is completely satisfactory. Women must be carefully examined and be followed for prolonged periods because of the association between genital warts and cervical cancer. Sexual partners must be contacted and examined for possible treatment.

A serologic test for syphilis is also a prudent part of therapy.

Trichomonas Infections

Trichomoniasis is caused by the protozoan, *Trichomonas vaginalis*. In women it is one of the most common causes of vaginitis, characterized by frothy, greenish-yellow discharge, soreness of the vaginal area and thighs, painful urination *(dysuria)*, and pain with intercourse. Men are usually asymptomatic carriers, although they may experience burning with urination and a slight frothy discharge from the penis, most evident in the morning.

Treatment. A single dose of metronidazole is usually curative for women; men are treated for seven days. All sexual partners should be contacted and examined for treatment. Intercourse must be avoided until the condition is cured.

Acquired Immunodeficiency Syndrome (AIDS)

We come now to that most feared of all of the sexually transmitted diseases, AIDS. Although the total number of AIDS victims is far less in any given year than, for example, the number of gonorrhea victims, the consequences are so devastating (usually fatal), the treatment so expensive and prolonged, with cure nonexistent, that this disease has become one of the most significant worldwide health problems we face today.

The AIDS Virus

The cause of AIDS is a *retrovirus* known now as the human immunodeficiency virus, HIV. The virus has an outer shell surrounding a protein core that protects its genetic material, RNA (ribonucleic acid). To infect a cell, the virus attaches to the cell surface, enters the cell, sheds its outer coat, and releases its RNA. Retroviruses contain an enzyme called *reverse transcriptase* that then converts the viral RNA into DNA (deoxyribonucleic acid) within the infected cell. In addition, the virus can cause the DNA thus formed to attach itself to the host DNA. There are two consequences of this insidious capability. First, every cell produced by the ongoing division of the infected, transformed cell carries the viral DNA. Second, at some point (still largely unknown), the cells containing the viral DNA can begin making new copies of the virus particles. In effect, the cell then becomes a factory for producing new viruses. These viruses then instruct the cell to give them a new protein coat and leave the cell (in the process destroying it) to invade new host cells and repeat the destructive cycle.

Retroviruses also have the ability to transform infected cells into cancers, presumably by stimulating the host cell's oncogenes (cancer-causing genes found in every cell).

The principal cell that HIV attacks is the white blood cell, the T-4 lymphocyte, also known as a "T-4 helper" cell. This cell is one of the first line defenses against invading diseases. It is responsible for forming antibodies to such foreign substances as viruses and bacteria. The key to the success of HIV is its ability to destroy the very cell that marshals the body's defense against it. In effect it knocks out the command center first. HIV also invades macrophages (the immune cells responsible for attacking and engulfing invading bacteria). In fact nearly all branches of the immune system are affected by HIV.

Other cell types attacked by HIV are neural cells in both the brain and spinal cord, the loss of which causes some of the most devastating symptoms of AIDS.

Spread of AIDS

HIV is transmitted when infectious body fluids of an infected person pass directly into another's bloodstream. In effect, any body fluid that contains lymphocytes can contain HIV. These include blood, semen, tears, saliva, mother's milk, and vaginal secretions. However, transmission through tears or saliva has not actually been demonstrated. In the United States the factors responsible for transmitting AIDS have largely been receptive anal intercourse among homosexual and bisexual men, and shared needles among intravenous drug abusers. However, heterosexual transmission is increasingly the principal mode of AIDS transmission, as it has always been in Africa.

Transmission by accidental needle stick has been documented, although it appears to be much less likely than transmission of hepatitis B virus by this means. HIV can be transmitted across the placenta in pregnant AIDS victims, and during delivery. HIV has been demonstrated in breast milk, and though rare, this too is a possible means of transmission.

Transmission of AIDS though undetected virus in blood transfusions is discussed on p. 40.

Signs and Symptoms of AIDS

The incubation period between infection and development of full-blown AIDS is highly variable, in some cases longer than seven years. In transfusion-related AIDS, the average time from transfusion to diagnosis is about 20 months for children and 30 months for adults.

Among homosexual men, the risk of developing AIDS following infection with HIV varies from 2 to 35% per year. It is now believed that most individuals who become serologically positive (those who have demonstrable HIV antigen or antibodies to HIV in their serum) will sooner or later develop AIDS. Some people are known to develop an *acute nonspecific viral syndrome* within 2–4 weeks after infection. This syndrome consists of fever, malaise, rash, joint pain, and swollen lymph nodes, lasting 3–14 days. It is followed in 1–3 months by *seroconversion*, i.e., the point at which the blood tests positive for HIV antigen or antibody.

AIDS-Related Complex (ARC)

ARC is a variable group of signs and symptoms that include weight loss, fever, malaise, weakness, swollen lymph nodes, diarrhea, anemia, and night sweats. Not all of these findings will be present at any one time, and their course and duration may also be variable and episodic.

The Full-Blown AIDS Syndrome

Any and all of the above signs and symptoms may be present. In addition victims develop opportunistic infections, Kaposi's sarcoma, or lymphoma. The term "opportunistic" means that the particular infection occurring does not ordinarily strike healthy humans, but only does so when they are debilitated, or when their immune systems are compromised, as in AIDS. Such opportunistic infections include *Pneumocystis carinii* pneumonia, cryptosporidiosis, toxoplasmosis, candidiasis, cryptococcosis, histoplasmosis, tuberculosis, and herpes simplex virus infections.

Kaposi's sarcoma is a tumor of blood vessels that involves the skin and other organs. In AIDS victims the skin tumors are deep pink to purple lesions that may appear anywhere on the body, including the mouth. They usually increase in size and number rapidly, adding to the patient's general disability and are often fatal.

The neurologic disorders associated with AIDS include meningitis, weakness of the limbs and loss of coordination, seizures, hallucinations, and progressive dementia. Neurologic involvement occurs in 30–50% of AIDS victims. Blindness usually results from CMV (cytomegalovirus) retinitis.

Diagnosis. Two common serologic tests for AIDS are currently in use. Both test for the presence of HIV antibody. Currently, direct tests for the presence of the virus itself are technically difficult. The most common screening test is an *enzyme-linked immunosorbent assay* (ELISA) in which the serum of the person tested is placed in contact with beads coated with HIV antigen. If antibody is present in the serum, the resultant *antigen–antibody reaction* produces a color change that is read by a sensitive light detector. The ELISA test detects 99% of those people who have been infected more than three months. The test will probably be falsely negative for very recently infected individuals because sufficient numbers of antibodies require time to develop in response to infection. This test produces *false positive* results (i.e., a positive test in a person who has no infection) in only about 0.2% or about 2 in 1000 persons tested. An ELISA result is not deemed to be positive unless a repeat test on the same serum sample is also positive.

What do these statistics mean? They mean essentially that the test is very accurate in a population with a moderate to high risk for infection, e.g., intravenous drug users in New York City. The test is also relatively inaccurate in a low risk population, e.g., heterosexual women in Kansas.

Ordinarily a positive ELISA is confirmed by a second test, the Western blot test. This is also a test for serum antibody, but is less subject to the false positive errors arising in the ELISA test. The Western blot is an immunologic procedure that is quite labor-intensive and requires considerable skill and experience to run and to interpret.

When both ELISA and Western blot tests are performed, the chance of a false positive result is only about 1 in 10,000 individuals tested. At the same time, the Western blot will fail to confirm about 2% of ELISA positive samples. Thus, though these tests are relatively accurate, they are by no means perfect, especially in a low-risk population.

Treatment. There is currently no effective treatment for AIDS, except that directed at opportunistic infections, the associated cancers, and other complications. This great challenge in finding either a cure or an effective means of prevention is posed by an organism whose genes become an integral part of the host cell's genetic framework. Once this occurs, there is little likelihood of getting rid of the virus.

Currently most of the antiviral AIDS drugs are targeted at the point where RNA is converted to DNA, where they attempt to block the

Prevention of AIDS

The High-Risk Group. Since there is no cure for AIDS, a nation-wide education program has been undertaken to modify behavior and slow the dissemination of the disease. Central to preventing the spread of AIDS is understanding which individuals are at increased risk of having or acquiring AIDS. These are:

- Men who have had sex with another man since 1977
- Those who have shared needles when they inject drugs
- Male or female prostitutes and their sex partners. Anal sex is particularly likely to transmit HIV to the recipient
- Sex partners of people infected with the AIDS virus are at increased risk of infection
- People with hemophilia who have received blood clotting factor products before 1985
- Infants of high-risk or infected mothers

Important Meaures to Prevent Transmission

- Avoid sexual encounters with persons in high-risk groups
- Reduce your number of sexual contacts. A stable, mutually monogamous relationship with an uninfected person eliminates any new risk of acquiring HIV infection
- Avoid high-risk practices, especially anal intercourse, and use condoms. The use of condoms decreases the chance of contracting AIDS from an infected partner at least tenfold
- Recent studies have shown that condoms containing the spermicide, nonoxynol-9, *may* be effective in sterilizing HIV virus. This drugs also inhibits the growth of chlamydia, herpes simplex virus, *N. gonorrhoeae*, and syphilis
- Avoid sexual contact whenever a genital lesion (including inflammation) develops. It is now believed that a genital lesion promotes the entry of HIV into the body
- Since HIV may be transmitted across the placenta, persons testing positive for AIDS should avoid becoming pregnant.
- Persons belonging to a high-risk group should not donate blood even if they test negative for the presence of AIDS antibodies.
- Persons belonging to a high-risk category should consult their doctors about the advisability of being vaccinated against hepatitis B.

> ### PERSONS WHO TEST POSITIVE FOR HIV SHOULD
>
> - Inform prospective partners that they test positive for HIV
> - Protect their partners from acquiring HIV through unsafe sex practices.
> - Inform previous sex partners of the need to be tested for HIV.

action of reverse transcriptase. Of the pharmacologic agents tested thus far, AZT (zidovudine) and DDI (dideoxyinosine) are the only drugs approved by the FDA for treatment. AZT works by "tricking" the virus into incorporating the drug into DNA. When this happens, the DNA cannot make new copies of the HIV virus. Preliminary results suggest that zidovudine prolongs life and may also delay the onset of clinical symptoms in seropositive individuals. But thus far, the time bought is measured in months, not years, and there are many serious side effects associated with zidovudine therapy.

New drugs being developed are targeted at other stages of the infection cycle—where they can prevent the virus from entering uninfected cells or can interfere with assembly of new virus particles within the infected cells.

Secondary infections can in some cases be prevented. Nasal pentamidine is effective in preventing *Pneumocystis carinii* pneumonia. A new drug, Foscarnet, is effective in preventing CMV retinitis.

Presently no AIDS vaccine is available, although development efforts are vigorous. AIDS is difficult to prevent through vaccination because HIV appears to mutate easily, producing many slightly different strains. A vaccine developed against one strain may not be effective against another—much like flu vaccines. HIV may enter the body already encapsulated within lymphocytes, which vaccines cannot penetrate. On the other hand it is likely that vaccines can be developed to contain the virus even though entrance into the body cannot be prevented.

When Should You Be Tested For AIDS?

As I noted earlier, people at a very low risk of having been exposed to AIDS are the ones most likely to have a false positive test. At this time, if 100,000 people without AIDS are tested for the presence of AIDS antibodies, 10 people will have a false positive result from both the ELISA and Western blot tests. The potentially damaging consequences of such misidentification should not be underestimated. There may be a difficulty obtaining health or life insurance, even in getting a job, let alone the anxiety attached to the mistaken belief that you have a fatal disease.

If you are in a high-risk group, you should be tested in order to know whether you must change your sex practices.

Ultimately healthy people considering being tested for AIDS must balance at least three factors: (1) the psychological reassurance that, having possibly been exposed, you have escaped contact; (2) the anxiety of not knowing what your status is; and (3) the potentially devastating knowledge that you have contracted an incurable disease.

Two other factors must be kept in mind: If you think you may have been recently exposed and test negative, you should have a repeat test in about 3 months to allow for the interval between infection and serologic positivity. If you elect to be tested, seek an

---

WHAT DOES *NOT* TRANSMIT AIDS

1. Casual contact with an infected person. AIDS is transmitted through intimate sexual contact, or through any mechanism that injects the virus into the bloodstream. There is no evidence that AIDS has ever been transmitted by touching an infected person, through handshakes, sharing bathrooms, toilets, or bathing facilities. Nor is the virus transmitted through food and drink.
2. Playing with children with AIDS. One of the most explosive issues is the separation of children with AIDS from other school children. Contact among children poses no demonstrated risk of transmitting AIDS. Nor is the disease likely to be transmitted by an infected child biting another child, because the virus rarely appears in the saliva.
3. Being bitten by mosquitoes and bedbugs. No evidence exists that AIDS has been or can be transmitted by insect bites.
4. By donating blood. Since only sterilized needles are used and nothing is injected during blood donation, you cannot be infected by donating blood; you can only serve your community and help your fellowkind by doing so.
5. Receiving a blood transfusion. Now that blood is universally tested for the presence of AIDS and high-risk individuals have been discouraged from donating blood, the risk of contracting AIDS by having a blood transfusion in the United States is extremely low: less than 1 in 100,000.

institution that can provide counseling for you in the event of a positive result.

AIDS and Quackery

Throughout this book I have tried to alert you to worthless and foolish medical practices. It seems that few victims of disease are surer targets of quacks than those with AIDS. It is understandable that anyone with an incurable disease will be receptive to a new idea for treatment, however radical. But, please, be wary of anyone offering a new form of treatment. If the individual is not directly related to a medical school or nationally recognized medical institution, suspect a quack, for it is in these institutions, not a Mexican clinic, that honest and reliable advances against AIDS are going to be made.

Among the numerous fraudulent AIDS products and remedies listed recently by the FDA Consumer are blue–green algae (also known as "pond scum"; injections of hydrogen peroxide, the food preservative BHT, pills derived from mice that have been given the AIDS virus, lecithin tablets, and herbal capsules found to contain dangerous quantities of poisonous metal. Some "therapies" that have been advocated are: thumping on the thymus gland to produce white blood cells; massaging the skin with a dry brush; bathing the body in bleach solution, and exposing the genitals and rectum to the sun's rays at about 4 PM. Please do not rely on any of these.

For more information on AIDS, call the Public Health Service's toll-free hotline: 1-800-342-AIDS, or

National Sexually Transmitted Disease Hotline, American Social Health Association: 1-800-227-8922, or

AIDS Information Hotline/National Gay Task Force: 1-800-221-7044.

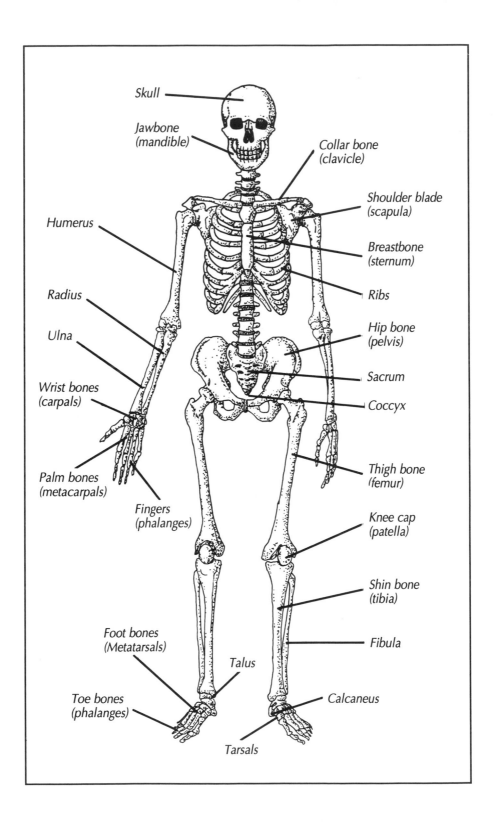

Skull

Jawbone
(mandible)

Collar bone
(clavicle)

Shoulder blade
(scapula)

Humerus

Breastbone
(sternum)

Radius

Ribs

Ulna

Hip bone
(pelvis)

Wrist bones
(carpals)

Sacrum

Coccyx

Palm bones
(metacarpals)

Thigh bone
(femur)

Fingers
(phalanges)

Knee cap
(patella)

Shin bone
(tibia)

Foot bones
(Metatarsals)

Fibula

Talus

Toe bones
(phalanges)

Calcaneus

Tarsals

Your Musculoskeletal System and Its Disorders

Bone Diseases

The skeleton is an actively metabolizing organ throughout life, not just during the period of growing to your adult size. It is a large reservoir of calcium, phosphorus, and proteins that is continually renewing and reshaping itself in response to stress. The diseases of bone involve primarily those conditions that interfere with bone metabolism. Bone marrow disorders are discussed on p. 222. Bone fractures are discussed on p. 71.

Osteoporosis

Osteoporosis means "porous bone." It is a disease in which bone substance and density is gradually lost, weakening the bone structure and predisposing it to fractures. Normally new bone is laid down at about the same rate that your old bone material is reabsorbed. In osteoporosis the resorption process is speeded up, so that new bone formation cannot keep up with continuing loss. The most common bone fractures associated with osteoporosis are in the spine, wrist, and hips. Though osteoporosis can occur as a result of immobilization, e.g., in a leg confined in a cast, or because of a low-protein diet, the most common cause is aging. As people age, new bone formation occurs more slowly than during youth and calcium is also absorbed less readily from the intestines. The result is that, in order to maintain calcium levels in the rest of your body, calcium is "borrowed" from its bone "bank."

Generally there are no symptoms of osteoporosis until a fracture occurs. Even then the fracture may result from a trivial injury. A common fracture is a "crush fracture" of one or more vertebrae, resulting in back pain and ultimately loss of height. If several of the thoracic vertebrae are involved, a "dowager's hump" develops. This is a rounded humping of the upper back caused by deformity of the spine through loss of height.

Your Risk of Osteoporosis

Who is at risk of developing osteoporosis? Several risk factors have been identified:

- *Being female.* Women are affected six to eight times more often than men, especially after menopause, when the protective effect of estrogens is decreased.
- *Early menopause.* Menopause before age 45 predisposes to osteoporosis, especially if it is surgically induced by removal of both ovaries.
- *Being white.* Caucasian women are at higher risk than black women, and white men are at higher risk than black men. Some estimate that by age 65, nearly one quarter of all white women have suffered one or more fractures from osteoporosis.
- *Sedentary life style*—yet another reason to keep moving.
- *Being underweight*—one of the very few adverse consequences of being seriously underweight.

Other possible risk factors include smoking cigarets, excessive use of alcohol, and a family history of osteoporosis.

Diagnosis. In very advanced cases, simple X-rays can detect the decreased density of the bones, and of course fractures and deformities are readily apparent. Early detection depends on more sophisticated imaging techniques. Computerized X-ray tomography (CT) scans can detect early loss of bone. Bone densitometry is also sensitive, and much less expensive. In the latter technique, gamma rays from a radioisotope source are beamed at especially vulnerable bones. The number of gamma rays that pass through the bones reflect its density.

Treatment and Prevention. The three principal measures by which osteoporosis is treated and/or prevented are adequate exercise, a diet rich in calcium, and hormone replacement after menopause.

Exercise appears is help keep your bones strong. Some of the best are low-impact exercises, such as swimming, cycling, gardening, and simply walking. Try to exercise for at least 30 minutes several times each week.

Your diet should provide an ample amount of calcium each day. The currently recommended amounts are 800–1200 milligrams per day for men and 1200–1500 milligrams per day for women. Good sources of calcium include low-fat dairy products, fish, and dark green vegetables. One 8-oz glass of skim milk contains about 300 mg. Ask your doctor whether you should take calcium supplements.

It is now recognized that the age at which you become "at risk" for developing the bone fractures of osteoporosis depends on the total bone mass you accumulate while you are young. For both men and women, "peak" bone mass occurs before the age of 30. Thus, a calcium-rich diet while you are young and growing will protect you from fractures well into advanced age. As you eat, so shall you prosper in age.

Most doctors now recommend that women take low-dose estrogen replacement after menopause, since calcium alone will not prevent bone loss. The protection against developing osteoporosis probably outweighs the other slight risks of estrogen replacement, especially when combined with small doses of progesterone (*see* p. 345).

Another hormone, calcitonin, which is produced by the thyroid gland, may be useful in arresting bone loss when administered as a nasal spray. Ask your doctor about it.

Osteomalacia *(Adult Rickets)*

Osteomalacia is a disease of bone softening caused by vitamin D deficiency. You get vitamin D from two sources: from foods, such as fish and dairy products, and from sunshine acting upon the skin. Vitamin D deficiency is rare in anyone with a normal diet, although it may occur in shut-ins who also have a very restricted diet. It can also occur in people with malabsorption syndrome (*see* p. 299) or with chronic kidney failure.

The chief symptom of osteomalacia is bone pain and stiffness. This pain is often mistaken for arthritis. In very severe cases, the bones may fracture easily, or become deformed, with bowing of the legs and loss of height as the vertebrae shorten.

Treatment and Prevention. Osteomalacia is rare in this country, since normal diets provide ample vitamin D. If your doctor finds through blood tests and X-rays that you have osteomalacia, he or she will prescribe vitamin D supplements. Do not attempt self-diagnosis and do not take vitamin D supplements without your doctor's advice—excess intake can cause vitamin D intoxication, manifested by nausea, weakness, nervousness, itching, and chronic thirst.

Paget's Disease

Paget's disease is a disorder of unknown cause in which localized areas of softened bone develop. Any bone may be involved, but those most commonly affected are the pelvis, femur, skull, arm bones, collar bone, skull, and vertebrae.

Often, Paget's disease is not symptomatic at all, but discovered incidentally on X-rays taken for other conditions. In other cases there may be localized pain that becomes worse at night. Headaches commonly occur when the skull is involved.

Deafness and skull deformity can occur. The bones may also develop local swelling at the site of the bone lesions and these may become warm and tender and fracture easily. If the lesions become very extensive, heart failure can result from the greatly increased blood flow within them.

Treatment. Pain can be controlled by analgesics, such as aspirin or ibuprofen. If the pain is especially severe, your doctor may prescribe the hormone, calcitonin, or the cytotoxic drug, mithramycin, to control the growth of Paget's lesions.

Bone Tumors

Most tumors found in bone have spread (metastasized) from cancers of other organs, such as the breast, lung, kidney, thyroid, or prostate. Most primary bone tumors are benign, such as *osteochondroma*, a mixed bone and cartilage tumor found mostly in young people, or *osteoid osteoma*, found mostly in long bones. These tumors may give rise to pain or weaken the bone, causing fractures. In some cases, surgical removal is required. Malignant tumors, such as *osteogenic sarcoma* and *Ewing's sarcoma,* are rare and often require amputation of the limb or excision of the affected bone in addition to cancer drugs.

Joint Disorders

Arthritis

Arthritis is one of the most common diseases known to man. We will all develop one type or another provided we live long enough. Arthritis literally means "inflammation of the joints." The condition is sometimes referred to as "rheumatism." It is not, however a single disease; the term is used to describe nearly a hundred different conditions that cause aches, pains, and stiffness in and around the joints.

The specific diagnosis of each particular type of arthritis may be difficult and is the special concern of rheumatologists, who specialize in joint and connective tissue disorders. By far the most common forms of arthritis are osteoarthritis, rheumatoid arthritis, and gout.

Osteoarthritis (Degenerative Joint Disease)

Osteoarthritis is the most common form of arthritis; nearly everyone over 50 years of age has some degree of degenerative joint disease. It has been around for a long time, since signs of the disease have been found in Egyptian mummies.

The cause of osteoarthritis is not known, but the disease affects the cartilage at the end of the bones, rather than the joint lining (*synovium*), as in rheumatoid arthritis. Joint cartilage acts as a shock absorber and frictionless surface between the joints. As the cartilage degenerates, its surface becomes thinned and eroded. Eventually bone grinds on bone as the cartilage is slowly destroyed, and this process in turn causes inflammation and pain.

Osteoarthritis is generally a disease affecting older people, although athletes and others who have sustained early joint trauma may develop symptoms before age 40. The most common symptoms are joint pain, stiffness, and swelling that begin gradually, especially after exertion. Some people have constant, nagging pain, even at rest. Often pain and stiffness result in decreasing use of the joint, and pain may then subside somewhat.

The most commonly affected joints are the hips, knees, spine, feet, and fingers, especially the joints closest to the fingertips. As the joint spaces narrow, bony "spurs" may develop where muscles and cartilage join bone. Such spurs on the fingertips are known as *Heberden's nodes*. Pain in the fingers is quite variable. Some people have considerable joint deformity with no pain at all.

Treatment. There is no cure for osteoarthritis, nor even any therapy that halts its progression, short of replacing the affected joint. Early in the disease's course, a carefully planned adjustment of habits and activities is useful in reducing later disability. Such measures include a combination of exercise to strengthen those joints particularly at risk, weight control to protect these joints, and the use of heat and analgesics.

Exercise is aimed at avoiding stiffness and muscle contractions that reduce the joint's useful range of motion. Building up muscles around joints helps absorb stress on joints during movement. A balance between rest and exercise is important to avoid overuse of joints and to avoid exhaustion, which has an adverse effect on the arthritis. A number of exercise programs, including "soft aerobics" (swimming, cycling, walking) are especially appropriate for arthritics. Ask your doctor for referral to a physical therapist experienced in home exercise programs.

Try to avoid soft chairs or recliners and pillows under your knees, all of which promote muscle contractions. Use a firm bed with a bed board beneath the mattress if necessary. Don't slump when sitting in a chair. When walking or standing, keep your back as straight as possible and pull your stomach in. All of these measures help reduce stress on joints.

Controlling your weight reduces the stress on joints. The more you weigh, the more pressure is placed on your weight-bearing joints (ankles, knees, hips, and spine). Losing weight is difficult when joint pain reduces some of your former exercise options. Ask your doctor for dietary recommendations. *See also* the section on obesity in this book, p. 313.

Applications of heat and cold also help reduce stiffness and relieve pain. The principles described below for rheumatoid arthritis also apply to osteoarthritis.

For the relief of pain, try aspirin or one the nonsteroidal anti-inflationary drugs (NSAIDs), such as ibuprofen (e.g., Advil, Nuprin, Motrin) first. Aspirin must be taken in fairly large doses (12–25 tablets per day) to have an anti-inflammatory effect. Such doses can cause irritation of the lining of the stomach (*see* Heartburn, p. 280). NSAIDs, though irritating to some users, may be less so than aspirin. Other NSAIDs, such as naproxen, fenoprofen, sulindac, and others can be prescribed by your doctor. Avoid the use of narcotics, because they are addicting, they have several unwanted side effects, and are almost never necessary if you are careful to adhere to more conservative treatment.

Try to avoid sedatives for sleep; you will soon become dependent on them and they can cause "rebound" depression. *See* p. 115 for tips on a good night's sleep.

If you have a restless sleeping partner, consider twin beds. Get the type that is joined so that motions are not transmitted, but emotions generated by physical closeness are not interrupted. The continuation of regular sexual relations is important in maintaining physical and emotional well-being.

Write for information about tips for the sexually active arthritic detailed in a pamphlet: *Living and Loving—Information about Sex* from the Arthritis Foundation, PO 1900, Atlanta, GA 30326.

Joint Replacement

If pain and disability become substantial, the diseased joint can often be replaced by an artificial joint made of metal or a combination of metal and plastic. Joint replacement is a rapidly advancing field and the number of successful joint replacements is ever increasing, although currently the most favorable results are obtained with replacements for the hip and knee joints. Ask your doctor for referral to an orthopedic surgeon for consultation.

Osteonecrosis

Osteonecrosis literally means "death" (necrosis) of "bone" (osteo) and is caused by interruption of the blood supply to a joint, usually the hip, shoulder, or knee, often caused by fracture, infection, sickle cell disease, or atherosclerosis. In many cases the cause is not known. Those at risk of developing osteonecrosis include:

- People with rheumatoid arthritis *(see below)*
- Those on large doses of corticosteroids
- Alcoholics
- Professional scuba divers who have suffered the bends

The chief symptom of osteonecrosis is pain. Small fractures develop in the dead bone. Since the bone lacks a blood supply, it cannot repair itself. Ultimately the dead bone becomes eroded from pressure within the joint and arthritis develops. This in turn induces muscle spasms and stiffness in and about the affected joint. Pain is commonly worse after standing or walking, which exerts stress upon the joints.

Treatment. The treatment is essentially the same as for osteoarthritis, described above.

Rheumatoid Arthritis

Rheumatoid arthritis is a disease of the *synovium* or joint lining, which becomes inflamed and swollen. The joints most often affected are the small joints in the hands and feet, especially the knuckles and toe

---

TREATING YOUR ARTHRITIS

Numerous drugs are effective in relieving the symptoms of arthritis. None is effective for all people and very few are effective during all stages of the disease in any individual. Your doctor may suggest any of the following:

- *Aspirin.* Aspirin is often the first drug to be prescribed, and is effective both in relieving pain and reducing inflammation. It is given in fairly large doses (10–25 tablets per day), with meals to minimize gastric upset. It may also be given in the form of buffered or enteric-coated tablets to reduce stomach irritation. Other forms of salicylates, such as sodium salicylate, salsalate, and choline magnesium salicylate, may cause fewer gastrointestinal side effects, but they are usually less effective in relieving arthritis.

- *NSAIDs.* Your doctor may recommend any one of several nonsteroidal antiinflammatory drugs, such as ibuprofen (Advil), fenoprofen, tolmetin, sulindac, naproxen, or piroxicam, among others. None of these has been found to be more effective than aspirin, although they may be better tolerated. *See* p. 120 for a discussion of NSAIDs.

  Other antiarthritic drugs include antimalarial drugs, such as hydroxychloroquine, gold compounds, indomethacin, and penicillamine.

- *Corticosteroids.* In severe cases, corticosteroids may be given when all else fails. Long-term use of steroids is prohibited by the many side effects of these powerful drugs.

- *Cytotoxic drugs.* Another class of drugs that may be effective in severe rheumatoid arthritis is those drugs that suppress the immune system. Those most commonly used are methotrexate and azathioprine. These drugs may also have serious side effects and must be carefully monitored by your doctor.

---

joints, although the wrists, knees, ankles, hips, and neck also become involved. Often more than one joint is affected at the same time.

Rheumatoid arthritis is an autoimmune disease, in which the body appears to make antibodies against its own tissues, in this case the synovium that lines the joints. However, the eyes and blood vessels can also be affected in rheumatoid arthritis.

The course of the disease is highly variable, but it is common to have periods of relief followed by sudden flareups. Muscle stiffness is most prominent in the mornings and after long periods of inactivity. Most often the same joints on both sides of the body are affected in a kind of symmetrical distribution.

Other symptoms associated with rheumatoid arthritis include fatigue, mild fever, inflammation of the eyes, chest pain (pleurisy), and lumps under the skin, particularly about the elbows. These "rheumatoid nodules" don't usually cause problems, although they may become sore or infected. Joints may ultimately become deformed, causing severe crippling. Stress and anxiety worsen arthritis' symptoms.

This disease affects about 1% of all adult Americans, three out of four of whom are women. It is most commonly a disease of middle age, although it can occur at any age. The cause is unknown. Perhaps the production of antibodies is triggered by an initial viral infection.

Diagnosis. Early in its course, rheumatoid arthritis may be difficult to distinguish from other causes of arthritis. Usually the diagnosis rests upon several factors, including joint stiffness, tenderness, swelling, and the symmetrical distribution of involved joints. Your doctor will also take blood tests and may biopsy a rheumatoid nodule if present.

REST AND EXERCISE

Regular periods of rest are essential in limiting the number and intensity of arthritic flareups. Avoid becoming overly tired; learn to pace yourself. Regular exercise is important in preventing joints from becoming stiff and contracted. Don't sit or lie too long in one position. In some cases your doctor may recommend special splints that keep joints from becoming contracted, painful, and useless. A physical therapist can be helpful in developing a system of exercise for you, as well as in recommending household aids, such as long-handled reachers, oversized pencils, pots and pans with built-up handles, devices to help you dress and to otherwise permit independence and reduce frustration from an often immobilizing disease.

HEAT AND COLD

The application of heat to stiff joints is a time-honored treatment for all types of arthritis. A hot shower in the morning when stiffness is worst always seems welcome. Other means of applying heat include hot packs, heat lamps, blown hot air, and paraffin wax treatments.

Cold may also help relieve the pain of arthritis. Apply cold compresses or ice bags to hot, tender joints to lessen pain.

Avoiding Medical Quackery

A word of caution in an area of medicine rife with abuse—

Avoid any doctor who tells you that you can be cured of your rheumatism by following some "revolutionary," "newly discovered," or "ancient" medical program. Such frippery as Dr. Fenby's Formula X, Groff's ArthroTone, ArThry-Go Tablets, Ring's Golden Herb Tonic, and Elmore's Rheumative Goutaline are just a few of a long list of charlatans' nostrums that will promise you relief. The only thing such medicines will relieve you of is your money. Oh, yes, add snake venom to the list. Some doctors in Florida are actually injecting highly poisonous snake venom into arthritis victims. Don't buy it. If a treatment has not been endorsed by the Arthritis Foundation, be wary. You may call them at their local office in your telephone directory.

For information, write to: Arthritis Foundation, 1314 Spring Street, NW, Atlanta, GA 30309.

Surgery

Several surgical procedures have been devised to reduce pain and lessen joint deformity. The swollen synovium may be removed surgically *(synovectomy)* if joint motion becomes severely limited. Contraction deformities may be relieved by arthroplasty to increase use of the hands and feet. Total joint replacement may be indicated in advanced disease. Replacements are most effective with the hip and knee joints. In some cases, small joints may be fused. This eliminates joint motion, but usually relieves pain.

A still experimental therapy for rheumatoid arthritis entails injecting small amounts of short-lived radioisotopes into the joints to destroy the inflamed synovium. Ask your rheumatologist about this therapy.

Gout

Gout is a particular type of arthritis caused by the deposit of uric acid crystals in the joint tissues and joint fluid. Uric acid crystals irritate the joint lining, causing pain, inflammation, and swelling.

The cause of gout is excess uric acid in the blood. This in turn is caused by either excess production of uric acid, or less commonly, by decreased excretion of uric acid by the kidneys. In either case, the arthritis develops when the buildup of joint crystals initiate joint inflammation.

Gout is mostly an hereditary condition that occurs chiefly in men between 40 and 50 years of age. It usually develops in a single joint and may spread to other joints in time. The most common joint involved is in the great toe. The symptoms appear without warning, especially at night. The attack may be precipitated by injury, overindulgence in rich foods or alcohol, fatigue, emotional stress, or by drugs, such as diuretics, insulin, or penicillin. These characteristics help explain the classic Hogarthian portrait of the gout victim as a corpulent gentleman (able to afford red meats and other foods high in the purines from which uric acid is formed in the body) with his foot bandaged, elevated on a pillow, and a look of anguish writ large upon his face.

The acute attack of gout is very painful. The joint is inflamed, with the skin tense, warm, shiny, and red or purple. The joint may be so tender that not even the pressure of a sheet can be tolerated. Other joints that are sometimes affected include the ankle, knee, wrist, and elbow.

The diagnosis of gout is often suspected by its sudden onset, although this may be confused with infectious arthritis or pseudogout (*see below*). Your doctor will take X-rays and blood tests. The demonstration of uric acid crystals in the joint fluid is diagnostic.

Treatment. Gout is treated quite effectively with drugs that your doctor will prescribe and carefully supervise. The acute attack is usually treated with colchicine, or if this is not well-tolerated, with a nonsteroidal anti-inflammatory drug (*see* p. 120) to control the inflammation. If treated promptly, the acute arthritis improves rapidly. Joint pain often begins to subside within 12 hours and may be completely gone in 36–48 hours.

Although gout symptoms are relieved rapidly with treatment, they usually recur in the same or different joints unless drug treatment is continued indefinitely. Drugs such as probenecid help promote the excretion of uric acid and allopurinol is effective in decreasing the production of uric acid. Your doctor will probably prescribe a combination of these drugs to prevent further attacks. Most victims of gout need to take medications for life.

DIET

The treatment of gout by medications is generally so effective that a relatively normal diet is generally possible. Some precautions are, however, prudent:

1. A high uric acid level in your blood greatly increases your risk of developing uric acid kidney stones. In fact, you are 1000 times more likely to develop kidney stones if you have gout. Consequently you should drink plenty of non-alcoholic beverages—a minimum of two quarts daily. You can drink coffee and tea. You can also have alcohol in moderation (no more than two ounces of hard liquor or its equivalent per day). Excess alcohol precipitates the attacks of acute gout.
2. You should lose weight if you are overweight (*see* table, p. 314). However, lose weight gradually, since fasting and sudden weight loss can precipitate acute gout. Ask your doctor for a diet tailored for you.
3. You may need to avoid foods containing large amounts of purines. Common foods high in purines include: liver, mussels, kidney, beer, brains, anchovies, sardines, wine, heart, legumes, sweetbreads, herring, salmon, gravies, seafood, and asparagus.

For more information about gout, contact the Arthritis Foundation at the address above.

Pseudogout (Crystal Deposition Disease)

Pseudogout is another type of acute arthritis that resembles gout, except that it is usually less severe and occurs in people over 60 years of age. In pseudogout, the deposits that form in the joints are calcium pyrophosphate dihydrate crystals. The cause of crystal deposition is not known. In fact it has only been recognized as a disease distinct from gout since 1962. The condition is diagnosed by demonstrating the specific crystals within the fluid removed from an inflamed joint.

The severity of pseudogout varies greatly. In some, it may start as acute arthritis with a warm, tender swelling in one or more joints that lasts several days. In others the symptoms are merely chronic pain without swelling that resembles osteoarthritis (*see* p. 409). The usual course is one of recurrent attacks with symptom-free periods of remission.

Treatment. Pseudogout is usually treated first with aspirin or one of the NSAIDs (*see* p. 120). Colchicine is also effective, although it is associated with more side effects than other NSAIDs. The symptoms usually subside within 3–10 days. The decision to continue regular medication to prevent further attacks must be made by your doctor.

Ankylosing Spondylitis

The name of this arthritis, *ankylosing spondylitis,* tells the story: the spine *(spondyl)* becomes fused *(ankylosed)* because of inflammation *(itis).* The disease begins as an inflammation of unknown cause that involves the ligaments surrounding the vertebral joints. This inflammation causes a bony growth into the ligaments that ultimately fuses the vertebrae together. The sacroiliac joints, hips, and ribs may also be involved.

The early symptoms of spondylitis are constant hip and low back pain with stiffness that lasts for more than three months. If the vertebrae become fused, deformity and loss of movement of the spine can result. If the ribs fuse to the spine and breastbone, breathing becomes difficult.

Treatment. Relief of pain is achieved with aspirin and NSAIDs. Hot showers and other applications of heat help reduce stiffness. Appropriate exercises help prevent spinal deformity and breathing problems. In severe cases, a corset and braces may be required to support the spine.

A good source of additional information is the Ankylosing Spondylitis Association, PO Box 5872, Sherman Oaks, CA 91403, 1-800-777-8189.

Reiter's Syndrome

Arthritis is only one aspect of *Reiter's syndrome* (a symptom complex). Others include conjunctivitis, inflammation of the urethra (the small tube down which urine passes from the bladder), enteritis (an inflammation of the bowel), and lesions of the skin and mucous membranes. In women the cervix may also become inflamed *(cervicitis),* although Reiter's syndrome is chiefly a disease affecting men between the ages of 20 and 40. The cause of Reiter's syndrome is not known, although it often follows a bacterial infection of the genitourinary tract or of the bowel. Susceptibility appears genetically determined and the bacterial infection somehow triggers the syndrome. The arthritis may be mild or severe, usually occurring in the large joints of the legs and in the toes. The initial symptoms last for 3–4 months. In some half of all victims, the arthritis recurs over several years.

Treatment. The most commonly prescribed drugs for Reiter's syndrome are the NSAIDs (*see* p. 120 regarding their proper use.) If

Reiter's syndrome follows sexual contact, your doctor will most likely prescribe an antibiotic. You will also be urged to use a condom with any new partner to prevent recurrences of the syndrome. The skin rash and conjunctivitis usually require no treatment.

Lyme Disease

Lyme disease is caused by small, spiral-shaped bacteria (spirochetes) called *Borrelia burgdorferi,* which are transmitted by the bite of the small deer tick. Lyme disease, like syphilis, has been dubbed "the Great Imitator" because at various times it can mimic several different diseases, one of which is arthritis. The disease is named after Lyme, Connecticut, where it was first identified in 1975. In fact, the disease has been known in Australia, Africa, and Europe for many years and was probably introduced into this country from Europe.

The first manifestation of Lyme disease is a small red pimple at the sight of the tick bite. This initial lesion may expand to form a ring-shaped rash, clear in the center, forming the shape of a bull's eye, ranging in size from that of a dime to several inches across. Multiple bull's eyes develop if there have been several tick bites. This rash is usually accompanied by flu-like symptoms, including headache, stiff neck, aching muscles, and fatigue.

If the disease is not treated with antibiotics, about half of those with Lyme disease will develop an arthritis that often resembles rheumatoid arthritis *(see above).* The knees especially are involved. Intermittent pain and swelling can last for years. Neurologic symptoms that resemble multiple sclerosis may also occur, with vague weaknesses, loss of pain sensation, and loss of muscle coordination. In a few individuals, dizziness, shortness of breath, and irregular heartbeat also occur.

The diagnosis of Lyme disease may be difficult, since not all those infected develop a skin rash, and the initial flu-like symptoms may be mistaken for another illness. Specific blood tests do not usually become positive until several weeks after the skin rash appears. Finding the tick and its bite are a sure clue that treatment is needed.

Treatment. Fortunately, Lyme disease is relatively easily treated with antibiotics once the diagnosis has been made. However, the best treatment is prevention. The deer tick, *Ixodes dammini,* is found along the eastern seaboard from New Hampshire to North Carolina, and in Minnesota and Wisconsin. On the Pacific coast, the disease is carried by a close relative, the tick *Ixodes pacificus.* These are very small ticks, measuring only about an eighth inch in diameter. They are active from early spring through summer. After coming in from the woods, you should examine yourself carefully and gently remove any ticks with tweezers, taking care not to squeeze the tick's body. Apply an antiseptic, such as rubbing alcohol, to the bite, and save the tick in a jar for later identification if you develop any Lyme disease symptoms. If you find such ticks, do not be alarmed, since they require two or three days of feeding to transmit the spirochete, but be alert for symptoms, especially the insignia bull's eye rash.

Other Types of Arthritis

Arthritis is associated with several other diseases:

1. Inflammatory bowel diseases, including Crohn's disease and ulcerative colitis (*see* p. 297).
2. Sjögren's syndrome (*see* p. 270).
3. Gonorrhea and other bacterial infections.
4. Psoriasis (*see* p. 460).
5. Hemophilia (*see* p. 219).
6. Sarcoidosis (*see* p. 263).
7. Thyroid disease.
8. Raynaud's disease (*see* p. 203).
9. Systemic lupus erythematosus.

Other Types of Rheumatism
(Bursitis, Tendinitis, and Fibromyalgia)

Most joint aches and pains are not caused by arthritis, i.e., an inflammation of the synovium lining the joint, but rather by inflammation or injury of tissues surrounding the joint. These include the bursas, tendons, and tendon sheaths.

A *bursa* is a small, fluid-filled cavity located around a joint where friction occurs, or where tendons and muscles pass over bony prominences. The function of the bursa is to facilitate movement and decrease friction between tissues. *Bursitis* results when the bursa becomes inflamed, usually because of trauma or overuse, but also from infection, gout, or rheumatoid arthritis. With inflammation, the bursa becomes tender, warm and reddened from increased blood flow, and swollen with excess fluid.

Tendons are the fibrous cords that serve to attach the ends of muscles to bones. Surrounding the tendon is a tendon sheath, which acts like a bursa to reduce friction between the tendon and surrounding structures. When the tendon becomes inflamed, usually by stretching or overuse, *tendinitis* results. Inflammation of the tendon sheath is known as *tenosynovitis*. Usually the two conditions occur together.

Fibromyalgia, also known as *myofascial pain,* occurs when a muscle is strained or improperly used. The result is pain, tenderness, and muscle stiffness. Fibromyalgia differs from bursitis and tendinitis in that the pain is often worse at rest, and does not prevent movement. In fact, gentle motion of the affected muscle often eases the pain.

All three of these conditions occur either in response to acute injury or to stress, or in response to repetitive motion.

Because of the latter, they are frequently encountered as occupational injuries, where they are known as "repetitive motion injuries." Such injuries are common among clerical typists, computer operators, slaughterhouse workers, and grocery checkout clerks, all of whom develop hand, wrist, or elbow pain from the repetitive motions required in performing their jobs. Usually these conditions are temporary. However, if the acute conditions are not alleviated by rest or changes in work habits, such crippling complications as *carpal tunnel syndrome* (see p. 424) can develop.

Shoulder and Arm Syndromes

The shoulder is a complex joint formed by the articulation of the upper arm bone *(humerus)*, the shoulder blade *(scapula)*, and the collar bone *(clavicle)*. The shoulder joint is surrounded by the deltoid and rotator cuff muscles that unite to form a muscular cuff around the upper end of the humerus. The rotator cuff itself consists of the tendons of five muscles that attach to the upper humerus to rotate the arm laterally.

SHOULDER BURSITIS

This condition is characterized by pain and tenderness at the outside tip of the shoulder. You may have difficulty lifting your arm away from your side or to turn (rotate) your arm outward. Combing your hair or putting on a jacket may be impossible without assistance. Usually the tendons of the rotator cuff that lie beneath the shoulder bursa are also inflamed (tendinitis). The inflammation is caused by the wear and tear of repetitive motion of the arm or by acute strain or injury. Shoulder bursitis is common in sports in which the arm is used in an overhead motion, such as in swimming, tennis, golf, and baseball. If the bursitis is not treated, a frozen shoulder may result, with permanent loss of shoulder motion.

Treatment. Rest your shoulder as much as possible, and try to avoid the activity that started the problem, or any activity that renews the pain. If the pain is severe, your doctor may recommend a sling. Apply an ice bag (over a towel) to your shoulder twice daily for 30–60 minutes.

The pain and inflammation are often relieved by one of the nonsteroidal anti-inflammatory drugs (NSAIDs), such as ibuprofen (*see* p. 120). To prevent immobility, you should also gently exercise your shoulder. One such exercise is the "pendulum" exercise in which you bend forward from the waist and swing your arm to-and-fro, side-to-side, and rotate your hands. Do this several times each day. Your doctor can recommend other exercises if the pain persists.

For more severe conditions, your doctor may inject your shoulder with a combination of corticosteroid and an anesthetic.

If X-rays show deposits of calcium *(calcific tendinitis)*, the calcium may have to be removed surgically. With treatment, your chance of a complete recovery is good.

BICIPITAL TENDINITIS

Wear and tear of the biceps tendon as it passes through the bicipital groove on the front aspect of your upper humerus may cause inflammation of the tendon and tendon sheath, with resulting pain, especially when lifting. This condition, known as *bicipital tendinitis*, is often recognized by "point" tenderness over the upper front side of your humerus. The treatment is similar to shoulder bursitis.

ROTATOR CUFF TEAR

Rotator cuff tear occurs when the rotator cuff tendons that surround the shoulder joint become torn or split. Extreme pain results and you may be unable to move your arm away from your body. Such tendon tears are usually brought about by trauma or extreme exertion. Should this happen, you should see your doctor, who may order arthrograms of your shoulder joint to detect torn ligaments. Complete tears may require surgical repair, although most partial tears can be treated by immobilization in a sling, followed by gradually increasing exercises.

SHOULDER FIBROMYALGIA

Shoulder fibromyalgia is a deep muscular pain or aching between your neck and shoulder. The cause of shoulder fibromyalgia may be repeated movement of the arm backward or behind your back. Such activities as holding a telephone between your head and shoulder or sleeping on bunched-up pillows may cause this pain.

Treatment. Apply heat, take frequent hot showers, take one of the NSAIDs, such as ibuprofen, to reduce inflammation, and avoid the kind of activities that trigger the pain. Try sleeping with a single pillow or none at all. If you do not obtain prompt relief, see your doctor.

SAGGING SHOULDER

Sagging shoulder is a shoulder pain syndrome, similar to shoulder fibromyalgia, that is caused by pinching or compression of the nerves and blood vessels between your neck and shoulder. This condition is also called the *thoracic outlet syndrome*. The causes include slumping your shoulders through poor posture, having heavy breasts, sleeping with your arms overhead (called "Saturday night palsy"), or awkward work postures. Carrying a heavy backpack or load upon your shoulders can also cause this syndrome. The most common symptoms are aching in the shoulders and arms and numbness and tingling in your hands and fingers.

Treatment. The best treatment is *prevention*. Try to recognize and avoid the condition or activity that causes the pain. Women with large breasts gain relief by wearing support bras.

Shoulder–Hand Syndrome

Also known as *reflex sympathetic dystrophy, causalgia,* or *Sudek's atrophy, shoulder–hand syndrome* is a poorly understood pain syndrome of unknown cause. It often follows an injury to major nerves, bones, muscles, ligaments, or tendons. Surgery to the bones or soft tissues, as well as fractures and other injuries, can be the cause of this problem. The upper extremities are usually involved, but the legs and feet may also be affected.

Pain in the shoulder and hand are the main symptoms. The hand may become weak and stiff. There is often a burning sensation in the hand. The arm and hand may become swollen, and flushing and sweating of the arm results from dilation of blood vessels in the extremity. Other symptoms include rapid growth of the nails and hair of the affected limb. If the condition remains untreated, the skin becomes drawn and shiny, and the muscles may become wasted (atrophy) and contracted.

Treatment. Your doctor will most likely recommend an analgesic for the pain and an exercise program to overcome the stiffness. Some therapists use biofeedback techniques in which you are taught to attempt to control the blood flow to your arms and hands. Another approach involves *transcutaneous electrical nerve stimulation* (TENS). This is done with a small battery-driven device that relieves pain by blocking nerve impulses, and can be self-regulated. For more resistant cases, oral corticosteroids, anesthetic nerve blocks, acupuncture, or surgery to the local nerves may be required.

You may obtain more information from: Reflex Sympathetic Dystrophy Syndrome Association, 822 Wayside Lane, Haddonfield, NY; 1-609-428-6510.

Tennis Elbow

Tennis elbow is another "repetitive-motion injury," here caused by repeated twisting motions of the forearm or by opening and closing the fists. It is by no means limited to tennis players. Carpenters suffer from tennis elbow and politicians are reported to develop tennis elbow by too much handshaking. The usual symptoms are pain in the outer aspect of the elbow when lifting the elbow or clenching the fist, in which pain is caused by strain on the tendons of the muscles that bend back the wrist. These tendons insert on the outside bony prominence of the elbow (the *lateral epicondyle*). Pressure applied to this bony point almost always elicits sharp pain. Strain on these tendons is common during the tennis stroke (especially an improperly executed stroke), and hence the name.

A related condition is known as "golfer's elbow," except that this involves the tendons that flex downward and rotate the wrist. In golfer's elbow, the pain is felt on the *inside* of the elbow.

Treatment. Rest your elbow temporarily. Stop playing tennis or golf, and avoid lifting and repeated handshaking. Only rarely is a sling necessary. Apply ice packs (over a towel) to your elbow two or three times daily for 30–60 minutes. You can reduce the pain and inflammation by taking one of the nonsteroidal anti-inflammatory drugs (NSAIDs), such as ibuprofen. Periodically stretching your wrist will help prevent stiffness. Your doctor can recommend appropriate exercises to help prevent recurrence. Tennis elbow splints, which can be purchased at most sporting goods stores, may be helpful in preventing recurrences; or ask your doctor to prescribe a wrist splint, since bending the wrist in the wrong way often causes tennis elbow. Steroid injections may also reduce pain temporarily. Improvement is gradual, and weeks or months may be required to relieve pain. Surgery is necessary only in rare cases to "release" muscle attachments.

Ulnar Palsy

The ulnar nerve supplies the little finger and the outer half of the ring finger. This nerve runs close to the skin's surface as it passes the inner side of the elbow. Pressure on this nerve, as a result of leaning on your elbows, or pressure against your mattress while lying on your back, can cause the numbness and tingling in your little and ring fingers known as *ulnar palsy*. A similar numbness, and even weakness, in these fingers can develop after prolonged bicycling as a result of pressure from the handlebars to the nerve that runs through the palm of your hand.

Treatment. The approach to ulnar palsy is prevention. You can usually avoid pressure to your elbow once you know that the problem arises in the elbow rather than in the hand. If you develop palsy while riding a bicycle, use padded gloves and change your grip frequently while riding to relieve pressure on the palm.

Hand and Wrist Syndromes

Carpal Tunnel Syndrome

Carpal tunnel syndrome is a common condition that causes pain in the wrist and forearm, and numbness and tingling in the palm and fingers. The cause is pressure on the *median nerve* as it passes under the carpal ligament in the wrist. This condition occurs in workers whose jobs entail repetitive motions that flex (bend down) the hand, e.g., garment workers, butchers, grocery checkers, assembly workers, typists, musicians, packers, cooks, carpenters, computer operators, and housekeepers. Such repetitive motion causes wear and tear and subsequent swelling of the structures that lie close to the nerve, compressing it in its narrow "tunnel." In some cases, tapping the under side of your wrist can invoke the pain; this is known as *Tinel's sign*. Interestingly, carpal tunnel syndrome can also occur in such conditions as pregnancy, diabetes, thyroid disease, and other conditions unrelated to repetitive motion.

Usually the dominant hand is involved, but both hands may be affected. You may notice an increased tendency to drop things as weakness in the fingers becomes apparent. If left untreated, some of the thumb muscles may shrink (atrophy).

Treatment. Carpal tunnel syndrome is treated with rest and avoidance of activities that flex the wrist. Your doctor may prescribe a wrist splint that prevents wrist flexion, thus relieving pressure on the median nerve. Nonsteroidal anti-inflammatory drugs (NSAIDs) are useful (*see* p. 120). If the syndrome is resistant to conservative measures, your doctor may recommend corticosteroid injections or surgery to decompress the nerve.

In most cases, carpal tunnel syndrome can be prevented by avoiding the repetitive motions that cause it. This may require redesign of the tools you use, your workstation, or the sequence of tasks you perform. Frequent breaks are often effective in resting the wrist and thus avoiding extended nerve pressure.

deQuervain's Wrist

Another of the "repetitive motion" injuries that causes pain in the wrist and thumb is known as *deQuervain's wrist*. It is a type of *tenosynovitis* caused by inflammation and subsequent thickening and narrowing of one of the wrist ligament compartments through which pass two of the ligaments that raise the thumb. The symptoms may be brought on by prolonged writing, by the use of scissors, or by other activities that involve repeated pinching type motions. You can usually elicit the pain by grasping your thumb and pulling down, thus stretching the tendons through the narrowed tendon sheath. This is known as *Finkelstein's test*.

Treatment. Rest and avoidance of pinching and grasping motions usually eliminates and prevents the pain. Apply ice packs two or three times daily for 30–60 minutes. Use of a nonsteroidal anti-inflammatory drug (NSAID), such as ibuprofen, relieves pain (*see* p. 120). Your doctor may also recommend a splint that limits thumb motion. In severe cases, injections of corticosteroids or surgical relief of the narrowed compartment may be recommended.

Trigger Finger and Thumb

Trigger finger and thumb are types of tenosynovitis (inflammation of a tendon and tendon sheath) that affect the function of the thumb or index finger and sometimes other fingers. Repetitive use causes a nodule to form in the tendon that flexes one of these digits. The tendon nodule irritates the sheath surrounding the tendon, causing inflammation and narrowing of the sheath. If the tendon sheath becomes so narrowed that the nodule cannot pass through it, the involved finger may lock in either the flexed or extended position. This condition is both painful and debilitating.

Treatment. The treatment is similar to that of the treatment for deQuervain's wrist above. In severe cases, surgical release of the narrowed sheath may be necessary to unlock the finger.

Dupuytren's Contracture

Dupuytren's contracture is a condition involving any of the fingers, although most often the little or ring finger. The tendons in the palm that flex the fingers become thickened and contract, eventually causing permanent contraction of the finger. The cause of the thickening is unknown, but it is thought to be in part hereditary and occurs predominantly in men. President Reagan had this condition. Initially the thickening bands are tender, but as contraction increases, tenderness subsides.

Treatment. Early in the course of contracture, X-ray therapy or corticosteroids may be prescribed. Unfortunately, there is not much that can be done to halt progress of the contracture. The condition should be followed by an orthopedic surgeon. Early surgery is not recommended because the trauma of surgery may worsen the growth of fibrous tissue and increase the deformity. On the other hand, surgery should be performed before marked deformity develops in order to ensure complete surgical repair.

Ganglions

These are fluid-filled cysts that develop in the joint capsules of the wrist bones. The buildup of fluid causes weakening and bulging of the joint capsule, forming a hard, painful nodule that usually flares up and subsides at unpredictable intervals. At times pain may be so severe as to interfere with lifting and other use of the hand. Pressure over the nodule elicits acute pain.

Treatment. Conservative treatment with rest is usually recommended. Take one of the nonsteroidal anti-inflammatory drugs (*see* p. 120) for pain. If the condition becomes chronic surgical removal may be required, although there is a chance that the ganglion will recur after surgery.

Leg, Knee, and Foot Syndromes

Hip Bursitis

The trochanter (pronounced *tró*-kanter) is an enlargement at the upper end of the femur to which numerous leg muscles attach. It is the bony prominence that you feel easily at the side of your hip. Between the trochanter and the muscle tendons lies a fluid-filled bursa that reduces friction between the bone and tendons. If this bursa becomes inflamed, you may experience pain while walking, or even while at rest. The condition, known as *bursitis,* can be distinguished from the more common condition of osteoarthritis of the hip by the fact that pressure applied over the bony prominence elicits pain in bursitis, while such pressure does not cause pain in osteoarthritis.

Treatment. Treatment consists of rest, heat, and nonsteroidal anti-inflammatory drugs, such as ibuprofen (*see* p. 120).

Leg Cramps

Leg cramps are muscle spasms, sometimes called charley horses, most often in the calves and feet. They occur most frequently at night and usually affect middle-aged and elderly persons. Their cause is not known, although they may be caused by poor arterial circulation, as well as by varicose veins. Persons taking diuretic drugs (to lose water) or corticosteroids that alter body mineral content may discover that they are more prone to leg cramps.

Treatment. Leg cramps often develop when you stretch your legs while the toes are pointing downward. When this happens, point your toes up toward your head and stretch your legs out from that position. This usually brings prompt relief. Try to sleep in a position that avoids downward pointing of the toes.

A regular program of stretching your calf muscles may be helpful: Stand about 12 inches from a wall. Keeping your heels touching the floor, lean forward, and touch your chest to the wall. Do this 10 times twice daily.

Two tablets of benadryl taken at bedtime may prevent leg cramps. Another over-the-counter preparation that contains quinine, Q-Vel, may also be effective. Be aware that the latter drug may cause skin rashes, ringing in your ears, and visual disturbances, and should not be taken during pregnancy. Hot water bottles and heating pads increase leg circulation and may be soothing. If these simple remedies are not effective, your doctor may prescribe a tranquilizer, such as Valium, or an antispasmodic drug, e.g., Flexaril.

Shin Splints

Shin splints are injuries of the muscles and tendons that insert into the front of the leg bones. In some cases they are caused by pulled tendons or microfractures of the bone. They are common among runners and basketball players. The most common symptom is pain in the shins when walking, running, or jumping.

Treatment. You need to reduce the level of your activity for several days or weeks to give the bone or tendon time to heal. Take one of the nonsteroidal anti-inflammatory drugs, such as ibuprofen (*see*

p. 120) for pain. Make sure you wear proper sports shoes. Throw away worn or ill-fitting sport shoes. If pain persists, ask your doctor to refer you to an orthopedic surgeon or a sports medicine specialist.

Restless Leg Syndrome

Restless leg syndrome is a relatively uncommon problem that may be quite discomfiting to those who suffer from it. It is most often described as an uncomfortable sensation, a "creeping" or "crawling" within the muscles, that comes from deep within the leg, usually between the knee and ankle, or in the feet or thighs. It usually comes on during times of relaxation or during the night and often forces the person to get up and walk around to dispel the unpleasant sensation.

Restless leg syndrome is thought to be a disturbance of the local nerves. It may be associated with alcoholism, iron deficiency anemia, diabetes, or other disorders. Because of this you should see your doctor, who will check for a serious underlying cause. Prescription drugs such as carbamazepine (Tegretol) or clonazepam (Klonopin) may bring partial or complete relief.

Knee Pain

The knee is the largest joint in the body and is held together by a number of ligaments, cartilage, and tendons. Since the joint must often bear your entire body weight on its relatively small surface area, it needs, in addition to these attachments, the help of strong surrounding muscles to support it. It follows that an important part of any rehabilitation of the knee following injury or surgery must involve strengthening the muscles of the leg.

Approximately one-fourth of all sport injuries involve the knees. Of these, meniscus tears and ligament injuries are the most important. There are two meniscus cartilages, medial and lateral, that separate and cushion the femur and the tibia. The two pairs of ligaments that serve primarily to stabilize the knee joint are the *collateral* and the *cruciate* (cross-shaped) *ligaments*.

Injuries to the collateral ligaments often result from direct blows to the knees. The medial collateral ligament will often heal with supervised rehabilitation alone. Injuries to the cruciate ligaments, particularly if combined with meniscus tears, more often require surgery.

Usually knee cartilage and ligament repairs can be made by arthroscopic surgery in which small nicks are made in the joint capsule and narrow tubes inserted. While the surgeon is observing through one tube, the repairs can be made through another. Such surgery imposes minimal trauma to the joint, greatly reducing complications and recovery times.

Following a ligament injury, there is pain, difficulty bearing weight, and swelling within 1–2 hours. Such injuries should be immobilized with a snug elastic bandage, elevated, and ice-packed to limit swelling during the trip to the orthopedic surgeon or emergency room. If the knee swells, keep ice packs on for the first 24 hours to reduce pain and swelling.

The knees can be protected against injury by developing strength in the quadriceps, the large muscle group on the front of your thigh. This is best accomplished by leg-raising exercises and by cycling (make sure your seat is set at the proper height, at the bottom of the cycle stroke, your knee should be only slightly bent). Make sure your shoes fit well. If you ride over your heels, or are knock-kneed, you may need orthotic shoes. See your orthopedic surgeon for this and for any chronic knee pain.

Runner's Knee

With the popularity of jogging, runner's knee is a common sports injury. The most common symptoms are pain at the front of the knee, often accompanied by swelling. It is probably caused by small sprains of the knee ligaments. X-Rays are usually negative.

Treatment. Apply ice to the sore knee and avoid the activity that caused the pain and swelling. An anti-inflammatory drug, such as ibuprofen, helps relieve both pain and inflammation. Avoid deep knee bends and calisthenics that place strain upon the knee. Since runner's knee is usually caused by improper training, reduce your level of exercise and then gradually increase, if desired, as your muscular strength improves. You may also want to consult your local sports authority. Consider switching to bicycling.

Foot Problems

Flat Feet

Also known as "fallen arches," *flat feet* are marked by an absence of an upward curvature, or arch, on the bottom of the foot. The lack of this arch does not in itself cause pain or an instability of the foot, since several races naturally have flat feet. It is when flat feet are combined with an inward angling of the ankle that pain with walking or running develops.

Treatment. Ask your doctor to refer you to a podiatrist, who can prescribe orthotic devices to be worn in your shoes that will correct your foot problem.

Plantar Fasciitis (Painful Heel)

The *plantar fascia* is a thick, fibrous band on the bottom of the foot that extends from the toes forward to the bottom of the heel behind. This fascia serves as a kind of bowstring to maintain the upward curvature of the arch of the foot. When stress is placed on this inflexible fascia through excessive or unaccustomed exercise, it may place undue tension on the narrow attachment to the heel. This results in inflammation and pain.

Plantar fasciitis is a common condition in people who run, who are active in sports, or who suddenly increase their level of exercise. It is characterized by pain in the heel with walking or running and may progress to a dull or sharp persistent pain. It is usually worst when first getting up in the morning or after resting. The condition may be brought on by running on the toes (hill running) or running in soft terrain, such as sand. Poorly fitting shoes are another culprit.

Treatment. Initially you should rest your heel, letting the pain be your guide. Ice packs to the heel for 30–60 minutes several times a day reduces inflammation and pain. Take one of the nonsteroidal anti-inflammatory drugs, such as ibuprofen (*see* p. 120). Heel pads of felt or sponge placed in your shoe may cushion the heel while walking. You may cut out a circle in the heel pad where it meets the pressure point of your heel to further reduce pressure on the point of inflammation. You can obtain these heel pads in most medical supply or sporting-goods stores.

Exercises also help relieve the pain and prevent recurrences. Stand one foot-length away from a wall with your hands against the wall. Keeping your heels flat on the floor, lean forward to touch your chest to the wall. You should feel a stretching in your calf muscles. This exercise stretches the Achilles tendon (the big heel tendon behind your ankle) and relieves tension on the plantar fascia. Do 10 repetitions 2–3 times daily.

If these measures do not help, ask your doctor to refer you to an orthopedic surgeon. In rare cases a bony heel spur may have developed that must be corrected surgically.

Morton's Neuroma

Morton's neuroma is an overgrowth of tissue around the nerve that supplies the third and fourth toe. When the neuroma becomes large enough, it can compress the nerve, often causing exquisite pain. The pain is usually quite characteristic. You will usually have no pain when walking barefoot, but with any shoe on, particularly a tight-fitting one, you may experience a sudden severe pain with tingling of the toes. If you then take your shoe off, the pain quickly subsides as pressure on the neuroma is relieved.

Treatment. A special foot pad, known as a Morton's pad, often will relieve pressure on the neuroma when wearing your shoes. However, the neuroma may later become so large that only surgical removal will relieve the pain. Ask your doctor for referral to a podiatrist.

Bunions

Bunions are bony growths at the base of the great toe. The condition stems from a hereditary weakness of the toes, known as *hallux valgus*. This causes the base of the toe to deviate toward the opposite foot, and the tip of the toe to point outward. Pressure of the joint against the shoes results in bony overgrowth and a painful bursitis. If the condition persists untreated, the deviated great toes will press and override the adjacent toe, while calluses develop at various pressure points with your shoes. The condition is more common among women and is made worse by high-heeled and tight-fitting shoes.

Treatment. You can relieve the pain relatively easily by cutting a hole out of an old pair of shoes at the site of the pressure point while the acute bursitis is healing. Ice packs for 30–60 minutes several times daily helps relieve inflammation. Take one of the non-steroidal anti-inflammatory drugs, such as ibuprofen (*see* p. 120) to relieve pain and inflammation. Wear comfortable shoes that fit well, but do not place pressure on your toe joint. If these measures do not help, ask your doctor to refer you to a podiatrist, who may recommend one of several procedures to correct this condition surgically.

Hammertoes

A *hammertoe* is a painful deformity that most often involves the second toe. The toe becomes clawlike in appearance because of mis-

---

PREVENTING LOW BACK PAIN

Protect your back by developing good back habits—

1. When you lift heavy objects, keep your back straight and bend your knees so as to let your legs do the work. Do not stoop over to pick up objects.
2. Wear low-heeled, comfortable shoes. The higher your heels, the more they force your back into an unnatural position.
3. When sitting, select a firm chair with arm rests. Keep your upper back straight and your shoulders relaxed. Keep your knees slightly higher than your hips (use a footstool or book under your feet if necessary). Keep your feet flat on the floor.

   If you are tired, avoid slumping in your chair. Instead, lie down with your knees bent so that your lower back touches the floor. When you are sitting or standing for prolonged periods, restore the normal *lordosis* (lower back curvature) by periodically stretching your shoulders backward until you feel a slight pressure on your lower back and pelvis.
4. When standing, stand with your weight equally on both feet. Avoid locking your knees. Keep your back straight by tightening your stomach muscles and buttocks.
5. Maintain your weight at a desirable level (*see* table, p. 314). Obesity increases stress on your back.
6. Sleep on a fairly hard mattress or put a bed board under your mattress. Remember that mattresses wear out. When yours begins to sag, throw it out and buy a new firm one.
7. Avoid high-risk sports and exercising, such as football, rowing, diving, bowling, fast or downhill running, and weightlifting. Low-risk, high-gain exercises include brisk walking, bicycling, and swimming. These are low-impact exercises that avoid large forces on or awkward positions for back muscles.

---

alignment of the joint surfaces, along with shortening and weakening of the toe and foot muscles. Diabetics are especially prone to developing hammertoes because of the vascular and nerve injuries they sustain.

Treatment. Ask your doctor to recommend shoe orthotics to relieve and redistribute the pressures on your feet. In some cases surgery may be required to relieve severe deformity. Analgesics help relieve pain. *See* p. 202 for proper foot care.

Miscellaneous Foot Conditions

Plantar warts are discussed on p. 454. Corns and calluses are discussed on p. 461. Proper care of the feet in diabetes and peripheral vascular diseases is discussed on p. 202.

Backaches

There are numerous causes of low back pain. Gynecological causes include endometriosis, uterine fibroids, pelvic infections, and displacement of the uterus. Neurogenic causes include herniated disc (displacement or rupture of the gelatinous cushion between two vertebrae) or a tumor that encroaches upon one of the spinal nerves. There are several bone abnormalities that cause low back pain, including degenerative arthritis (*see* p. 409), displacement of a vertebra (*spondylolisthesis*), congenital spine malformations, vertebral collapse (common in osteoporosis), tumors, and of course, injuries to the back.

The great majority of backaches, however, are nonspecific; that is, they have no obvious cause, or appear after vigorous exercise or lifting. Such backaches may develop slowly or suddenly, as when you lift a heavy object. The pain is then usually persistent, increases with bending and twisting the back, and is associated with stiffness after lying or sitting. These backaches are caused usually by "strain" of muscles and ligaments, and you can usually treat them yourself.

Treatment. Total bed rest on a firm mattress may be necessary for a severe back pain, but usually intermittent rest is better for you and all that is needed. When resting, either lie on your back with a pillow placed under both your knees and your calves, or lie on your side with your knees pulled up toward your chest and a pillow held lengthwise between your knees and calves.

Immediately after an acute injury, place an ice bag (protected by a towel) over your back, or ask someone to gently massage your back. Later, when stiffness develops, heat may be more effective. Moist heat from a hot bath or whirlpool is more effective than a heating pad.

Mild analgesics, such as aspirin or ibuprofen (*see* p. 120) help relieve pain. Avoid taking muscle relaxant drugs unless specifically prescribed by your doctor.

You should see your doctor about your low back pain if:

1. Pain persists for more than 3–4 days.
2. You have weakness, numbness, or tingling in your feet or legs.
3. You develop sciatica. This is a sharp pain that runs down the back of your leg. This is caused by pressure on the sciatic nerve, often by

a herniated disc. The pain is usually made worse by coughing or
sneezing.
4. You have a fever with back pain.
5. You have loss of bladder or bowel control, either incontinence or
difficulty urinating (possible spinal nerve injury).

Avoiding Sports Injuries

Most of the injuries that occur during exercise result from unusual
demands that you put on your bones, muscles, and other musculo-
skeletal tissues. The most common of these are sustained by those
who exercise infrequently and "make up" for idle time by going all
out. Novice runners who struggle to complete self-determined running goals are also candidates for injury. Here are some prudent
measures to guide your exercising:

1. Warm up before exercising. Devote a minimum of 5–10 minutes to
   stretching and loosening your muscles. The increased blood flow
   induced by such warming up reduces the tension in your muscles,
   improves their range of motion, and may even increase your level
   of performance. All of these measures help reduce the chances for
   tearing or straining your muscles.
2. Select a sport that is really suited to you. If you have a painful hip
   or knee, jogging and tennis are probably not for you. Consider
   swimming, walking, and cycling. Before embarking on a new exercise program, consult your doctor to determine that you've got what
   it takes—literally.
3. Pace yourself so that your exertion is spread more or less evenly
   over the time you allot to your exercise. Develop a program that
   allows your body to become conditioned to the activity you call
   upon it to perform. Increase exercise levels gradually.
4. Cool down after exercising. Muscles used during workouts have
   contracted, and most repetitive activities also cause them to become
   shortened. Stretching after exercise helps restore length and balance, and prevent you from "stiffening up."
5. If you sustain an injury, stop and take care of it. Don't continue
   exercising—especially in competitions that dispose you to neglect
   reasonable caution! You can often worsen an existing injury and
   expose yourself to additional injuries by weakening your musculo-
   skeletal support.

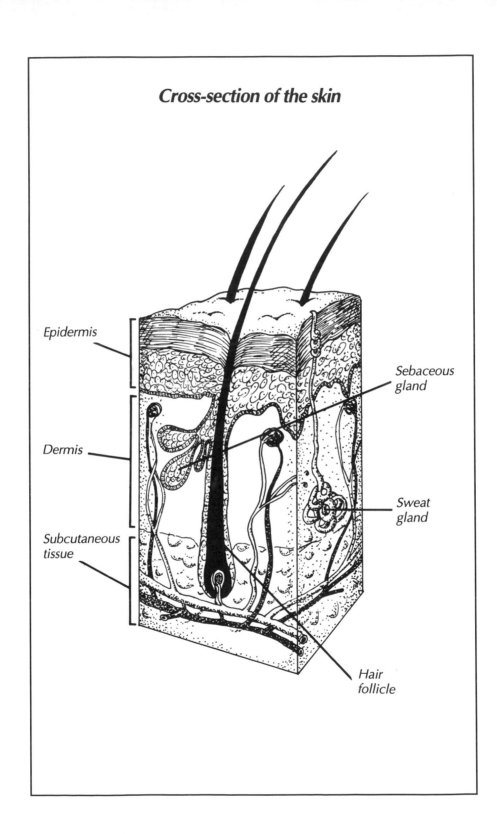

Cross-section of the skin

Epidermis

Dermis

Subcutaneous tissue

Sebaceous gland

Sweat gland

Hair follicle

Your Skin, Hair, and Nails

Anatomy and Physiology

Skin is not usually thought of as an organ, yet it is indeed the largest organ of the body, totaling one-seventh of normal body weight and covering nearly two square yards of surface area. The skin is complex, and includes several smaller organelles that have many specialized functions beyond serving as the protective covering of the body. Among the skin's functions are:

- Physical protection of the underlying structures
- Prevention of dehydration
- Regulation of body temperature
- Manufacture of essential nutrients (Vitamin D)

Itching

Montaigne wrote that, "Scratching is one of the sweetest gratifications of nature and as ready at hand as any." No one knows exactly why we itch. Itching, also known as "pruritus," is akin to pain and is probably the body's signal that *something*, if only scratching, needs to be done.

Localized Itching

Itching is associated with most primary skin lesions and is an almost invariable accompaniment to all forms of contact dermatitis. For itching associated with organs, e.g., itchy ears, please refer to the index or chapter heading under that particular organ.

Generalized Itching

Generalized itching is often a complex problem, one that is associated not only with various skin diseases and with dry skin, but with several systemic diseases. In the case of primary skin diseases, there is almost always an associated rash that indicates the source of the itching. In the cases of dry skin and systemic diseases, however, no other sign or symptom may be apparent.

GLOSSARY OF SKIN-RELATED TERMS

Many skin rashes, to the casual eye, look alike. Yet on more careful inspection there are often differences in the appearance of individual skin lesions. A knowledge of these differences will help you better understand much of the text that follows. Brief descriptions of common skin disorders are given for reference.

PRIMARY LESIONS

These are the first lesions to appear when the skin is involved in disease or trauma.

- *Macule.* A flat, nonraised, discolored spot, usually less than one-half inch in diameter. Examples are freckles and nonraised moles. A spot larger than one-half inch is referred to as a "patch."
- *Papule.* A raised lesion less than one-half inch in diameter. Examples are small warts, hives, and insect bites. Larger raised lesions are referred to as "plaques."
- *Nodules.* A solid lesion that can be felt in, on, or beneath the skin, usually larger than one-half inch in diameter. Examples are small lipomas (benign fatty tumors) and lymph nodes.
- *Vesicle.* An elevated lesion containing clear fluid, usually less than one-fourth inch in diameter. Larger lesions are called "blisters." Vesicles and blisters are often associated with poison ivy, insect bites, sunburn, and contact dermatitis.
- *Pustule.* A lesion similar to a vesicle or blister that contains pus. Pustules often form when blisters become infected.
- *Wheal.* A temporary raised lesion (a "hive") caused by local swelling (edema), usually from an allergic reaction, e.g., insect bites or drug eruption.

SECONDARY LESIONS

When primary skin lesions change, e.g., either by natural evolution or by trauma, secondary lesions form.

- *Scales.* These are heaped-up piles of dried epithelium that result from chronic inflammation. They usually have a rough, whitish appearance. The most common cause is a chronic dermatitis in which primary lesions form on top of one another because of the persistent irritation.
- *Scab.* The crust on a lesion formed by dried serum, blood, or pus.
- *Ulcer.* Loss of skin layers, usually because of trauma to or infection of the primary lesion.

TOPICAL SKIN PREPARATIONS

The following are commonly used preparations for the treatment of skin disorders:

- *Ointments.* These preparations contain very little water and feel greasy. Vaseline is an example. They are used to lubricate the skin, especially when scales, crust, or thickening has developed. They are best applied over damp skin to help retain moisture. Ointments are often more acceptable than creams if the skin is open, as on ulcers.
- *Creams.* These are emulsions of oil and water that vanish when rubbed into the skin. They often feel better than ointments, because they lack greasiness.
- *Lotions.* These are suspensions of either powders (e.g., Calamine lotion) or oils (e.g., corticosteroid lotions) in a water or alcohol base. Lotions are cooling and help dry your inflamed skin.
- *Solutions.* Homogeneous mixtures of two or more liquids. They are drying if they contain alcohol.

SYSTEMIC DISEASES

There are several systemic diseases associated with generalized itching for reasons that are little understood: poorly controlled diabetes, kidney disease, jaundice, hyperparathyroidism, hypothyroidism, lymphoma, and polycythemia vera. Psychological disorders underlie many cases of itching, but the above treatable diseases should be carefully ruled out before an itch-maddened wretch is packed off to the psychiatrist.

DRY SKIN

Everyone has dry skin, or "xerosis" at some time or another. Fortunately it can be successfully treated with simple home remedies. Dry skin most often occurs in wintertime, when a combination of low humidity and high indoor temperatures dehydrate the outer layers of your skin. When this happens, the outer skin begins to flake off, almost like dandruff. Areas most affected are the arms and legs.

Dry skin is especially a problem for the elderly, whose skin gradually produces less and less moisturizing oil, and for people who bathe too often or swim frequently, thus removing their natural skin oils.

TREATMENT OF DRY SKIN

1. *Raise indoor humidity* if dry skin develops only during winter. This can be done by installing a central or room humidifier, or simply by placing long pans of water over radiators.
2. *Take less frequent baths.* People who believe that cleanliness is next to godliness may be in for an unholy problem. Few people get so dirty that they need to bathe oftener than every two or three days during winter. If you feel you must get into water, try taking a brief, lukewarm shower.
3. *Try changing soaps.* Most bar soaps contribute to dry skin by their detergent action, which removes natural skin oils. Some soaps that minimize detergent action are Dove, Alpha Keri, Neutrogena, Aveeno, Oilatum, Eucerin, and Basis.
4. *Apply a moisturizer* such as Eucerin, Keri lotion, Lubriderm, or Aquaphor after bathing and patting yourself dry with a soft bath towel. Ointments and heavy creams are best. Vaseline and lanolin may also be used, if you don't mind a somewhat greasier product. In a recent test comparing several products, petrolatum relieved dry skin more quickly and for a longer time than any other product. Lanolin was second, although some people develop contact dermatitis to lanolin *(see below)*. Ointments like Vaseline and lanolin are most effective if applied while the skin is still damp.
5. *Use cool water for your baths and showers.* Cool water is less drying and irritating than hot water. Try using a bath oil if you itch all over, but *please* be careful with slippery tubs. During cool weather, use soap only on areas in which skin rubs against skin, such as armpits, genital areas, under breasts, and between toes.
6. *Avoid woolens and scratchy clothing* that irritate the skin.
7. *Avoid hot drinks, food, and alcohol.* Be aware that itching is made worse by dilation of skin blood vessels.
8. *Avoid stress*, which makes itching worse. Though most of us are poor at stress management, it is something to think about.

If the above measures don't bring relief within 7–10 days, you should consult your doctor about the possibility of a more serious, systemic condition as a cause of generalized itching.

Icthyosis

Icthyosis is an especially severe type of dry skin characterized by extremely dry, scaly skin, especially on the hands. It is an inherited condition. The affected skin is often broken up into diamond-shaped areas that resemble fish scales, hence the name icthyosis. Cold weather worsens this condition; thus you should make certain your offspring are well protected in winter.

Dermatitis

The term dermatitis is quite nonspecific and is used to describe a superficial skin inflammation characterized by itching, redness, and often vesicles early in its course, followed by swelling, oozing, scabs, and scaling, particularly if scratched. "Eczema" is a commonly used term when vesicles are prominent.

There are numerous causes of dermatitis. The most simple classification divides the causes between internal and external:

Classification of Dermatitis

Internal causes	External causes
Atopic	Contact
Seborrheic	Direct irritant
Nummular	Light sensitivity
Exfoliative	
Stasis	Allergic
Pruritus ani	Physical substance
Pruritus vulvae	Light allergy
	Drug eruption

Contact Dermatitis

This is an eruption characterized by the appearance of multiple small vesicles and is caused by direct contact with some offending substance. The reaction may be highly localized, affecting only that skin that has come in contact with the agent, for example, as in watch-strap dermatitis. On the other hand, such irritating substances as soap that contact large areas of the body may result in generalized dermatitis. There are three mechanisms that produce contact dermatitis: irritation, sensitization, and photosensitization.

Direct Irritant

Irritation dermatitis is a rash or redness of the skin that develops within minutes or hours after contact with the irritant. An example is propylene glycol, often added to cosmetics to make them feel silky smooth. A classic case cited by Alexander Fisher in his text, *Contact Dermatitis*, involved a man who developed massive penile swelling after intercourse using K-Y Jelly, which contains propylene glycol.

Sensitization (Allergic) Reactions

These involve development of an actual allergy to a sensitizing substance. Following the initial sensitization, each subsequent contact will initiate an acute allergic dermatitis. Examples abound:

1. *Rubber.* Synthetic rubbers contain a variety of antioxidants, preservatives, and vulcanizers to help retain their elasticity. It is these additives rather than the natural latex that cause contact dermatitis allergies. Such problems have been traced to wet suits, swimming caps, nose clips, and earplugs. Rubber used in shoes may provoke a dermatitis across the top of the foot. Other rubber-containing apparel include trousers with rubber waistbands, bras, underpants, gloves, and even condoms. The dermatitis associated with these items occurs only when the article is worn or used.

   Interestingly, the type of "jock itch" associated with wearing elastic jock straps or tight-fitting underwear is not usually caused by a reaction to the rubber itself. Rather, bleach used in washing them reacts with the rubber to produce an irritating deposit on the fabric. To avoid this type of jock itch, buy a new jock strap and separate it from your bleached clotheswash.

2. *Nickel.* More people are allergic to nickel than any other metal. It is found in necklaces, rings, bracelets, and watchbands. Even some eyeglasses contain nickel. The typical rash that develops is highly localized to the area of skin contact, which is the usual tipoff. Chrome, mercury, and their compounds may also cause contact dermatitis.

3. *Topical medications.* Many ingredients in topical medications can cause contact dermatitis. Among the more common are certain antibiotics [neomycin (e.g., Neosporin), sulfonamides, penicillin]; antihistamines (diphenhydramine, promethazine); anesthetics (benzocaine); and antiseptics (thimerosal, hexachlorophene).

4. *Poison ivy, oak, and sumac.* These plants contain a substance, known as urushiol, in the sap of the leaves, roots, stems, and flower parts.

Insects chewing on the leaves allow escape of the sticky urushiol, so that touching even an apparently intact plant can cause an intense dermatitis. Within 12–48 hours of contact, redness and swelling develop, followed by vesicles over the area of contact. Intense itching is invariable. After a few days the vesicles crust over and the dermatitis clears up after about 10–14 days.

If you come into contact with poison ivy, oak, or sumac, wash the contacted area with soap and lots of water as soon as possible. This will prevent the sticky urushiol from being spread to other parts of the skin, and may prevent some penetration. If you act promptly enough, you may prevent the rash altogether. The weeping fluid from the rash itself does not spread the rash, but you should avoid scratching and breaking the vesicles in order to avoid secondary infections.

The best way to get rid of poison ivy plants is to spray with an herbicide, or pull them up wearing rubber or vinyl gloves and long sleeves. Put the plants in plastic bags for disposal. Do not burn them since the urushiol is released in the smoke; breathing the smoke can then cause a dermatitis over your entire body that may require hospitalization. Remember, too, that if you have pets that come in contact with these plants you can develop the rash from petting and nuzzling an innocent beast that is itself quite unaffected.

Certain trees of the Anacardiaceae family are related to poison ivy, including mangos, the Japanese lacquer tree, and cashew trees. If you are allergic to poison ivy, you will also be allergic to these trees. There are dozens of folk remedies for poison ivy, but the simple remedies described below for all forms of contact dermatitis are best.

5. *Other common substances.* The list will never be complete, but some commonly allergenic substances are: formaldehyde in new durable press clothing (always wash thoroughly before wearing), tanning agents in leather, bubble bath, industrial dyes, adhesives, cutting oils, hair-waving ingredients (glyceryl monothioglycolate), hair dyes, nail polish, nail polish remover, eye makeup, and lanolin.

Treatment. Avoidance of the offending substance is the only way to prevent contact dermatitis. This of course supposes that the sensitizing agent has been recognized. Often a complicated sleuthing problem confronts you and your dermatologist. In some cases, such as nickel-containing jewelry, the cause is obvious and avoidance is simple. However, gold-plated jewelry is a common and often unrecognized cause of dermatitis once the micrometer-thin layer of gold wears through.

In the acute vesicle or blister stage (e.g., poison ivy) applying a compress soaked in cool water for 30 minutes 4–6 times a day is soothing and stops the itching. Dilute aluminum acetate (sold as Burrow's solution), saline, or sodium bicarbonate (baking soda) solutions may also be effective in drying the blisters.

Topical cortisone cream is not effective during the acute blister stage, but may hasten healing during the crusting stage. Antihistamines are of no help, except that they are sedating and may induce sleep and reduce itching at night. Scratching may result in secondary infection, in which case a topical antibiotic such as bacitracin should be used.

Extensive or severe rashes, especially those occurring on the face and genital regions, should be treated by your doctor, who will probably prescribe an oral corticosteroid such as prednisone to reduce inflammation. Follow directions precisely, because corticosteroids are heavy-duty medications that must be taken exactly as prescribed.

Photosensitizing Reactions

Certain skin rashes are caused by the sun's ultraviolet rays, which may interact with an otherwise innocuous substance to produce a toxic or allergenic product. When this breakdown product comes in contact with your skin, contact dermatitis results. Common photosensitizing substances include aftershave lotions and perfumes. You may use any of these products with impunity indoors, but when exposed to sunlight, watch out!

Atopic Dermatitis

The cause of atopic dermatitis is not known. It occurs in individuals with a personal or family history of allergies, such as asthma or hayfever. It is a chronic superficial, itching rash located on the face, scalp, and extremities. It usually begins during early childhood, but may appear during young adulthood. The dermatitis usually clears up after age 3–4 years, but may recur for several years. In older individuals the rash may be confined to the inside of the elbows, back of the knees, wrists, and neck.

Atopic dermatitis is a wretched condition, because of the recurrent itching and the many environmental factors that make it worse: high temperature and humidity, woolen clothing, and secondary infections. Because it is common to apply numerous creams and lotions in an attempt to stem the itching, the sufferer comes in contact with

---

TREATMENT OF ATOPIC DERMATITIS

Since there is no specific preventative or cure for atopic dermatitis, general measures and common sense apply.

1. Select a physician experienced in the treatment of atopic dermatitis who will also expend the necessary time to become familiar with you or your child's pattern of dermatitis in order to avoid prescribing sensitizing medications.
2. Bathing should be minimized if it is found to have a drying and irritating effect upon the skin. Nondrying soaps should be used (*see* Dry Skin *above*). Oils and moisturizers should be applied after the bath, while the skin is still damp, then patted dry.
3. Fingernails should be kept short to minimize trauma from scratching.
4. For children, an antihistamine, such as diphenhydramine (e.g., Benadryl, Sominex) or doxepin (Adapin, Sinequan), may be given at bedtime for its sedative effect in reducing scratching.
5. Secondary infections should be treated promptly by a doctor.
6. Oral steroids are very useful in treating severe atopic dermatitis, but must be carefully administered. Prolonged use by children may stunt growth, induce osteoporosis, and have other serious side effects. The appropriateness of ultraviolet B therapy should be discussed with your doctor.

---

many substances that actually *promote* the contact dermatitis to which they are especially prone. Thus the two types of dermatitis may be difficult to distinguish.

Individuals with atopic dermatitis may also develop cataracts at an early age, and they are especially prone to herpes simplex.

Seborrheic Dermatitis

Seborrheic dermatitis is another chronic inflammation and scaling of unknown cause that affects areas of skin in which there are many sebaceous (oil) glands. The most commonly affected areas are the scalp, sides of the nose, eyebrows, and the skin behind the ears and over the sternum (breastbone). There is often confusion about the difference between dandruff, seborrhea, and seborrheic dermatitis.

Dandruff is a condition associated with excess scaling of the scalp. Though it is often accompanied by itching, there is no inflammation with dandruff alone.

Seborrhea is a term used to describe excessive oiliness of the skin and scalp. Again there is no associated skin inflammation.

Seborrheic dermatitis occurs in three age groups: infants, middle age, and the elderly. In infants, seborrheic dermatitis may take the form of a thickened, yellowish, crusting scalp lesion called "cradle cap." This condition is often associated with unusually severe diaper rash and disappears after about eight months of age. Though the disease in adults is easily treated, it tends to recur.

Treatment. Simple dandruff in adults is usually well-controlled by daily application of shampoos containing selenium sulfide (Selsun), sulfur (e.g., Sebulex, Vanseb), or pyrithione zinc (Danex, Head & Shoulders). Coal tar and salicylate shampoos (Denorex, Tegrin, Vanseb-T) are also effective. Once under control, use of a medicated shampoo twice weekly is usually sufficient for maintenance. If inflammation develops, topical corticosteroids can be rubbed into the scalp and other affected areas as your doctor directs. Infantile and childhood seborrheic dermatitis should be treated by your doctor.

Recent studies have suggested a causal relationship between seborrheic dermatitis and a common skin yeast, *Pityrosporum ovale*. For resistant cases, ask your doctor about such topical anti-yeast preparations as imidazole.

Nummular Dermatitis

This type of chronic dermatitis appears as red, scaly, itchy coin-sized lesions on the extremities, buttocks, and trunk. The cause is not known. They are often treated with topical corticosteroids or cortisone-impregnated tape. You should consult a dermatologist.

Stasis Dermatitis

This dermatitis appears on the legs and is commonly associated with leg edema and varicose veins. It is characterized by persistent inflammation and dry, scaly skin with a tendency to develop permanent patches of brown pigmentation. If left unattended, chronic ulcerations develop that are slow to heal.

Treatment. Elevate your legs periodically above the level of your heart to promote venous drainage and reduce leg edema. A variety of dressings for leg ulcers have been developed; these must be prescribed by your dermatologist. Avoid nonprescription creams and ointments; they may complicate the condition with contact dermatitis (*see* p. 441).

Scratch Dermatitis

This is a localized itching of unknown cause that is more common in women than in men. It occurs most often on the back of the head, arms, legs, and ankles. It is the scratching that causes the characteristic rash, which is localized, dry, scaling, and irregular. If the condition becomes chronic, increased pigmentation may appear. Other names for this rash are "lichen simplex" and "neurodermatitis." Stress and tension appear to increase the amount of scratching, which may become an unconscious habit.

Treatment. It is important to realize that scratching and rubbing produce the skin changes. As scratching diminishes, the lesions themselves begin to disappear, which in turn may serve as a positive reinforcement to stop scratching. Hydrocortisone cream (e.g., Cortaid) may be helpful. Your doctor may prescribe a cortisone-impregnated tape applied morning and evening, as well as oral medications to relieve the itching sensation.

Anal and Vulvar Itching

When scratch dermatitis is limited to the anus or vulva, it is known as *pruritis ani* or *pruritis vulvae*, respectively. The treatment is the same as described above, but your doctor will need to rule out other causes of this localized itching, including pinworms, yeast infections, hemorrhoids, anal fissures, venereal warts, and contact dermatitis.

Drug Eruption

The skin reactions caused by a drug allergy or sensitivity can be quite varied, from a mild rash to a toxic sloughing of the skin (called *pemphigus*). The onset may be sudden (e.g., the rash after penicillin) or delayed for hours or days. The rash may begin as small papules, especially on the arms and trunk, or as small vesicles on the skin and mucous membranes. Scratching, of course, modifies the appearance of the rash. Common drugs associated with skin eruptions are penicillin, sulfonamides, ampicillin, erythromycin, nitrofurantoin (Furadantin), barbiturates, hydantoin, iodides, INH, methyldopa, hydralazine, and ethambutol. Often a fever will accompany the rash.

Treatment. The rash usually disappears when the drug is stopped and requires no other treatment. However, some reactions develop *after* the drug has been stopped (e.g., with ampicillin). If several drugs are being taken simultaneously, all may have to be stopped and restarted individually to discover the offending drug. Antihistamines are helpful in relieving itching. Skin lubricants may be used if the skin is dry. If the drug must be continued, oral corticosteroids may be prescribed to reduce inflammation.

Skin Infections

Boils *(Furuncles)*

Boils are acute, tender, reddened nodules caused by the common skin bacterium, *Staphylococcus aureus*. They occur in and around hair follicles and rapidly point up to form pustules from 1/4 to 1-1/2 inches in diameter. They often develop blackened centers and drain pus or bloody pus. They occur most often in healthy young individuals. They are most tender just before rupturing and when they involve skin closely attached to bone, such as that on fingers or shins. They may afflict several individuals when people live in close quarters and practice poor hygiene.

Clusters of boils are known as *carbuncles*. They occur most frequently in boys, often on the nape of the neck. When the infection is deep and extensive, fever may develop. Carbuncles are usually slower to heal than boils.

Infection of hair follicles in the hair and beard is known as *folliculitis* and may involve single or multiple hair follicles.

Treatment. Single boils can be treated with periodic application of warm, moist towels until they point up and drain. Surgical incision should generally be avoided because of the danger of spreading the infection. To contain the drainage from boils, cover them with a light gauze dressing that is changed two to three times daily to prevent saturation. Boils in the nose and on the face should be treated with antibiotics by your doctor.

Folliculitis is best treated with oral antibiotics, usually a penicillinase-resistant type, such as cloxacillin. Carbuncles should be cultured by your doctor to determine the most appropriate antibiotic.

If you develop skin infections, give careful attention to personal hygiene. Take care not to use others' towels and washcloths. Use liquid soap to help prevent spreading infection through bar soap. Wash your hands thoroughly after cleansing and changing bandages.

Infections in the axilla and groin are often caused by inflammation of the *apocrine* glands, the glands responsible for the distinctive sexual scent of mature men and women, and which many feel we could do without entirely. These infections are treated by frequent, gentle cleansing and avoidance of antiperspirants. If severe, the infection should be treated with antibiotics.

Hot Tub Rashes

In well-maintained hot tubs, high chlorine or bromine levels and filters keep bacterial levels in check. With high usage and infrequent maintenance, skin rashes caused by the bacterium *Pseudomonas* may develop within eight hours to several days after bathing. Typically, an itchy red rash (a folliculitis) occurs in the armpits and trunk regions. You should consult your doctor for treatment. Steroid creams make this rash worse.

Ringworm

Ringworm on the body *(tinea corporis)* is caused by a fungus, *Trichophyton,* that grows on the dead layers of the skin, but causes an inflammation in the deeper, living skin layers. The lesions start as scaly macules that expand slowly outward in a ring shape while the center heals. Ringworm occurs mainly in children and in adults who become debilitated by chronic illnesses. Itching is often not intense. Ringworm of the scalp *(tinea capitis)* is usually found in children and may be highly contagious. In adults patchy baldness may result.

Treatment. The generic drug tolnaftate (Tinactin) is a synthetic anti-fungal agent that can be purchased over-the-counter and is usually effective in clearing ringworm in 4 weeks. Apply morning and evening and continue for 2 weeks after the lesions clear to prevent recurrence.

If the above treatment is ineffective, your doctor may prescribe one of the imidazole or ciclopirox creams. Again these antifungal drugs should be applied until 7–10 days after the lesions disappear. In cases of multiple lesions, your doctor will prescribe oral griseofulvin. Some doctors recommend that children with ringworm of the scalp receive oral griseofulvin in addition to the antifungal creams. Humans often contract ringworm from pets, so check your animals for the presence of a rash and have them treated if necessary.

Jock Itch

This condition is known medically as *tinea cruris* and may be caused either by a fungus or yeast organism. Ring-shaped lesions may or may not be identified among the lesions that appear in the folds of the groin extending down to the upper inner thighs. Recurrence is common, especially during summer when moisture favors growth of the organisms. Tight clothing and obesity also favor growth.

Treatment. The treatment described for body ringworm also works for jock itch. To reduce moisture, apply talcum powder to the affected area twice daily and before going to bed. Continue treatment for at least two weeks after the lesions disappear. If improvement is not noted within two to three weeks, consult your doctor.

Athlete's Foot

This is another form of ringworm *(tinea pedis)*, caused either by a yeast or fungus. The infection develops on the soles of the feet and in the webs between the toes, particularly between the third and fourth toes, which are anatomically close together and prone to retain moisture, the fungus' favorite environment. The skin cracks and the outer layers of skin peel off, resulting in itching and or burning. If secondary bacterial infection develops, redness, swelling, and oozing result. In severe cases the toenails become involved, appearing thickened, yellow, and crumbly; this greatly complicates treatment.

Treatment. Two common over-the-counter preparations are effective in uncomplicated cases of athlete's foot: tolnaftate (Tinactin, Aftate, generic tolnaftate) and undecylenic acid (e.g., Desenex). Apply twice daily, in the morning and just before bed. These products are available as liquid, creams, powders, and sprays; some believe liquids are preferable because the cream-base products are thought to retain moisture. I have had consistent success using tolnaftate cream.

These products should be applied to the affected areas for at least four weeks. Thereafter, periodic application of the medicated powders to shoes and sneakers will prevent recurrence. Infections that do not clear after four weeks treatment should be seen by your dermatologist to exclude such conditions as psoriasis, eczema, and allergic contact dermatitis that may mimic athlete's foot.

Bacterial infections heralded by redness, swelling, pus, and swollen lymph nodes requires saline soaks and antibiotics, and should be supervised by your doctor. Toenail infections are notoriously resistant to treatment, often requiring surgical removal of the toenail and prolonged medication.

Prevention is the best approach to athlete's foot. Dry well between your toes after showering. Don't put your socks on immediately; air drying is more effective than mere toweling. Shoes that "breathe," made of leather and canvas, will keep the feet drier than those of rubber and plastics. Use absorbent socks—cotton and, especially, the newer, thick acrylic socks that "wick" moisture from the feet are preferred to wool or cotton, which retains moisture. Regular use of medicated powders (tolnaftate) is advised.

Fat Fold Rashes *(Intertrigo)*

Rashes that occur between fatty folds of skin and beneath the breasts (intertriginous infections) are most often caused by the yeast, *Candida albicans*. Treatment with topical nystatin, the imidazoles, or ciclopirox (all prescription drugs) is usually effective. Apply three or four times daily. Pat the area thoroughly dry after bathing. After applying medication, sprinkle with talc to keep the inner skinfolds dry.

Sun Spots

Common in young adults, sun spots first appear as tan, brown, or white, slightly scaling lesions on the chest, neck, and stomach. They are called "sun spots" because they do not tan, but appear as white spots against the background of tanned skin. Medically they are known as *tinea versicolor*. They are caused by a yeast, *Pityrosporom orbiculare*. Itching is not common unless the skin becomes hot and moist. The lesions are distinguished from freckles by the raised, scaling appearance.

Treatment. Apply selenium sulfide shampoo (Selsun) undiluted over the area of the lesions as well as the scalp for 7 days at bedtime and wash off in the morning. If this is irritating, try applying for 20–60 min and then wash off. Continue for two weeks.

Scabies

Scabies is caused by the female "itch mite," *Sarcoptes scabiei*, which burrows into the skin and lays her eggs. The eggs induce an intensely itching allergic response. The burrows produce fine wavy dark lines up to 1/2-inch long, found mainly on the wrists, finger webs, elbows, armpits, breasts, and male genitals. The burrows are often difficult to find, particularly if scratching or secondary infection has obscured them. Then the diagnosis must be made by your dermatologist who will identify the mites under a microscope.

Scabies are most commonly found in crowded households, especially when children sleep together. Often several members of the family will contract the mites.

Treatment. Cure is rather simple, but your doctor will have to prescribe the 5% permethrin cream (Elimite), which is applied over the entire body from the head down, including the soles of the feet at bedtime. Leave the lotion on overnight and shower completely the next morning. Itching may persist for 1–3 weeks while the body's reaction to the mites subsides, but this does not mean that retreatment is necessary unless new mites (most likely through reinfestation) can be demonstrated. All clothing, towels, and bedding should be washed in a washing machine, or dry-cleaned. Fumigation is not necessary.

Lice

Though lice are usually associated with poverty and undesirable living conditions, they can infect members of all classes, particularly head lice in children. Lice come in three varieties: head (*Pediculosis capitis*), body (*Pediculosis corporis*), and pubic (*Pediculosis pubis*, or "crab") louse.

Head lice are most common among school children and older people living in crowded quarters. They are transmitted by personal contact and by such objects as combs and hats. The eggs are called "nits" and are found as small grey ovoids attached to the shafts of hairs. Less frequently, the lice can be found on the back of the head and behind the ears. Itching is intense and secondary scratch dermatitis is common.

Body lice are usually found among people living in crowded, unhygienic conditions. The nits are found on body hairs, but the adult lice live in the seams of clothing. The small red bites are most often found on the shoulders, buttocks, and stomach.

Pubic lice are relatively large, being the size of small ticks and dark brown to black in color. The nits are easily found at the base of pubic hair shafts. Transmission is usually venereal.

Treatment. The preferred treatment for all types of lice is 1% permethrin cream rinse (Nix, Rid, Triple X), which can be purchased over-the-counter. This is used as a rinse after shampooing or bathing, left on for 10 minutes, and then rinsed off. Removal of the nits is not necessary. Remember that recurrence is likely unless the lice and nits in the clothing and bedding are destroyed by laundering. All members of a household should be treated at the same time. Sexual partners should definitely be treated, otherwise reinfestation is very likely.

Milia

Milia are small pinhead-sized white or yellow cysts that appear on the face, especially the eyelids and forehead. They are thought to be caused by blockage of the skin pores. These small cysts are entirely benign and can usually be removed with a comedo extractor; see your dermatologist about its proper use.

Warts

Warts are small, slightly contagious growths caused by more than 35 types of human papilloma virus (HPV). The virus causes the infected epidermal cells to multiply rapidly, forming a lump of heaped-up skin. Some warts, particularly those on the anal and genital region, and on the larynx, are associated with the development of malignant tumors.

Warts occur in all shapes. Common warts *(verruca vulgaris)* are usually small, from 1/16- to 1/2-inch in diameter, with raised, irregular, cauliflower-like surfaces. They are firm and vary in color from flesh-colored to tan, yellow, gray, or brown. These warts occur around areas subject to trauma: face, hands, elbows, knees, and the fingernails of people who bite their nails. They are most common in children and rarely are found in the elderly.

When warts occur on pressure-bearing surfaces, such as the palms and soles of the feet (plantar warts), they grow inward. Frequently they are found in clusters known as *mosaic warts.*

Flat warts *(verruca plana)* can occur anywhere, but are frequently found on the backs of the hands and on the face. These tend to grow in great profusion, so that 25–100 may be present. If they grow in the beard region, shaving may become difficult because it produces myriad lesions through nicks and self-inoculation.

Are warts contagious? They almost certainly are, but the long delay between contact and their appearance makes the person responsible almost impossible to determine. Susceptibility to warts varies greatly among individuals. Those given to allergies seem to be prone to "catch" warts. Since doctors use no special care in handling warts, it is usually thought that contagion is low and that people with warts surely need not be given wide berth. This is not true of genital warts though, which are highly contagious venereal infections and are discussed more completely on p. 395.

Treatment. Most warts will disappear spontaneously in 6–24 months. It is probably this characteristic that has given rise to so many mythical folk cures. Recall that Huckleberry Finn espoused the handling of dead cats (possibly their 102nd use!) and Tom Sawyer swore by spunk water. This worked only when the stump was approached in a certain way and just the right incantations were offered.

Nevertheless, home remedies generally do not work. If you want to treat common warts yourself, you can purchase a product called Wart-Off, which contains salicylic and lactic acids in a collodion solution. This is applied daily (never on the face) for several weeks until the wart disappears. Follow the directions carefully and avoid contact with surrounding normal skin. If you have any doubt about whether you are dealing with a wart, consult your dermatologist.

Never cut warts off with a knife or razor blade. This just asks for bleeding, infection, and spread of the warts. Also avoid biting your nails, since this only increases the chance of the warts spreading.

There are several treatments your doctor can offer, including, freezing, caustic agents, laser therapy, and surgery. Plantar warts, which are often very painful and interfere with walking, are usually treated with caustic agents, followed by freezing and other destructive remedies. Small flat warts are often successfully treated with tretinoin (Retin A), otherwise used for acne. You will have to see your doctor for a prescription.

Herpes Simplex

The herpes simplex virus (HSV) causes blister-like sores primarily around the mouth, nose, and genitals, although lesions can appear anywhere. There are two HSV strains, HSV-1 and HSV-2. HSV-2 is responsible for genital herpes and is discussed on p. 394. The Herpes family is relatively large. Other herpes strains cause infectious mononucleosis (Epstein-Barr Virus), chicken pox (varicella), and shingles (herpes zoster).

The sores of HSV-1 are also called "cold sores" and "fever blisters," because secondary infections often erupt during or after a cold or high fever. Typically the sores are tiny, clear, fluid-filled blisters on the face. They develop from 2 to 20 days after exposure to an infected person and last from 7 to 10 days. The number of blisters varies from one to a cluster of several small blisters. These blisters break and scab over before disappearing without scarring.

Although the primary infection clears, the virus migrates to nearby nerve cells where it lies dormant, often forever. In many, however, the virus will reactivate and blisters reappear, often in response to stress, exposure to the sun, certain foods, menstruation, or fever. Frequently the trigger mechanism is unknown.

Treatment. Herpes simplex is extremely widespread in the United States; if a vaccine were available, it would be widely recommended.

Unfortunately there is none. Gentle cleansing with soap and water is useful, as are compresses moistened with Domeboro solution. Apply bacitracin ointment if infection develops. Towels, clothes, and other personal items should be strictly separated from those of other household members to prevent the spread of infection. In severe cases your doctor may prescribe acyclovir.

For a discussion of the treatment of genital herpes, please *see* p. 394.

Chicken Pox (Varicella)

Chicken pox is caused by another of the herpes virus group, *varicella zoster*. It is most common in young children, although adults who have not had chicken pox during childhood are susceptible as well. The rash begins 10–14 days following exposure. Often there will be other children in the family or community with chicken pox. In some cases children contract chicken pox from an adult suffering from herpes zoster, which is caused by the same virus. Usually there is a mild fever and achiness 1–3 days before onset of the blisters, which begin on the face and trunk primarily. They are usually quite itchy and crust over in 2–5 days, during which time more are forming on the arms and legs. If the blisters become infected, they may leave depressed scars upon healing. The lesions are usually less itchy in adults, although fever and constitutional symptoms are usually more severe than in children.

A single bout of chicken pox confers lifelong immunity. Like the *herpes simplex* virus, the varicella virus retires after the initial infection to reside in the nerve ganglia. If they later reemerge, it is as *herpes zoster* (shingles).

Treatment. The fever may be treated with acetaminophen (do *not* give aspirin to children). Treat itching with an antihistamine (Actifed, Benadryl, Dimetane, and the like) . If the itching is severe, give soothing baths of lukewarm water and oatmeal powder (e.g., Aveeno Bath). Adults are treated with oral acyclovir. Vaccines are currently being developed to immunize against chicken pox. Ask your doctor.

Herpes Zoster (Shingles)

The characteristic lesions of shingles are small vesicles, each with a central indentation and all aligned along a peripheral nerve. They most commonly occur on the back and trunk. Before the eruption, the skin may be sensitive to touch, itch, tingle, or be associated with sharp pain. Until the vesicles erupt, the pain may be mistaken for a heart attack, peritonitis, or acute arthritis.

The herpes zoster virus eruption follows an initial chicken pox infection, often decades later. A severe illness, cancer, or immunosuppression may be the precipitating event that heralds the viral emergence. A severe and prolonged localized pain (post-herpetic neuralgia) may follow an acute bout of shingles.

Treatment. Since there is no specific treatment for the virus, treatment is directed at the symptoms. Analgesics are administered for pain. Domeboro compresses applied to the eruption are soothing. If the lesions are broken and oozing, apply bacitracin ointment to cover them. Oral acyclovir may be prescribed by your doctor. Corticosteroids may also be prescribed to lessen the pain of postherpetic neuralgia.

Rocky Mountain Spotted Fever

Rocky Mountain spotted fever is a disease caused by rickettsia, a tiny microscopic organism intermediate in size between bacteria and viruses. Transmitted by tick bites, it is more common in the Carolinas, Massachusetts, and on Long Island than in the western mountain region from which it derives its name. The symptoms include abrupt onset of severe headaches, muscular aches, weakness, chills, and high fever approximately two days after the tick bite. On about the fourth day, a rash consisting of flat red spots or splotches appears on the ankles, wrists, palms, and soles, and gradually moves on to the rest of the body.

Treatment. Prompt treatment with tetracycline will prevent serious damage to the kidneys, liver, lungs, and blood that occurs in the absence of treatment. Prevention consists of carefully checking for, and removal of, ticks after exposure to the woods and fields they inhabit. If you discover a tick firmly attached to your skin, remove it as described on p. 64 and see your doctor at once to determine whether prophylactic antibiotics are recommended.

Acne

Acne vulgaris, that bane of so many teenagers, is a disease of the sebaceous glands, the small glands surrounding hair follicles that produce skin oil (sebum). Acne begins at puberty, when increased secretion of androgens stimulates the activity of the sebaceous glands. At the same time changes in the cells lining the hair follicle may plug

TREATING ACNE

Several general principles for treating acne apply to both superficial and deep acne:

- *Wash the affected area daily* with ordinary soap and water. Expensive antibacterial and medicated soaps have no proven value. Do not scrub vigorously; a simple washcloth will do. Do not use abrasive soaps or granular facial preparations. The object of washing is to remove excess oil and to soften and remove the sebaceous plugs that lead to pimples and cysts.
- *Use drying lotions,* especially those that contain benzoyl peroxide, kill bacteria, and stimulate peeling along the hair follicles, thus opening up sebaceous glands. Preparations that contain salicylic acid and alcohol (Stri-Dex, Clearasil Astringent, Noxzema Clear-Ups, etc.) are also useful drying agents. Ofter they can prevent swollen sebaceous glands from rupturing to form pimples.
- *Get some sun.* Sunlight causes mild drying and may be beneficial. However, you should avoid excessive exposure and sunlamps, which promote long-term skin damage.
- *Avoid moisturizing creams and lotions;* they often contain substances that promote the formation of blackheads. Women who develop acne after their teens often do so because of these preparations. Avoid oily hair tonics and wear your hair off the face.
- *Avoid makeup.* If you must use it, select water-based makeup.
- *Do not scratch, pop, squeeze, or pick at your face.* Removing the natural crust that forms over pimples often leads to secondary infection and scarring. Though most dermatologists doubt their value, you may ask your doctor about using a blackhead extractor available at most drugstores. Extractors should be used only after 5–10 minutes of hot water compresses to loosen sebaceous plugs. Be sure to keep the instrument meticulously clean.

the outlet of the sebaceous glands. This results in "whiteheads" if the plug is below the surface and "blackheads" if the plug is at the surface. Whiteheads and blackheads are known as *comedos,* composed of sebum, keratin (from the follicle cells), and bacteria, particularly *Propionibacterium acnes.* Enzymes (lipases) from *P. acnes* break down triglycerides in the sebum to form free fatty acids. These fatty acids irritate the sebaceous gland lining, causing the gland to swell. Eventually the gland ruptures, resulting in an inflamed lesion that everyone knows as a "pimple."

Acne has a variable course; it tends to improve during summer, possibly because sunlight is beneficial. Despite the fact that many acne sufferers believe that foods like chocolate, nuts, and cola worsen acne; there is no scientific evidence for this. Neither masturbation nor constipation causes acne, as some would have it. Though acne vulgaris is mainly a disorder of teenagers, it affects from 6–8% of adults as well. The eruptions usually cease spontaneously, but no one can predict when this will occur.

Acne is generally classified as either "superficial" or "deep." Superficial acne consists of blackheads, whiteheads, and pimples, mostly confined to the face. Occasionally pus-filled cysts develop, especially after traumatic attempts to squeeze pimples.

Deep acne is more severe and widespread, often affecting the neck, upper back, and shoulders. Pus-filled cysts are common and scarring frequently follows healing.

The gentler the measures you use in skin care the better. Acne will disappear in time. Make sure you are left with as few reminders as possible.

Deep Acne

For deep or *cystic acne*, more rigorous measures must be adopted to prevent scarring. Topical preparations are generally not effective. Among the therapies dermatologists may use are:

- Drying masks containing sulfur (e.g., Vlemasque) are often useful in treating the pustules, abscesses, and cysts of more severe inflammatory acne.
- Oral and topical antibiotics, including tetracycline, minocycline, or erythromycin. Tetracycline can diminish the effectiveness of certain types of birth control pills, and must not be given during pregnancy because of possible effects on the fetus.
- Oral isotretinoin (Accutane) is effective in patients who do not respond satisfactorily to antibiotics. This drug should only be used by doctors experienced in its use because of the many serious side effects. These include:

  1. Dryness of the skin and mucous membranes in 90% of patients. Symptoms include anogenital dryness and irritation, itching, peeling, sun sensitivity, and problems wearing contact lenses.

2. Joint pain in about 15% of patients.
3. High blood cholesterol and triglyceride levels.
4. Extremely high likelihood of birth defects when used in undiagnosed pregnancy. Use of Accutane during pregnancy is a probable cause for abortion. A pregnancy test should be obtained in women of child-bearing age before use is begun.

- For isolated deep lesions, incision and drainage often prevent scarring. If scarring occurs, surgical dermabrasion is sometimes a useful restorative.
- Estrogens are prescribed for some women who do not respond to other treatment. However, there are potentially serious side effects with estrogen therapy and most dermatologists are reluctant to treat the whole body for the sins of the face.

Acne Rosecea

Sometimes referred to as "adult acne," or simply as "rosacea," this disease usually commences after the age of 30. The cause of acne rosacea is unknown, although some theorize that its occurrence is caused by the microscopic skin mites, *Dermodex folliculorum*.

Acne rosacea has many of the characteristics of acne vulgaris, including pimples and pustules, but because this is not a disease of the sebaceous glands, blackheads and whiteheads are not found. Also unlike acne, this disease worsens with time and may be affected by such foods as alcohol, spicy foods, and caffeine. If untreated, tissue overgrowth may result, particularly around the nose, giving rise to a W. C. Fields-type nose called *rhinophyma*.

Treatment. The usual treatment for acne rosacea is oral and topical antibiotics, including tetracycline and metronidazole. Short-term treatment with topical cortisone may be useful. Plastic surgery can improve the appearance of rhinophyma should it develop. No cures are currently available, but supervised care can usually keep the disease under control.

Sebaceous Cysts

As described above, the sebaceous glands are the tiny glands associated with hair follicles that produce natural skin oils. When the gland's outflow becomes obstructed, it will fill with a thick, "cheesy" substance that slowly accumulates and produces a painless subcutaneous nodule. They occur singly, most often on the scalp and around the upper back. If they become infected, they will form boils.

Treatment. Since these cysts are harmless, most people simply tolerate them. If they become infected, they should be treated as boils (*see* p. 448). If you wish to have a sebaceous cyst removed, your doctor can do so in a simple outpatient operation with a local anesthetic.

Discoid Lupus Erythematosis (DLE)

This is a chronic skin disorder of unknown cause associated with an itchy, scaling rash typically on the bridge of the nose and cheeks, known as a "butterfly" rash. Circular patches of rash may occur on other parts of the body.

DLE may occur in association with systemic lupus erythematosus (SLE), which is an autoimmune disorder associated with inflammation of connective tissue in many parts of the body, affecting the joints, muscles, skin, blood vessels, heart, and lungs. At times, the disease may mimic rheumatoid arthritis.

Treatment. In severe DLE, your doctor may prescribe topical or oral steroids, or possibly chloroquine. Since sunlight tends to worsen DLE, protection with a sunscreen of SPF 15 or higher is recommended. SLE, a much more serious disease, is treated symptomatically and with systemic steroids.

More information can be obtained from: National Lupus Erythematosus Foundation, 5430 Van Nuys Boulevard, Suite 206, Van Nuys, California 91401.

Psoriasis

Psoriasis is a chronic skin disease characterized by well-circumscribed, pink plaques covered by silvery or opalescent scales. The disease may vary from one or two asymptomatic plaques to extensive skin involvement associated with a crippling arthritis. The cause is not known; some body substance (estrogens?) may stimulate localized overproliferation of skin, which causes the piled up, scaling plaques.

Psoriasis is common, affecting 2–4% of Caucasians; far fewer Asians and blacks are affected. The usual onset of disease is between 10 and 40 years of age. The lesions commonly occur behind the ears, on the knees, elbows, the back, and the buttocks. In more extensive disease, the skin of the stomach, anogenital area, armpits, and nails may be involved. Stress and anxiety may worsen old lesions and stimulate new ones. Certain drugs, such as malaria pills, lithium, propranolol, and systemic corticosteroids, often worsen the disease. Sun exposure is beneficial, but sunburn may have the opposite effect. The disease sometimes clears during pregnancy, only to recur after childbirth. In severe cases, psoriatic arthritis may also occur.

Treatment. When psoriasis is suspected, you should consult a dermatologist to distinguish it from other skin diseases that have a different prognosis and treatment: lichen planus, pityriasis rosea, fungal infections, skin cancer (in older individuals), and localized scratch dermatitis.

In mild cases involving limited sites, simple lubricants (e.g., white petrolatum), and over-the-counter keratolytic ointments (e.g., Balnetar, Carmol, Fostex, Noxzema, Pernox, etc.) may be all that is required. Your doctor may prescribe a corticosteroid in either ointment or in the form of impregnated tape, or anthralin in either cream or ointment. Anthralin may be irritating and should not be used on the face, genital areas, or between folds of skin.

In cases that are resistant to conservative treatment, the use of ultraviolet B light, and occasionally psoralens and ultraviolet-A (PUVA), therapy may be indicated. In the most severe cases, methotrexate, an anticancer drug may be effective. All of these agents are used to control psoriasis; none is curative.

Keloids

A keloid is a scar that grows excessively large or deforms the skin. It is more common among blacks and occurs for no known reason. Keloids usually develop from surgical scans, but they can occur after minor injuries, such as earlobe piercing and scratches.

Treatment. Keloids are harmless and only require treatment if they become cosmetically objectionable. They are treated with steroid injections or with X-rays, after which they may shrink, if not disappear. Some keloids disappear spontaneously. They cannot be simply cut out, because of the likelihood of the new scar also developing a keloid. In some cases they can be surgically removed while treating with steroids or X-rays during the healing process to prevent reformation.

Corns and Calluses

Calluses are areas of thickened skin caused by repeated pressure or friction. They usually develop on the hands and feet, but they may occur anywhere. An often-cited example of unusual calluses are those that form under the jaws and over the collar bones of violinists.

Corns are painful areas of built-up, cornified skin occurring on the toes, usually caused by ill-fitting shoes. "Hard" corns occur on the outer toe surfaces; "soft" corns develop between the toes.

Treatment. The simplest means of removing corns is by rubbing them with a pumice stone during the bath. They can also be filed down with a nail file. The use of a sharp knife is to be discouraged because of the danger of cutting too deeply and introducing infection. They can also be removed by keratolytic drugs such as a 20% salicylic acid in collodion (e.g., Wart-Off, Compound W Gel) or with 40% salicylic acid plasters.

Corns can usually be prevented by avoiding heels that are too high and shoes that fit too tightly. Spike heels and cowboy boots are frequent culprits. The advice of a podiatrist should be sought if you are on stage or screen and must wear ultra "stylish" shoes.

Alterations in Skin Pigmentation

Hypopigmentation

Post-inflammatory hypopigmentation occurs as small areas of skin lacking pigmentation following trauma or inflammation. It may develop after acne clears, following burns, in scars, after infection, or from excessive sun exposure. The light spots that follow acne and infections usually disappear after several months or years. The cause is a local absence of melanocytes, the skin cells responsible for producing pigment.

In *vitiligo*, pale irregular patches of skin appear for no apparent reason. They may occur symmetrically on both sides of the body. They may shrink or enlarge with time and are entirely harmless, except for possible cosmetic reasons.

Treatment. For all of these conditions the best treatment is a coverup cosmetic tanning preparation that does not come off on clothes (e.g., Dy-O-Derm). These areas sunburn easily and should be covered with a sun screen with SPF of 15.

Universal absence of pigmentation is a rare genetic disorder known as *albinism*. Albinos are very prone to skin cancer and thus must take meticulous care to avoid sunlight, wear sunglasses, and use a high SPF sunscreen during daylight hours.

Hyperpigmentation

Regionally increased pigmentation occurs in a variety of forms—from freckles and "age spots" to the universally increased pigmentation seen in some cases of Addison's disease (failure of the adrenal glands). Local darkened areas may follow infection, trauma, and excessive sun exposure.

A special type of local hyperpigmentation known as *melasma* is a dark, sharply defined, symmetric pigmentation of the face and cheeks that occurs mainly during pregnancy (the "mask of pregnancy") and in some women taking birth control pills. This condition usually abates after pregnancy or stopping the hormone pills.

Treatment. The standard treatment is a "fading" cream with 2% hydroquinone in an alcoholic glycol base (e.g., Esoterica, Eldopaque). Applied twice daily, these areas often fade away. Be careful about applying hydroquinone to your face since it may cause a skin reaction or may lighten the skin too much. Apply a "test patch" behind your ear to see whether it causes irritation. Your doctor may prescribe use of 0.1% tretinoin (Retin-A) on alternate days to increase the effectiveness of hydroquinone. Use a high-SPF sunscreen on hyperpigmented areas, because their response to sunlight is exaggerated.

Problems of Sweating

We come here to a delicate area for many people, especially those who are hypersensitive to the social aspects of sweat, and whose polite conversation even eschews the Anglo-Saxon word "sweat," preferring to camouflage this most common of bodily functions in more genteel Latin word, perspiration.

The purpose of sweating, of course, is to reduce body temperature. When the "core body temperature" (the temperature of the deep organs and of blood) rises above 98.6 degrees Fahrenheit, the hypothalamus, which lies deep in the brain, signals the blood vessels in the skin to dilate and the heart to beat faster. This sends more blood to the outer parts of the body, where heat can be lost to the atmosphere—provided that the air temperature is lower than body temperature. At the same time the sweat glands secrete water. Usually this water evaporates before visible moisture accumulates, and so is called "insensible" perspiration because the skin remains dry.

As the need to lose heat increases, because of either increased metabolic rate or high ambient temperature, the hypothalamus stimulates the sweat glands to secrete larger amounts of water in what is called "sensible" perspiration, or sweating. Thus, as moisture evaporates, heat is carried away from the skin by the "heat of evaporation."

Under cool conditions water loss through sweating varies from negligible up to about two quarts per day. Heat, fevers, and physical exertion can increase this output to 5–10 quarts per day. Factors such

---

NIGHT SWEATS

There are many causes of night sweats and consequently they are quite common. Among the causes:

- *Exercising before bedtime* may result in continued sweating for as long as two hours.
- *Aspirin and acetaminophen* both act to lower body temperature. One of the principal mechanisms the body uses to accomplish this is sweating.
- *Alcohol* impairs the body's ability to regulate heat. Night sweats are common after a night of overindulgence. This also may be a sign in heavy drinkers of alcoholic liver disease.
- *Pregnancy* causes about 60% of women to experience night sweats.
- *Common diseases* associated with night sweats include tuberculosis, lymphoma, cancer, and AIDS.

Occasional night sweats are probably no cause for alarm. However, if they are accompanied by a fever, if you have drenching sweats after a chill, or if you have sweats occurring at a time of unexpected weight loss, you should see your doctor.

---

as sex, race, age, and temperature conditioning also determine the amount one sweats. For a discussion of heat exhaustion and heat stroke, *see* p. 84.

Excessive Sweating

Very heavy sweating *(hyperhidrosis)* occurs in a small number of people. Usually the sweating is confined to the armpits, or to the palms or soles, and is stimulated by emotions, stress, anxiety, or exercise. Generalized hyperhidrosis may be caused by an underlying infection, hyperthyroidism, or an endocrine disease.

When localized, the use of topical antiperspirants is usually sufficient to control excessive sweating. A potent antiperspirant is a 20% solution of aluminum chloride in absolute ethyl alcohol (DrySol). This is usually applied at bedtime and covered with saran wrap. In the morning the saran wrap is removed and the area washed free of salts. A treatment once weekly is often adequate.

The sweat glands can be removed surgically, but this should only be performed as a last resort by an experienced surgeon. In resistant cases, the nerves supplying the affected region may be severed surgically *(sympathectomy)*.

Body Odors

Unpleasant body odor (BO) is usually considered more a matter of personal hygiene than a medical problem. After all, no one ever got sick from smelling bad—although a person downwind might. Most body odor comes not from the type of sweat glands found on the face, limbs, and trunk, but from a special set of *apocrine* glands found in the armpits, nipples, naval, and genital regions. These are essentially atavistic organs that serve little purpose in modern society. For primitive man they no doubt served to identify familiar clan members, warn against strangers, and possibly served as the human equivalent of pheromones in sexual attraction. No doubt Tarzan would immediately recognize Jane's and Cheetah's scents.

Bacteria break down the apocrine secretions and cause the human aroma, which may vary with the particular population of bacteria. Although many people are not repelled by the normal apocrine scent (indeed many are turned on by it), most find the bacterial component a little too gamey, if not outright repellant.

"Good" hygiene, by which we mean frequent cleansing and changes of clothing, usually is sufficient to keep body odor in check. For those who feel secure only with "added protection," deodorants and antiperspirants abound.

Deodorants usually contain an antibacterial component (benzalkonium, methylbenzenthonium, etc.) along with fragrances that mask all but the most flagrant odors. Deodorants, however, do not reduce perspiration.

Antiperspirants contain an ingredient that enters sweat glands and reduces perspiration (aluminum chlorohydrate, aluminum–zirconium chlorohydrate), along with a fragrance and/or antibacterial agent.

The most frequent problems with both antiperspirants and deodorants are allergic reactions and skin irritation. Usually this problem can be overcome by trying other products after the initial reaction disappears. For the truly intolerant, daily or twice-daily showers suffice. Indeed, most of the world's population gets along quite well with neither deodorant nor antiperspirants.

Other Body Odors

Some systemic diseases are associated with distinctive odors that may even serve as signals of the underlying malady. One of the most common of these is a "mousy" smell *(fetor hepaticus)* associated with liver failure, so named because it smells like caged laboratory mice.

Certain lung infections, such as tuberculosis and lung abscess, cause a putrid breath, as does severe gingivitis. Patients with diabetes out of control (ketoacidosis) give off a kind of cloying sweetish or fruity odor. Severe kidney failure (uremia) is associated with an ammonia-like odor. Certain rare metabolic disorders of children are associated with smells resembling fish, cat's urine, and maple syrup. Any persistent body odor that is not eliminated by bathing and freshly washed clothes should prompt a visit to the doctor.

Prickly Heat

Also known as *miliaria*, this is an acute eruption caused by obstruction of the ducts in which sweat is retained, forming minute vesicles that itch severely. Prickly heat is most common among fair-skinned individuals in warm, humid climates. Unfortunately there is little to be done, except to cool and dry the skin and to avoid conditions that promote sweating. Getting to an air-conditioned room is ideal. Needless to say, sufferers of prickly heat do well to avoid the tropics.

Cellulite

Cellulite (pronounced *cell-u-leet'*) is mentioned here, not because it is a medical entity at all, but rather to help debunk a popular myth that it represents an abnormal collection of fat that demands special treatment, surgery, lotions, potions, and pills. Cellulite is a concept invented by European spas to convince women that they needed help that only spas could give. The term refers to the irregular, lumpy, orange peel-appearing subcutaneous fat distribution found on women's hips, thighs, and buttocks.

Actually there is nothing more to cellulite than normal excess fat. When there is excess fat, it has to be stored somewhere and in women it is characteristically in the breast, hips, and thighs. In men the spot of choice is in the abdomen. The reason that this excess fat has a lumpy appearance in women and seldom has in men lies in the underlying nature of the subcutaneous fibrous structures. The connective tissue beneath women's skin creates large, rounded, fat-cell chambers. In men, on the other hand, the chambers tend toward a polygonal shape that prevents the more noticeable bulges characteristic of "cellulite." Too, the epidermis of women is thinner then men's, thus offering less resistance to surface bulges and indentations.

There is a simple way (notice I don't say *easy*) of eliminating cellulite: diet and exercise. Where there is no excess fat, there is no cellulite. Losing weight is seldom easy for any of us, but don't be taken in by sensational (and false) advertisements trumpeting revolutionary (and expensive!) methods to get rid of the bulges. These often include strange techniques, such as electric shocks that stimulate regional muscle contractions, and that are advertised to make exercise effortless and take away local body fat. Such methods rarely work, robbing clients of the beneficial effects they would gain if they engaged in aerobic exercising.

The Effect of Sunlight on the Skin

The skin normally reacts to sunlight by stimulating the pigment-producing cells (melanocytes) to form melanin, which gives you a suntan and provides protection against further exposure. Uneven distribution of melanin results in freckles, particularly in light complected people. Acute overexposure to sunlight results in sunburn, whereas in the long run, excess exposure to sunlight causes chronic changes that include loss of elasticity (wrinkles), hyperpigmented spots, actinic keratoses (*see* p. 470), and skin cancer in some.

Sunburn

Ordinary sunlight varies in wavelength from about 280–2900 nanometers (nm). The sunburn-producing rays, called ultraviolet-B (UVB) are the shortest, varying between 280 and 320 nm. These short rays are filtered out completely by ordinary window glass and largely by smoke and smog. However, they pass through fog and light clouds and up to about three feet of clear water. Water, snow, and sand accentuate exposure to UVB through reflection.

A sunburn appears 3–24 hours after exposure and can vary from mild redness to second-degree burning with blisters, swelling, fever, chills, weakness, and shock.

Treatment. Mild sunburn usually requires no treatment. There is no evidence that preparations containing aloe are more soothing or promote faster healing than simple moisturizing creams. If the burn hurts, cold water compresses are soothing. Topical anesthetics such as benzocaine also relieve the pain temporarily, though many doctors believe that all of the "-caine" anesthetics should be avoided because in some people these drugs cause allergic reactions. Preparations that contain lidocaine especially should be avoided because they are absorbed through the skin and can cause a toxic reaction. Topical corticosteroid ointments are of little value in relieving sunburn.

If you develop a second-degree sunburn (i.e., there is blistering, swelling, tenderness, and pain), see your doctor. In such cases corticosteroids may be given to decrease the inflammation. Don't put anything on a second-degree burn. Don't break the blisters or peel damaged skin. Try to keep the burned skin meticulously clean.

Sunburn Prevention

The vast majority of all sunburns result simply from imprudence. When you're having fun in the sun, its hard to stop and cover up. But that of course is what you must do. Hats, long-sleeved shirts, and long pants or skirts are sensible. Don't rely on a T-shirt in the water; the rays go right through wet cotton. More tightly woven, dyed fabrics have a higher "sun protection factor" (SPF) than loosely woven white cloth. Denim, for example has a SPF of about 1000! This means that the denim-protected skin would receive in 1000 hours the same amount of sun radiation that the unprotected skin would receive in one hour. Denim is rather warm and not very comfortable in hot weather, but you get the idea.

The use of sunscreens is essential. There are two general types of sunscreens:

- "Physical blockers," which are opaque pastes, usually containing zinc oxide or titanium dioxide, that completely block the sun's rays. They are applied to the nose, lips, tops of feet, and other particularly sensitive areas. The older white products were rather unfetching, but new products (e.g., Le Zinc from Manhattan Ice Inc.) have a myriad of brilliant Day-Glo colors that make a statement as well as being protective.
- "Chemical blockers," which absorb the sun's rays and reflect them at a wavelength that does not cause sunburn. Of the many active sunscreen ingredients, the most common is para-aminobenzoic acid, or PABA, and its derivatives. These compounds provide great protection against the ultraviolet-B rays that are responsible for sunburns and skin cancer. On the other hand, they let through most of the ultraviolet-A (longer) rays responsible for aging the skin.

If you are allergic or sensitive to PABA, other sunscreen ingredients can be substituted. Look for benzophenones (oxybenzone and sulisobenzone), cinnamates (octylmethyl cinnamate and cinoxate), and salicylates (homomenthyl salicylate). Remember that substances like petrolatum and Chapstick have no sun protection at all, unless special formulations include a sunscreen agent.

Chemical blockers must remain on the skin in order to be effective. Therefore they should be applied in generous quantities and reapplied frequently. Some preparations, e.g., Sundown, have a longer retention time than others and are therefore more effective. Apply your sunscreen before going into the sun to allow it time to penetrate the outer layer of skin. Choose a product with an SPF of 15 or higher. If you go into the water or sweat a lot, reapply after toweling off. There are newer products (e.g., Bullfrog Amphibious Sunblock by Chattem Inc.) that is reported to provide an SPF of 18 even after six hours of swimming. There is no indication that PABA taken orally has any protective effect.

If you insist on a tan, begin tanning gradually. Many light-skinned individuals require 10–14 days to tan fully. Forget about so-called "tan accelerators," advertised to make you "tan faster" or give you a "longer-lasting tan." Their only affect is on your pocketbook. Wear a sunscreen even in the shade because reflected ultraviolet rays can still burn. Remember, the sun's rays are brightest from 10 AM to 3 PM. The closer you get to the equator, the more intense the sun's rays are. It has been estimated that the long-term risks of skin cancer double with every 300 miles nearer the equator you go. Altitude also determines ultraviolet ray intensity, which is greater at higher elevations. So when vacationing in Quito, Ecuador, take along plenty of sunscreen.

The older you are, the more sensitive you become to sunlight. This happens because the number of melanocytes decreases with age. Cell loss is estimated at about 15% per decade.

Chronic Effects of Sunlight

Years of overexposure to the sun have many effects upon the skin; none are good and some, like skin cancer, can be fatal. The four principal effects on the skin caused by prolonged sun exposure are discolorations arising from alterations of pigmentation, actinic keratoses, premature aging, and skin cancer.

Discolorations (Solar Lentigos)

Solar lentigos, erroneously called "liver spots" or "age spots," are the small yellow, red, tan, or brown patches located in areas of greatest sun exposure: the face, backs of the hands, upper arms, shoulders, and upper back. They are formed from local overproduction of melanocytes, the pigment-producing cells. They range in size from one-eighth inch to about one inch, and can be round, oval, or irregularly shaped. They always have sharply defined borders and like freckles, which they resemble, they are not raised. Unlike freckles they usually do not become darker with exposure to sunlight. Nor do they respond predictably to the so-called "fade creams." These discolorations probably got the name "liver spots" because they were once thought to be associated with liver disease; they are not, however, nor are they precancerous. The spots are common over the age of 40, more common among fair-skinned individuals, and most prominent among sun worshipers; they develop very gradually. If you notice rapid changes, or if any become raised, see your doctor. Recently it has been shown that the acne drug tretinoin (Retin-A) can be effective in eliminating liver spots if applied over several months. Although the drug is not approved for this purpose, ask your doctor about it. Otherwise the only thing to be done about these spots is to cover them with long sleeves and high collars—a recourse which, if adopted early in life, would have prevented them in the first place.

Actinic Keratoses

The word "actinic" means "of the sun." These lesions are usually red to tan in color, firm to the touch, somewhat scaly, and slightly raised, with sharply defined borders. They increase in size and number with age, and develop on areas of the body most exposed to sun. You should consult your dermatologist who will distinguish them from seborrheic keratoses (*see* p. 445).

Treatment. These lesions can develop into skin cancer. When they are few in number, the preferred treatment is "cryotherapy" using liquid nitrogen to freeze them. If the lesions are too numerous for cryotherapy, they can be treated with topical 5-fluorouracil, a cancer chemotherapy drug, but this takes longer and causes inflammation and some discomfort.

Premature Aging

Although wrinkles may not seem like a medical problem, they are the most visible sign of aging and they motivate people to spend vast sums for cosmetic surgery and potent drugs to get rid of them. Dermatologists now believe that most signs of aging skin are caused by long-term exposure to the sun. Even the elderly would have younger looking skin if they avoided the sun. For example, compare the skin on the face of someone over fifty with the skin on the inner arms. Quite a difference, isn't there? Sun-exposed skin thickens with time and the skin can only fold (wrinkle) or sag to accommodate the excess tissue. As skin ages, it also becomes drier.

The sun's rays that are believed responsible for this "photoaging" are the longer UVA rays that penetrate more deeply into the lower layers of the skin where "collagen" and "elastin" lie. It is collagen that gives skin its tone, whereas elastin is responsible for its elasticity. Remember too, that unlike UVB rays that cause sunburn and peak at midday, UVA rays are strong all day long, and all year long. Even on cloudy days! Up to 80% of UVA rays penetrate through clouds.

What used to be considered the "normal aging process" is now thought to be the accumulated effects of sun exposure. The skin is like a time machine: it has a memory. Each hour of sun exposure is added to that of last week and last decade to determine the cumulative effect upon the skin's basic structure. Children should be taught early that sunshine is healthy, but too much exposure will have unfortunate long-term effects.

What Can Be Done for Aging Skin?

Mark Twain quipped, "When your friends begin to flatter you on how young you look, it's a sure sign you're getting old." But that was the 19th century when a majority of folks spent most of their waking hours outside. These are different times. To avoid wrinkles, you must limit sun exposure. This can be done by covering up when you go out (rediscover the parasol), or by the use of sunscreens. Select a broad spectrum sunscreen that blocks both UVB and UVA. Among the brands that protect against UVB, plus some UVA rays, are Photoplex, Bain de Soleil 15, PreSun 15, Sundown 25 (this product has superior retention), Clinique 19, Elizabeth Arden 15, and Estee Lauder sunscreens. Many cosmetics are now being made with sunscreens.

Apply a sunscreen each morning after showering and reapply after swimming or vigorous exercise.

Avoid tanning salons. This is surely one of the most pernicious industries to develop since the use of X-ray machines in shoe stores. Though salon owners may tell you that their tanning lamps don't produce harmful rays, it's not true. These sunlamps carry the same risks of skin burns, eye damage, cataracts, premature skin aging, and skin cancer as any other sunlamp that promotes tanning. Ultraviolet rays from any source should be avoided.

Watch out for "tan accelerators" and "tanning pills." There are no pills that promote tanning. They only tan your wallet's hide.

Stop smoking. Smoking not only causes lung cancer and a host of other chronic diseases, it leads to "smoker's face." This is a combination of "crow's feet" wrinkles about the eyes, linear wrinkles perpendicular to the mouth, and a grayish tinge of the skin—not pretty.

No over-the-counter or cosmetic preparation marketed today has the least effect on aging skin, except to moisturize it. No royal jelly, no antiwrinkle or anti-aging cream, no moon drops, no expensive crème (if its got a French name, hold onto your cash), no exotic glandular or cellular extract has any but a moisturizing effect. Vitamin A capsules taken orally don't work either, despite lavish claims for them—and they are toxic if taken in large doses.

But there may be hope. The prescription drug tretinoin, marketed as Retin-A for the treatment of severe acne, has been shown in preliminary studies to retard the development of aging changes in skin and may even reverse some. The drug appears to work by stimulating growth of thicker epidermis, the outer layer of skin. This process appears to fill in wrinkles and cover some "age" spots.

Retin-A does have side effects, however. In most subjects studied so far, it causes redness, irritation, and peeling of skin. This is usually only temporary, and most have noticed clearer, younger looking skin after 4–6 months use. On the down side, continual use is required to sustain these apparent effects.

Before you run off to your doctor to beg a prescription, you should know that the Food and Drug Administration has not yet approved Retin-A for treatment of wrinkles, or any sun-induced changes for that matter. The FDA and most dermatologists agree that many more long-term studies must be done before recommending it as an antiwrinkle drug. For one thing, its possible role in producing skin cancer is unknown.

Skin Cancer

Certainly the most dreaded long-term effects of over-exposure to sunlight are skin cancers. They are among the most common cancers today and fortunately most are curable if discovered and treated early. There are three types: basal cell carcinoma, squamous cell carcinoma, and malignant melanoma. They occur most often in sun-exposed skin. For example, women are more apt to develop a skin cancer on the legs than men. People who drive a lot tend to develop cancers on their left arms in countries that drive on the right and on their right arms in countries that drive on the left.

Basal Cell Carcinoma

This is the most common skin cancer in light-skinned individuals—about 500,000 new cases will be diagnosed this year in the United States. This is also the most easily cured skin cancer because it seldom metastasizes (spreads to distant organs). Most commonly the tumor begins as a small shiny lump that enlarges slowly, gradually developing raised, well-defined borders and a central indentation or ulcer. Crusting and bleeding are common because the cancer traumatizes easily. Basal cell carcinomas most commonly develop on the head, neck, and hands. They are very rare in dark-skinned people.

Squamous Cell Carcinoma

This is the next most common skin cancer. It occurs often on the rim of the ear, the lips, face, and in the mouth. The cancer may begin in normal skin or in a pre-existing actinic keratosis (*see* p. 470), often starting as a small, red, scaly patch. As the lesion grows, it becomes nodular, invades surrounding tissue, and often ulcerates. Unlike basal cell cancers, squamous cell cancers can metastasize. Nevertheless the cure rate is about 95% if found early and treated properly.

Malignant Melanoma

This is by far the most dangerous skin cancer. Of the 30,000 new cases each year in the United States, about 6000 victims, or 22%, will die of their disease. Melanomas arise from the pigment-producing cells in the skin, the melanocytes. Consequently, these cancers are frequently pigmented; some grow out of pre-existing moles. The appearance of melanomas is highly variable; they have irregular borders and may appear in mixed shades of tan, brown, red, blue, pink, and black. The most common locations are the upper back, torso, head, neck, and lower legs, but they can occur anywhere. The incidence of melanoma is increasing rapidly in this country because Americans for many years have favored the "bronzed" look. The increase is greatest in the Sun Belt states. There are several other risk factors for developing malignant melanoma listed below.

Kaposi's Sarcoma

Kaposi's sarcoma, a cancerous condition, is characterized by skin tumors heavily infiltrated by blood vessels. It typically appears in three different forms: (1) a slow-growing form characterized by nodu-

---

RISK FACTORS FOR DEVELOPING MALIGNANT MELANOMA (IN ORDER OF DECREASING IMPORTANCE)

1. *Persistently changed or changing mole.* Pigmented moles that change in color (becoming darker or lighter), size, borders (becoming irregular), and surface (becoming elevated) should prompt a visit to your doctor. A mole that bleeds, itches, or becomes painful is also suspicious.
2. *Adulthood.* Melanoma is chiefly a disease of adults. The chance of developing a melanoma increases with each decade of life.
3. *One or more large, irregular, pigmented moles.* Large pigmented moles present at birth are more likely to become malignant than those acquired after birth.
4. *Occupation.* You are at increased risk if you are exposed to coal tar, creosote, pitch, arsenic compounds, or radium in your work.
5. *Caucasian race.* Whites have a 12 times greater chance of developing melanoma than blacks and a 7 times greater chance than Hispanics. When melanoma occurs in nonwhites, there is a greater likelihood of it developing on the palms, soles, nailbeds, or mucous membranes.
6. *Previous melanoma.* There is a greater likelihood of developing a melanoma if you have had one previously.
7. *Family history.* If you have a parent, child, or sibling with melanoma you are at increased risk.
8. *Immunosuppression.* Long-term steroid medication, or other cause for immunosuppression (e.g., AIDS) increases risk.
9. *Sun sensitivity.* If you sunburn easily, you are at increased risk.
10. *Excessive sun exposure.* Excessive sun exposure, particularly during childhood, seems to be an important risk factor for melanoma.

---

lar plaque-like lesions; (2) a lymphatic form, which is disseminated and aggressive, involving lymph nodes, viscera, and occasionally the gastrointestinal tract; and (3) a form associated with AIDS, in which the lesions are widely disseminated in the skin, mucous membrance, lymph nodes, and viscera. In the early stages of this cancer, the lesions appear to be colored between red and purple. As the cancer progresses, the lesions appear between brown and black.

Treatment. All skin cancers are treated by specialists experienced in cancer surgery and chemotherapy. When found early, the usual treatment is biopsy, microscopic examination, and surgical removal. Basal cell and squamous cell cancers may also be treated by liquid nitrogen cryosurgery. Metastases are treated using chemotherapy.

Prevention. Since all skin cancers, except Kaposi's sarcoma, are related to sun exposure, the precautions used in preventing premature aging and sunburn also apply to skin cancer, especially in light-skinned individuals. In addition, periodic self-examination is a key element in early discovery. Examine your entire body at regular intervals using a full length mirror and a hand-mirror to view your buttocks, back, and the back of your neck. Older people in particular are at risk because their thinner skin is more susceptible to a form of rapidly spreading melanoma.

If you have a family history of malignant melanoma, examine yourself carefully every month. The average body has about 25 moles. You should be thoroughly familiar with yours. Examine them every month or so. An enlarging (or changing) mole should be seen by your doctor immediately.

Moles

Everybody has moles; many have 40 or more. Moles may be large or small; flat or raised; regular or irregular; pigmented or flesh-colored; smooth, hairy, or warty. Many moles appear in childhood. During adolescence and pregnancy, new moles often appear and old ones frequently darken or enlarge. The average life of a mole is about 40 years. Most gradually fade with time, although since the process is so slow, you will only notice this with large, dark moles.

There would be little to concern yourself with about moles except that some, fortunately quite few, can become malignant. There are two types of moles that should be watched carefully for signs of change. Large moles present at birth occur in about 1 in 100 infants. When more than about 8 inches in diameter, there is a greatly increased incidence of their becoming malignant and thus they must be examined frequently for any changes.

A second type of mole, known as "dysplastic nevus" may also become malignant. These moles have the following characteristics:

- They are asymmetrical, i.e., one half does not match the other.
- They have irregular borders; often these edges are slightly lighter than the centers.

- The color varies from tan to brown to black; sometimes white, red, or blue. Within a single mole, two or more colors may be present.
- They have a diameter larger than 1/4 inch (about the diameter of a pencil eraser).

Such moles should be examined by your doctor, especially if they undergo any noticeable change. Moles that become irritated, bleed, itch or become painful should also be examined.

Treatment. Become familiar with all of the moles on your body. You can examine yourself best in a full-length mirror and use a hand-held mirror to view your back and buttocks. Moles that rapidly enlarge, become raised, change shape or become multicolored should be brought to the attention of your dermatologist. The vast majority of moles are benign and require no medical attention. Suspicious lesions will be biopsied or removed by your dermatologist. In some cases moles may be objectionable for cosmetic reasons. These may be "shaved off," or removed surgically.

Moles with unsightly hair can either be themselves removed, or your dermatologist can permanently remove the mole's hair follicles.

You should not be concerned about irritating moles on your face when shaving. There is no evidence that this induces cancer. If moles in the beard interfere with shaving, they probably ought to be removed, merely for convenience. Makeup can also be cleverly applied to disguise moles, though if you can convince yourself that they add "character" to your face, you will be spared a lot of needless concern.

Skin Tags

These are small, elongated, fleshy growths that usually grow on the neck, armpits, or groin. They appear as if they were attached to the skin by a narrow stalk. They are often multiple and may or may not be pigmented. They are completely benign, but sometimes become irritated by friction from clothing. They may be treated by your doctor by freezing with liquid nitrogen or merely snipped off with scissors. They can be avoided by wearing looser clothing.

Lipomas

Lipomas are small, benign, fatty growths that appear as soft, freely movable nodules under the skin. They occur more often in women than men; they may be multiple; and they are found most commonly on the trunk, back of the neck, and forearms. They do not require treatment unless they become painful, become fixed to surrounding tissue, or begin to enlarge. "Lumps" that develop in the armpits, groin, and neck should be examined by your doctor.

Angiomas

These are local overgrowths of blood vessels just beneath the skin and may be cosmetically objectionable. There are several types; most are present at birth or appear shortly afterward. One congenital angioma, known as a "port wine stain" because of its pink or purplish color, often occurs as a large, flat, pigmented lesion on the neck. Recent advances in the use of lasers offer new ways of treating these tumors when they occur on exposed skin.

"Strawberry hemangiomas" are raised blood vessel tumors that appear at or shortly after birth. They are bright red in color and usually disappear within 2–5 years. Treatment is not ordinarily necessary, but depending on their location they may be removed surgically or by use of a laser.

"Spider angiomas" are tiny, bright red lesions consisting of a central blood vessel surrounded by spider-like red arms. If you press on the central vessel, the lesion disappears, only to reappear when pressure is released. Spider angiomas are common on the face, chest, and arms of patients with cirrhosis of the liver. They may also occur during pregnancy or while taking oral contraceptives. They are not symptomatic and usually disappear within a year after pregnancy or discontinuing contraceptives. If treatment is desired for cosmetic reasons, consult your dermatologist.

Nails

Fingernails

The nails are actually another form of skin, made up of a tough protein called keratin. Each nail is formed from a specialized layer of cells under the base of the nail near the cuticle. Part of this layer is visible as a pale crescent moon just beyond the cuticle. The nails adhere closely to the skin below and are kept growing straight by the skin folds along the sides the the nails and the cuticle. When these folds are injured, the nail plate becomes distorted.

The nails themselves are translucent. Their color reflects the color of the skin below—darker in people with darker skins and pink (from the blood vessels) in people with light skin color.

Nail growth varies among individuals and from finger to finger. The nails of the middle fingers grow slightly faster than the nails of the thumb and little finger. The average growth rate is about one-eighth inch per month. Thus it takes 5–6 months to grow a new nail when one is lost due to injury. Men's nails grow faster than women's, possibly because their nail beds are larger. Hormones also play a role; e.g., growth rate increases during pregnancy and in hyperthyroidism. No foods, including the often touted gelatin, increases nail growth, although malnutrition definitely slows growth.

Other factors that slow nail growth are cold weather, major surgery, and severe illness. After a serious illness, a thin groove forms across the nail plate called *Beau's line*, after the French physician who described it. The position on the nail provides an estimate of when the illness occurred. An illness that occurred in June will still show in November.

Common Fingernail Problems

Brittle Nails

Brittleness is caused by drying (nails are more brittle in winter) and by chemicals interacting with sulfur molecules in nail proteins. Frequent immersion in water containing chlorine and detergents causes the nails to dry, weaken, and break. Use rubber gloves while washing dishes to avoid this problem. Nail polish should not be removed too often, because polish removers also dry the nails. It is usually recommended that polish be kept on for 5–7 days, then removed and reapplied at least two days later to allow the nails time to recover texture.

Ridges

The fine ridges that run the length of the nails are normal and do not indicate injury or illness, although injury to the nail bed may produce a single pronounced ridge. Ridges may appear in rheumatoid arthritis and the skin disease, lichen planus, and furrows may be associated with measles, and other severe infections, but they are not a sign of nail bed infection.

Warts commonly form along the nail folds, probably spread by nail biting. If these grow under the nail, they often distort the nail and must be removed by your doctor.

White Spots

Generally small white spots in the nails indicate minor injury. They do not signify a vitamin deficiency. White bands may occur after exposure to arsenic, which binds to nail proteins. The nails may become white and opaque with cirrhosis of the liver.

DISCOLORATION

The most common cause of brownish discoloration is cigaret smoking. The discoloration is limited to the fingers that hold the cigaret. Hair dyes and colored organic chemicals will dye fingernails, just as they dye hair. Exposure to copper or silver can turn the nails blue.

SEPARATION FROM THE NAIL BED

Separation may be caused by psoriasis (*see* p. 460) or by fungus infections. Allergy to ingredients in nail polish can also cause separation. This is a condition for your dermatologist.

BLOOD BLISTERS UNDER THE NAIL

Bleeding under a fingernail (hematoma) is usually caused by a blow to the nail or by catching the finger in a closing door or drawer. The result is a blue-red spot under the nail that turns black with time. The blood blister can also be very painful as the fluid pressure of the escaped blood separates the nail from its bed.

Treatment. The simplest treatment is to straighten a paper clip and heat the end until it glows. Then carefully place the hot tip of the paper clip over the center of the discolored area and let it burn through the nail, thus creating a tiny hole through which the blood escapes. Keep the entire nail clean to avoid infection as the nail grows and the hole migrates to the outer edge of the fingernail.

SPOON NAILS

Spoon nails result from a reversal of the normal curvature of the nails. It is usually associated with the iron deficiency syndrome in children. See your doctor.

TORN NAILS

Nails that are torn off or separated from the nailbed require special care. Try to save the nail so that it will continue to do its job of protecting the finger. Wash the nail and nailbed with running water. Place the torn nail in its original position over the nailbed. A small piece of gauze spread with vaseline or an antibiotic preparation should be placed on top of the nail and secured with adhesive tape. The vase-lined gauze prevents lifting of the nail fragment when the adhesive tape is removed.

HANGNAILS

Hangnails are cracked or torn cuticle around the nail that result from trauma, especially in those with dry skin. Torn edges can be cut off with cuticle scissors. Hangnails can be largely prevented by the use of moisturizing creams and lotions to prevent drying and by pro-

---

CARE OF ARTIFICIAL NAILS

Artificial nails come in package kits for self-application or can be sculpted to your fingernails by a manicurist. The following notes will help familiarize you with these products:

• Sensitivity to the materials in artificial nails is quite common. If you have any question about your possible sensitivity, have one nail done as a test and wait a few days to see whether any redness, swelling, or tenderness develops around the artificial nail.
• Never apply an artificial nail if the nail or tissue around it is infected or irritated; let the infection or inflammation heal first.
• If an artificial nail separates, dip the fingertip into rubbing alcohol to clean the space between the natural and artificial nails before reattaching the artificial nail. This will help prevent infection. Never use household glues for home repairs. Use only the products supplied for such use.
• Full-sized press-on or glue-on nails should be removed after 48 hours because they do not always fit tightly over the natural nail and may allow a space for bacteria to grow.

---

tecting the cuticles with gloves, especially when the hands are subjected to repeated immersion.

Fingernail and Toenail Infections

Infections around and beneath your nails (subungual infections), if minor, may be treated by applying a drop or two of dilute tincture of iodine after each washing and thorough drying of your hands. Any infection that does not heal promptly, or is associated with redness, pain, and swelling should be treated by your doctor at once. Nail infections are often caused by yeast or fungus and require prolonged treatment with specific antimicrobial agents.

Toenails

Most of the remarks made about fingernails apply to toenails as well, except that since they are covered most of the day, they are either out of harm's way or out of sight and mind. However there is one very common problem, which may be the most common of all foot problems: ingrown toenails.

Ingrown toenails usually affect the great toes only and have two common causes, ill-fitting shoes and improper trimming. If you develop ingrown toenails, wear low-heel shoes with ample toe room. Tennis and jogging shoes are ideal if you can get by wearing them.

Treatment. To relieve pressure on an ingrown toenail, soak your foot in water for 15–20 minutes twice daily to soften the skin around the toenail. Thoroughly dry your foot with a clean towel. Coat a small piece of gauze dressing with an antibiotic ointment and gently insert it under the toenail with an orange stick or a tongue depressor to raise the toenail slightly

In caring for your toenails, use heavy scissors to cut the nail neatly and straight across—do not round the cut. Contrary to popular belief, cutting a small V in the center of the nail does not prevent ingrown toenail. Avoid cutting the nail too close. Keep your feet very clean to avoid infection. If pus, bleeding, or painful swelling develops, see your doctor or podiatrist.

Hair

Normal Hair Growth

Hair growth occurs in two cycles: a growth phase lasting 2–6 years, and a rest cycle, lasting 2–3 months, after which the hair falls out and a new cycle begins. At any time about 15% of the hair is in the rest cycle, so that out of 100,000 or more hairs on the head, 70–100 fall out daily. As we age, the growth rate of many follicles begins to decline and some follicles cease functioning altogether. By age 25, hair in most individuals begins to thin and the hairline begins to recede. This process continues so that by age 65, about 65% of individuals experience significant hair loss.

Dandruff

The little white flecks that may fall upon your shoulders and look like a dusting of snowflakes on dark-colored clothing are merely small flakes of dead skin from the scalp. The most usual cause is mild seborrheic dermatitis (*see* p. 445). Dandruff is not a serious condition, but most people find it unattractive. For treatment, *see* p. 446.

Excessive Hair

Excessive body hair, or hirsutism, is often a familial problem, common among people from the Mediterranean region. Excessive hair in younger women and children may mean an endocrine problem, which

---

TREATMENT OF EXCESSIVE BODY HAIR

- Tweezing is acceptable for occasional hairs about the face, ears, and chin. They will reappear in 4–6 weeks.
- Shaving, contrary to popular myth does not make hair coarser, thicker, or grow faster. But, as most men well know, it must be done frequently, e.g., every 2–3 days for leg hair.
- Waxing is a popular method of hair removal that lasts 6–8 weeks. It is somewhat painful and initially should be done by a professional.
- If your hair is fine, bleaching is inexpensive and also lasts 6–8 weeks. As for any new product used on your face, apply a small amount of the dye or bleach in a "test" patch to make certain you are not sensitive to the chemicals.
- Chemical depilatories work by dissolving hair at just below the surface of the skin. Hair will reappear in 1–2 weeks. Again, apply the product to a test patch before using. Electrical depilatory appliances grab and pluck the hairs. The treatment may be painful. Hairs regrow at the same rate as they would following tweezing, about 4–6 weeks.
- The only safe, permanent hair removal process entails the destruction of individual hair follicles by electrolysis. The process is both tedious and expensive. Before making a selection, examine the electrologist's credentials, or, better, ask a dermatologist for a recommendation. Untrained operators can cause permanent skin damage. Regrowth is also possible if electrolysis is performed improperly.

---

only your doctor can diagnose. Among older women, the cause is usually an overabundance of male hormones, the androgens. As a woman's estrogen levels drop with increasing age, androgens may begin to assert themselves as unwanted hairiness. For treatment, see box on next page.

Baldness

The most common form of male baldness, or *alopecia* as it is known medically, is "male-pattern" baldness, an hereditary loss of hair that begins in the front and spreads back, or on top of the head and spreads fore and aft. The sides usually are spared longest. Young men look anxiously upon their fathers' glistening heads and fear their fate is before their eyes. Some of these search for any ray of hope to forestall their fate. They have not far to look, for charlatans' promises abound. More than $100 million is spent each year on fraudulent balding remedies.

What Can Be Done About Baldness?

Not long ago the drug, minoxidil, which is used to treat high blood pressure, was noted to stimulate hair growth in some men. This drug has recently been approved as a topical medication, marketed as Rogaine, and may offer hope of increasing hair density in people with early balding. Those men most likely to benefit from Rogaine include younger men who are just beginning to lose hair on the crown. Older men, and men with a longer history or greater degree of baldness, are probably poor candidates for Rogaine use. Rogaine has never been known to reverse a receding forehead.

There is some indication that Rogaine may be even more useful in "female-pattern" baldness. This is common in older women, marked by thinning of hair above the forehead and on the sides of the head. Ask your doctor about the drug if you feel a wig is not for you.

HAIR TRANSPLANTS

In some individuals (actually quite few) in whom hair loss is not extensive, hair transplants may prove effective. Small cores of skin are taken from normal hairy parts of the scalp and inserted into balding areas. Possible complications include swelling of the forehead and eyelids, as well as scalp numbness. The surgical scars may be observable.

In the end, a healthy resignation to the mandates of heredity is the happiest solution. And since vanity is the ultimate font of hair anxiety, men can take pleasure in the widespread notion that bald men are more virile.

Reversible Baldness

There are several common causes of hair thinning related to improper hair care. Excessive use of permanent waving, hair straightening, dying, and bleaching cause hair to become brittle and break. Excessive hair dryer heat, tight hair styles and compulsive brushing are other causes of hair thinning. The use of looser hair styling, gentle care and use of after-shampoo conditioners to coat and protect the hair are obvious good grooming practices. Swimmers especially need to wear caps and carefully condition their hair to prevent chlorine from turning the hair brittle.

In rare individuals a condition known as "toxic alopecia" may follow certain severe illnesses (e.g., scarlet fever). It also occasionally follows pregnancy and overdoses with such drugs as Vitamin A. Toxic alopecia is temporary and hair regrows when the precipitating condition ends.

Another form of regional baldness is "alopecia areata." This disease is of unknown cause, characterized by patchy areas of irregular hair loss on the scalp and beard. Dermatologists often treat this condition with injections of steroids into the bald patches.

Hair Pulling

A particularly insidious cause of patchy baldness is "trichotillomania," a neurotic habit that usually appears in children. One sign is that many shafts of hair surrounding the hair loss will be broken off and irregular new growth is evident. Hair pulling is resistant to psychological therapy, but may be treated by certain types of tranquilizing drugs.

Ingrown Hairs

Ingrown hairs have the wonderful medical name, "pseudo-folliculitis barbae." They are most common in black men and others who have stiff, curly hair. The stiff hair tips penetrate the skin before they reach the surface, or else they curl back to penetrate the skin and form a small pustule. The reaction is more a *foreign body reaction* than an infection. Nevertheless, their presence is irritating and makes shaving difficult and painful.

The best cure is to grow a beard, since it is the freshly cut hairs that cause the problem. For those in whom this is not acceptable, tweezing the hairs is probably the most common solution. Special razors are available and offer varying results. A number of preparations may be tried. Depilatory agents may be used every 2–3 days, although for many these are irritating. Tretinoin (Retin-A) is sometimes effective. It should be applied every other day to begin with because it is irritating. An over-the-counter preparation, 10% benzoyl peroxide, may be helpful.

Many people with fine hair develop asymptomatic ingrown hairs about areas that are repeatedly chafed by clothing, particularly about the buttocks, knees, and thighs. They appear as small papules with a central hair covered by a fine layer of skin. No treatment is usually necessary. Their presence can be greatly lessened by vigorously cleansing these areas with a coarse washcloth, which removes the tops and frees the hairs.

The Uncombable Hair Syndrome

I am not making this up. In rare individuals a defect in the hair shaft causes the hair to lie in random, unpredictable directions that makes normal combing impossible. Since this is a genetically determined condition, there is no cure except to wear very short hair or find an ingenious barber. Actually the look is very "punk," if you favor that look.

Appendix 1

Smoking

Only someone living on a mountain top or another planet for the last ten years is likely to be unaware of the health risks (to yourself and others) of smoking. We're talking about cigaret smoking here. Pipe and cigar smoking carry all these risks, and more; but they are less common—possibly because such smokers have discovered themselves increasingly becoming social pariahs.

If you smoke, you know it is hazardous, if for no other reason than you can read it (not that you do) printed plainly on each package of cigarets you buy. You are quite well aware that your habit increases your risk of developing lung cancer (one out of every 10 heavy smokers); chronic bronchitis (do you cough and spit in the morning?); emphysema (do you easily get short of breath?).

You also know that cigarets stain your teeth and fingers, make your hair and clothes stink, and befoul the room air. When did you last walk into a bathroom where someone had just been smoking?

But did you know about the following hazards of smoking?

- You have an increased risk of developing cancers of the mouth, throat, esophagus, bladder, kidney, pancreas, stomach, and cervix. In fact, 30% of all cancers are caused by smoking.*
- You have an increased risk (30%) of developing coronary heart disease. If you smoke a pack a day or more, you have two and one-half times the risk of nonsmokers and two to four times the risk of sudden cardiac death.** In fact, the American Lung Association estimates that the number of premature deaths due to smoking in the United States is 350,000 people each year. That is the equivalent of the total loss of 900 fully-loaded jumbo jets every year! This number is also higher than the combined death tolls from alcohol, illegal drugs, traffic accidents, suicide, and homicide.

*Surgeon General Report, 1982; American Cancer Society, Cancer Facts and Figures, 1986.
**Surgeon General Report, 1983.

- You have an increased risk of developing such dangerous vascular diseases as stroke (Cerebrovascular disease), atherosclerotic peripheral vascular disease (leg pain, gangrene), and aortic aneurysm.
- You are more likely to develop peptic and duodenal ulcers. Deaths from duodenal ulcers are two to four times more common in smokers than nonsmokers.*
- As a smoker, you have twice the likelihood of having an accident.
- You are more likely to take sick leave from work and retire early due to disability.
- You are more likely to cause a fire that results in significant property damage.**

Smoking and Your Children

Would you knowingly do harm to your children? Probably your answer is "No." But if you smoke and have children, you are very likely to do just that. Here are some provocative facts:

- Women who smoke during pregnancy have more stillbirths, spontaneous abortions, and premature deliveries than women who don't smoke. This is not surprising when you consider that a pregnant woman who smokes two packs a day blocks off the equivalent of 25% of the oxygen supply to her fetus.
- Babies of mothers who smoke during pregnancy are more likely to be born undersized and have a greater chance of dying soon after birth. There is even some evidence to suggest that "passive smoke," the smoke a mother inhales from others smoking, may affect birth weight.
- A University of Maryland study has shown recently that 3-year-old children of mothers who smoked while pregnant scored an average of 5 points lower on IQ tests than children of women who quit smoking while pregnant.
- Several studies have shown that infants under one year of age have significantly increased incidences of bronchitis and pneumonia than children in smoke-free environments.
- Most serious of all, your smoking greatly affects the chances your children will smoke when they get older, especially as teenagers. Almost one million teenagers take up smoking every year, and

*Kurata JH, et al.: Sex and smoking differences in duodenal ulcer mortality. *American Journal of Public Health* **76**:700, 1986.
Keistein MM: How much can business expect to profit from smoking cessation. *Preventive Medicine* **12:358, 1983.

among teenagers who smoke, most have parents who smoke. Girls tend to follow their mother's smoking behavior and disregard their father's. The percentage of teenage girls who smoke is now almost as high as for boys. And it as well known that the fastest growing incidence of lung cancer is among women. Both mothers and fathers have to ask themselves, "Do we want to do this to our children?"

How Is Tobacco Smoke Harmful?

Tobacco smoke contains thousands of chemical substances. The three most damaging are nicotine, tars, and carbon monoxide.

- *Nicotine* causes your blood vessels to constrict, reducing the blood flow to all of your body organs, and thus making your heart pump harder. Nicotine may also interfere with normal platelet function, causing blood clots to form more easily. Nicotine thus figures prominently in the development of brain and heart blood vessel diseases.
- *Carbon monoxide* binds tightly with hemoglobin, thus reducing the total amount of oxygen the red blood cells can carry. In patients with cardiovascular disease, such added stress can precipitate a heart attack.
- *Tars* are complex substances that adhere to the bronchial tissues. These are the substances that stain cigaret filters (as well as your lungs) a dark brown. They irritate the bronchial lining, causing bronchitis and, secondarily, emphysema. They are also responsible for causing lung cancer; more than 50 substances in tobacco tars have been found to be carcinogenic. For example, tobacco smoke contains radioactive polonium-210 and 214. These are breakdown products of radon, which are thought to be responsible for lung cancer among uranium miners.

What Are the Benefits of Quitting Smoking?

For one thing, you will probably find it easier to win new friends and keep the ones you have. If you are a smoker, you have undoubtedly experienced, more than once, a subtle barb or dirty look when you lit up in public. Believe me, it was only the beginning. Nonsmokers are becoming increasingly bold and aggressive. You can't smoke in most government buildings, except in a basement cubicle designed to repel you. In many cities you can't smoke in restaurants and in some you can't smoke in any establishment where you might encounter a nonsmoker.

There are lots better reasons to quit smoking:

- Within 12 hours after your last cigaret, your body begins to heal itself. Blood levels of carbon monoxide and nicotine decline rapidly.
- Within a few days, your sense of taste and smell begin to return. Your smoker's hack will disappear and your digestive system will return to normal.
- Within a week, you will feel more clear-headed, more full of energy. You will be able to climb stairs without becoming winded or dizzy. You are now beginning to feel really good about yourself.
- Within one year you decrease the risk of coronary heart disease. After two to seven years, your risk is the same as a never-smoker.
- Within 10–15 years, the risk of lung cancer approaches that of a never-smoker.
- In short, you add measurable years of healthy productive years to your life. And from the very beginning, you have freed yourself and those around you from the mess, smell, inconvenience, and expense of smoking.

How Do You Go About Quitting?

There is obviously no best method for all, just as there is no sure method for anyone. The first time I stopped smoking, I waited until I had a bad cold and cigarets tasted awful. Like most smokers, I made several attempts, each quietly agonizing, before stopping completely. (As Mark Twain is quoted as saying: "It's easy to stop smoking. I ought to know, I done it a thousand times.") When I did quit, it was "cold turkey," which I think is best. But it is not best for everyone, because nicotine is addictive and withdrawal symptoms may be intense at first. These include nervousness, irritability, depression, reduced attention span, and craving for a cigaret (by far the worst symptom).

Numerous programs have been devised and they are readily available to anyone determined—or who can be cajoled—to quit. Some of them are available from:

American Cancer Society
777 3rd Avenue
New York, NY 10017
(212) 371-2900

Office of Cancer Communications
National Cancer Institute
Bethesda, MD 20205
(800) 638-6694

American Heart Association
7320 Greenville Avenue
Dallas, TX 75231
(214) 750-5300

Smoke Enders (National Office)
37 North Third Street
Easton, PA 18047
(215) 250-0700

American Lung Association
1740 Broadway
New York, NY 10019
(212) 245-8000

Stop Smoking System
American Health Foundation
320 East 42nd Street
New York, NY 10017

Office of Smoking and Health
US Department of Health and Human Services
5600 Fishers Lane, Park Bldg, Room 110
Rockville, MD 20857
(301) 443-5287

Four-Week Do-It-Yourself Program

One popular program that is used in part by many successful smoke-ending clinics is a simple self-help plan that can be adapted to your particular needs:

- *First week.* Make a list of all the positive reasons why you want to quit smoking, and read the list daily. Wrap your cigaret pack with paper and tie it with rubber bands. Each time you smoke write down the time of day, what you are doing, how you are feeling, and how important that cigaret is to you on a scale from 1 to 5. Then rewrap the pack.
- *Second week.* Keep reading your list of reasons. Don't carry matches and keep your cigarets some distance away. Each day, try to smoke fewer cigarets, eliminating those least or most important, whichever works best for you.
- *Third week.* Continue with the second week's instructions. Don't buy a new pack until you finish the one you're smoking and never buy a carton. Change brands twice during the week, each time choosing a brand lower in tar and nicotine. Try to stop smoking for 48 hours sometime during the week.
- *Fourth week.* Continue the above. Increase your physical activity. Avoid situations you most closely associate with smoking. Find a substitute for cigarets—gum, celery, carrot sticks, toothpicks, and so on. Try deep breathing exercises whenever you get the urge to smoke.

What Not to Do

- *Don't switch to a pipe or cigars.* There is growing evidence that these are just as bad for you as cigarets. There is a strong tendency for former cigaret smokers to inhale small amounts of the smoke, a direct carryover from cigaret smoking. Not only do you not quit smoking, you substitute a much more toxic smoke. It is entirely possible to *increase* your risk of lung cancer and heart disease.

- *Don't switch to "smokeless tobacco."* As cigaret smoking becomes less popular, tobacco companies are fast at promoting chewing tobacco and snuff. Either way, they want to keep you hooked. To switch to oral tobacco, you merely trade one set of bad habits and risks for another. If the risk of lung cancer declines, the risk of oral and throat cancer increases; and the risk of heart disease and stroke remain the same. *Plus*, you assume all of the charms of bad breath, stained teeth, tooth loss, slow-healing mouth wounds, lowered sense of taste and smell, excessive salivation, and lots of spitting. This is very much like exchanging tuberculosis for leprosy: hardly a deal.
- *Don't switch to clove cigarets.* Also known as "kreteks" and imported from Indonesia, clove cigarets have become popular among young people who think they are safe because they are not tobacco. But in fact, clove cigarets are usually 60% tobacco and 40% ground cloves, clove oil, and other additives. Some scientists believe the combination is more damaging to the lungs than tobacco alone.
- *Try not to gain weight.* A major deterrent for many who want to stop smoking is the fear of getting fat. This reason is cited most frequently by women. For them it is little comfort to be told that the harm of gaining a few pounds is negligible compared with the benefits of stopping smoking (one estimate holds that a pack a day has the same deleterious effect as 75 additional pounds!).

  Nevertheless, you will probably have to make a conscious effort to avoid gaining weight. The reason for this is that smoking acts to increase the metabolic rate (the rate at which the body burns calories). When you stop, calories are burned a little more slowly. There is also a tendency to snack more often as a means of relieving the nervous tension generated by the unfulfilled habit. Consequently, the average smoker gains five to seven pounds when he or she stops. At 3500 calories per pound of body fat, that is a lot of exercise that must be added to keep body weight at the smoking baseline. You should limit your snacking to such things as raw vegetables, unbuttered popcorn, and fresh fruits. Fruits are a good way of relieving the craving for sweets that many ex-smokers report.

  Two books that may be useful if diet is your main consideration not to stop smoking:

- Ogle, Jane: *The Stop Smoking Diet*. New York, Evans, 1981.
- Solomon, Neil: *Stop Smoking, Lose Weight*. New York, Putnam, 1981.

What About Nicotine Gum?

A nicotine-containing chewing gum is marketed under the name *Nicorette*. It is promoted as helping alleviate the craving to smoke by supplying the drug in an alternative form. Relatively few controlled studies have been reported. However, it is generally agreed that this smoke-ending aid should not be prescribed (it does require a doctor's prescription) except in conjunction with a supervised behavior modification program. There are definite contra-indications to its use, such as in pregnant women and patients with heart disease. It may be worth a try when all else has failed. The same is probably true for nicotine patches.

Marijuana

Remember "reefer madness"? Before the 1960s we thought that only Indian fakirs and criminal low-lifes smoked marijuana, and little abiding thought was given to either. Then in the 1960s the drug culture mushroomed—some pun intended. Those too were the days when the concentration of THC (tetrahydrocannabinol) in the leaves and flowers of *Cannabis sativa* was maybe 0.5% and perhaps a few million were "given to the weed."

Time has changed things in more ways than one. With enhanced cultivation methods and the miracles of hybridization, street marijuana often contains 5% THC, the main mind-altering ingredient in "grass." That is enough to render a teenager (the biggest users) insensate after a few "hits." Smoking marijuana has reached epidemic proportions among school-aged Americans. A survey by the American Lung Association showed that nearly half of all 7th graders reported peer pressure to use marijuana. By the 9th grade almost 70% reported some peer pressure. The trend has long since reached the proportions of a major social problem.

Children are also the most susceptible to the many harmful effects of the drug. Few would argue that occasional social use by adults constitutes much of a problem. Indeed by contrast with the dangers of alcohol, the impact of marijuana might be compared to herbal tea among most adult users. Not so for kids.

Lung Damage

The smoke from burning marijuana contains over 2000 chemical compounds, including benzpyrene and bezanthracene, known to cause cancer, and acetone, acetaldehyde, and hydrocyanic acid, common lung irritants. Furthermore, these substances are found in significantly higher concentrations than in tobacco smoke. In terms of lung irritation, one "joint" is equivalent to about a pack of cigarets. Smoking marijuana daily for five years or more produces the kinds of lung tissue damage found in people who have been smoking tobacco for 10 to 15 years. This damage is the same as found in people who develop chronic bronchitis, emphysema, and lung cancer. Though a definite correlation between marijuana and lung cancer has not been incontrovertibly demonstrated, the association is suspected. After all, it took 40 years to adequately demonstrate the dangers of chronic tobacco smoking.

Brain Effects

Marijuana has both short-term and long-term effects on the brain. Short-term effects include acute intoxication. There is pronounced interference with memory, speech, reasoning, problem solving, learning, and motor skills. Some marijuana smokers experience acute anxiety reactions that include paranoia and abnormal fear. Long-term users are often dependent on the drug (even though it is thought not to be physically addicting) and these individuals often experience apathy and a loss of energy. What would you expect from people who spent a substantial portion of their waking hours "stoned"? They are certainly not apt to feel their best without the drug.

Like alcohol, marijuana interferes with hand–eye coordination and fine motor functions. Tests of marijuana-intoxicated drivers have shown that driving ability is impaired. When asked, however, they report a belief that they are performing at a higher level of proficiency.

Statistics show that marijuana users are much more apt to smoke tobacco, drink alcohol, and use cocaine. Since alcohol and marijuana have a potentiating effect, combined use greatly increases the risk of tragedy while driving.

Heart Effects

Marijuana increases the heart rate and lowers oxygen supply to the heart muscle. Among healthy users, this may be of little consequence. For a patient with heart disease, it may be truly dangerous.

Other Effects

In women, marijuana causes increased menstrual cycle abnormalities and interferes with ovulation. In males, marijuana decreases sperm production, sperm motility, and male hormone levels.

Because THC readily crosses the placenta, it quickly reaches the fetus. There is some evidence to show that marijuana contributes to birth defects, premature deliveries, and spontaneous abortions.

The Psychological Impact

Particularly among adolescents, there is a real danger that regular use of marijuana can lead to social and adjustment problems. Young men and women who spend time tripping out are not mentally available for other life experiences (recreation, study, moral and attitude development, etc.). Youths can get away with some of that, but in time, it catches up with them. They lose out; they become losers—both by their own and by other people's perceptions. When that happens, the loss to society is incalculable. It is for you, dear reader, to take cognizance of this, both for your own behavior and for the examples you create for those you love and are loved by.

Appendix 2

Drug Names and Their Generic Equivalents

Trade	Generic
A	
Anavar	Oxandrolone
Ancef	Cefazolin
Anspor	Cephradine
Antabuse	Disulfiram
Antepar	Piperazine citrate
Antivert	Meclizine
Anturane	Sulfinpyrarone
Apresazide	Hydralazine, hydrochlorothiazide
Apresoline	Hydralazine
AquaMephyton	Phytonadione
Aquatag	Benzthiazide
Aralen	Chloroquine phosphate
Arfonad	Trimethaphan
Aristocort	Triamcinolone acetonide
Arlidin	Nylidrin
Artane	Trihexyphenidyl
Ascriptin	Buffered aspirin
Atabrine	Quinicrine
Atarax	Hydroxyzine
Ativan	Lorezapam
Atromid-S	Clofibrate
Avlosulfon	Dapsone
Azo-Gantrisin	Azo-sulfisoxazole
Azolid	Phenylbutazone
Azulfidine	Sulfasalazine
B	
Bactocill	Oxacillin
Bactrim	Sulfamethoxazole, trimethoprim
Bancap	Acetaminophen; butalbital
Beclovent	Beclomethasone
Benadryl	Diphenhydramine
Benemid	Probenecid
Benisone	Betamethasone
Bentyl	Dicyclomine
Benzedrex	Propyl hexedrine
Betadine	Povidone–Iodine
Bicillin	Penicillin G
Blocadren	Timolol maleate
Bonine	Meclizine

Trade	Generic
Brethine	Terbutaline
Brevital	Methohexital
Bricanyl	Terbutaline
Bronkosol	Isoetharine
Bufferin	Buffered aspirin
Bumex	Bumetanide
Butazolidin	Phenylbutazone
Butisol sodium	Butabarbital
C	
Cafergot	Ergotamine tartrate
Calan	Verapamil
Calciferol	Ergocalciferol
Calcimar	Calcitonin-salmon
Calderol	Calcifediol
Capastat	Capreomycin
Capoten	Captopril
Carafate	Sucralfate
Catapres	Clonidine
Ceclor	Cefaclor
Cefadyl	Cephapirn
Cefizox	Ceftizoxime
Cefobid	Cefoperazone
Cefotan	Cefotetan
Centrax	Prazepam
Cephulac	Lactulose
Cerespan	Papaverine
Chenix	Chenodiol
Chlor-Trimeton	Chlorpheniramine maleate
Chloromycetin	Chloramphenicol
Choledyl	Oxtriphylline
Chronulac	Lactulose
Claforan	Cefotaxime
Cleocin	Clindamycin
Clinoril	Sulindac
Clistin	Carbinoxamine
Clomid	Clomiphene
Cloxapen	Cloxacillin
Cogentin	Benztropine
Colace	Docusate sodium
Colestid	Colestipol
Combipres	Chlorthalidone, clonidine

Trade	Generic	Trade	Generic
Compazine	Prochlorperazine	Ditropan	Oxybutynin chloride
Cordarone	Amiodarone	Diucardin	Hydroflumethiazide
Cordran	Flurandrenolide	Diulo	Metolazone
Corgard	Nadolol	Diuril	Chlorothiazide
Coricidin	Chlorpheniramine, aspirin	Dolobid	Diflunisal
Cortaid	Hydrocortisone	Dolophine	Methadone
Cortrosyn	Cosyntropin	Dopar	Levodopa
Cosmegen	Dactinomycin	Doriden	Glutethimide
Cotazym	Pancrelipase	Dulcolax	Bisacodyl
Coumadin	Warfarin	Durabolin	Nandrolone
Crystodigin	Digitoxin	Duracillin	Penicillin G procaine
Cuprid	Trientine	Duricef	Cefadroxil
Cuprimine	Penicillamine	Dyazide	Hydrochlorothiazide,
Cyclapen	Cyclacillin		triamterene
Cyclogyl	Cyclopentolate	Dymelor	Acetohexamide
Cyclospasmol	Cyclandelate	Dynapen	Dicloxacillin
Cytomel	Liothyronine sodium		

D

E

Trade	Generic	Trade	Generic
Dalmane	Flurazepam	Echodide	Echothiophate
Danocrine	Danazol	Edecrin	Ethacrynic acid
Dantrium	Dantrolene	E.E.S	Erythromycin
Daraprim	Pyrimethamine		ethylsuccinate
Darbid	Isopropamide iodide	Elavil	Amitriptyline
Darvocet-N	Propoxyphene napsylate,	Eldopaque	Hydroquinone
	acetaminophen	Eldoquin	Hydroquinone
Darvon	Propoxyphene	Elixophyllin	Theophylline
Decadron	Dexamethasone	E-Mycin	Erythromycin
Decapryn	Doxylamine succinate	Endep	Amitriptyline
Declomycin	Demeclucycline	Enduron	Methylclothiazide
Delalutin	Hydroxyprogesterone	Enactin	Triacetin
	caproate	Equagesic	Meprobamate; aspirin
Delatestryl	Testosterone enanthate	Equanil	Meprobamate
Delsym	Dextromethorphan	Erythrocin	Erythromycin stearate
Deltasone	Prednisone	Esidrix	Hydrochlorothiazide
Demerol	Meperidine	Eskalith	Lithium carbonate
Dendrid	Idoxuridine	Euthyroid	Liotrix
Depakene	Valproic acid	Eutonyl	Pargyline
Desferal	Desferoxamine	Exna	Benzthiazide
Desoxyn	Methamphetamine		
Desyrel	Trazodone		
Dexedrine	Dextroamphetamine		
	sulfate		
Dexatrim	Phenylpropanolamine		
DiaBeta	Glyburide		
Diabinese	Chlorpropamide		
Diamox	Acetazolamide		
Dianabol	Methandrostenolone		
Diapid	Lypressin		
Dibenzyline	Phenoxybenzamine		
Didronel	Etidronate disodium		
Dilantin	Phenytoin		
Dimetane	Brompheniramine maleate		
Diprosone	Betamethasone		
	dipropionate		

F

Trade	Generic
Fastin	Phentermine
Feldene	Piroxicam
Feosol	Ferrous sulfate
Fergon	Ferrous sulfate
Fiorinal	Butalbital, aspirin,
	caffeine
Flagyl	Metronidazole
Folvite	Folic acid
Fortaz	Ceftazidime
Florinef	Flumethasone pivalaate
Fluonid	Fluocinolone acetonide
Furacin	Nitrofurazone
Furadantin	Nitrofurantoin
Furoxone	Furazolidone

Trade	Generic
G	
Gantanol	Sulfamethoxazole
Garamycin	Gentamicin sulfate
Geocillin	Carbenicillin indanyl sodium
Geopen	Carbenicillin
H	
Halcion	Triazolam
Haldol	Haloperidol
Haldrone	Paramethasone
Halotestin	Fluoxymesterone
Halotex	Haloprogin
Hibiclens	Chlorhexidine
Hibitane	Chlorhexidine
Humatin	Parmomycin
Hydergine	Ergoloid mesylate
Hydrea	Hydroxyurea
Hydrocortone	Hydrocortisone
HydroDiuril	Hydrochlorothiazide
Hydromox	Quinethazone
Hydropres	Hydrochlorothiazide, reserpine
Hygroton	Chlorthalidone
Hyperstat	Diazoxide
Hytakerol	Dihydrotachysterol
Hytone	Hydrocortisone
Hytuss	Guaifenesin
I	
Ilosone	Erythromycin estolate
Imferon	Iron dextran
Imodium	Loperamide
Inderal	Propranolol
Inderide	Propranolol, hydrochlorothiazide
Indocin	Indomethacin
INH	Isoniazid
Intal	Cromolyn sodium
Intropin	Dopamine
Inversine	Mecamylamine
Ionamin	Phentermine resin complex
Ismelin	Guanethidine monosulfate
Isoptin	Verapamil
Isopto-Cetamide	Sulfacetamide sodium
Iordil	Isosorbide dinitrate
Isuprel	Isoproterenol
Ivadantin	Nitrofurantoin
K	
Kaochlor	Potassium chloride
Kaon	Potassium chloride
Kaopectate	Kaolin; pectin
Keflex	Cephalexin

Trade	Generic
Keflin	Cephalothin
Kefzol	Cefazolin
Kemadrin	Procyclidine
Kenacort	Triamcinolone
Kenalog	Triamcinolone acetonide
Kwell	Lindane
L	
Lanoxin	Digoxin
Larodopa	Levodopa
Larotid	Amoxicillin
Lasix	Furosemide
Levoprome	Methotrimeprazine
Librium	Chlordiazepoxide
Lidex	Fluocinonide
Limbitrol	Amitriptyline, chlordiazepoxide
Lincocin	Lincomycin
Lithane	Lithium carbonate
Lithonate	Lithium carbonate
Lomotil	Diphenoxylate, atropine sulfate
Loniten	Minoxidil
Lopid	Gemfibrosil
Lotrimin	Clotrimazole
Loxitane	Loxapine
Ludiomil	Maprotiline
Luminal	Phenobarbital
M	
Macrodantin	Nitrofurantoin
Mandelamine	Methenamine
Mandol	Cefamandole
Marezine	Cyclizine
Marinol	Dronabinol
Matulane	Procarbazine
Maxzide	Hydrochlorothiazide; triamterene
Mebaral	Mephobarbital
Meclomen	Meclofenamate sodium
Medrol	Methyl prednisolone
Mefoxin	Cefoxitin
Megace	Megestrol acetate
Mellaril	Thioridazine
Mesantoin	Mephenytoin
Mestinon	Pyridostigmine
Metandren	Methyl testosterone
Metaprel	Metaproterenol
Metatensin	Trichlormethiazide
Methosarb	Calusterone
Methicortelone	Prednisolone
Meticorten	Prednisone
Metrazol	Pentylenetetrazol
Micatin	Miconazole
Micro-K	Potassium chloride

Trade	Generic	Trade	Generic
Micronase	Glyburide	Oreton	Testosterone
Midamor	Amiloride	Orinase	Tolbutamide
Milontin	Phensuximide	Ortho Novum	Norethindrone,
Miltown	Meprobamate		ethinyl estradiol
Minipress	Prazosin	Otrivin	Xylometazoline
Minocin	Minocycline		
Mintezol	Thiabendazole	**P**	
Mithracin	Mithramycin	Panoxyl	Benzoyl peroxide
Moban	Molindone	Paraflex	Penicillin G potassium
Modane	Danthron	Parfon Forte	Chloroxazone;
Monistat	Miconazole		acetaminophen
Monocid	Cefonicid	Parnate	Tranylcypromine
Motrin	Ibuprofen	Pavabid	Papaverine
Mucomyst	Acetylcysteine	PBZ	Tripelennamine
Mustargen	Mechlorethamine	Pentids	Penicillin G potassium
Mutamycin	Mitomycin	Pen Vee K	Penicillin V potassium
Myambutol	Ethambutol	Percocet	Acetaminophen,
Mycelex	Clotrimazole		oxycodone HCl
Mycifradin	Neomycin sulfate	Percodan	Aspirin, oxycodone HCl;
Mycodan	Homatropin methyl		oxycodone terephthalate
	bromide, hydrocodone	Pergonal	Menotropins
Mycostatin	Nystatin	Periactin	Cyproheptadine
Mydriacyl	Tropicamide	Permitil	Fluphenazine
Mylicon	Simethicone	Persantine	Dipyridamole
Mysoline	Primidone	Pertofrane	Desipramine
		Phenergan	Promethazine
N		Placidyl	Ethchlorvynol
Naldecon	Nechlorin	Plaquenil	Hydroxychloroquine
Nalon	Fenoprofen	Plegine	Phendimetrazine tartrate
Naqua	Trichlormethiazide	Polaramine	Dexchlorpheniramine
Nardil	Pheneizine	Polycillin	Ampicillin
Naturetin	Bendroflumethiazide	Pondimin	Fenfluramine
Navane	Thiothixene	Pre-Pen	Benzyl
Nebcin	Tobramycin		penicilloylpolylysine
Neggram	Nalidixic acid	Presamine	Imipramine
Neosynephrine	Phenylephrine	Principen	Ampicillin
Neotrizine	Trisulfapyrimidines	Priscoline	Tolazoline
Nicolor	Niacin	Privine	Naphazoline
Nitrobid	Nitroglycerine	Pro-Banthine	Propantheline bromide
Nizoral	Ketocoazole	Procan	Procainamide
Noctec	Chloral hydrate	Procardia	Nifedipine
Nolvadex	Tamoxifen	Progelan	Progesterone
Noludar	Methprylon	Proglycem	Diazoxide
Norflex	Orphenadrine citrate	Proketazine	Carphenazine
Norinyl	Norethindrone, ethinyl	Prolixin	Fluphenazine
	estradiol	Proloprim	Trimethoprim
Normodyne	Labetalol	Pronestyl	Procainamide
Norpace	Disopyramide phospate	Propine	Dipivefrin
Norpramin	Desipramine	Prostaphlin	Oxacillin
Novrad	Levopropoxyphene	Prostigmin	Neostigmine
		Prostin E-2	Dinoprostone
O		Proventil	Abuterol
Ophthaine	Proparacaine	Provera	Medrox yprogesterone
Ophthetic	Proparacaine	Purodigin	Digitoxin
Oretic	Hydrochlorothiazide	Pyopen	Carbenicillin

Trade	Generic
Q	
Quaalude	Methaqualone
Quide	Piperacetazine
Quilbron	Theophylline; guiafenesin
Quinaglute	Quinidine gluconate
Quinamm	Quinine sulfate
Quinidex	Quinidine
Quinora	Quinidine sulfate
R	
Raudixin	Rauwolfia serpentina
Rau-Sed	Reserpine
Reglan	Metoclopramide
Restoril	Temazepam
Retin-A	Tretinoin
Rifadin	Rifampin
Rimactane	Rifampin
Riopan	Magaldrate
Ritalin	Methylphenidate
Robaxin	Methocarbamol
Robaxisal	Methocarbamol, aspirin
Robinul	Glycopyrrolate
Robitussin	Guaifenesin
Rufen	Ibuprofen
S	
Saluron	Hydroflumethiazide
Salutensin	Hydroflumethiazide, reserpine
Sanorex	Mazindol
Sansert	Methysergide
Seconal	Secobarbital
Sectral	Acebutolol
Seldane	Terfenadine
Selsun	Selenium sulfide
Septra	Sulfamethoxazole, trimethoprim
Serax	Oxazepam
Serpasil	Reserpine
Silvadene	Silver sulfadiazine
Sinemet	Carbidopa, levodopa
Sinequan	Doxepin HCl
Skelaxin	Metaxalone
Slow-K	Potassium chloride
Sodium Sulamyd	Sodium sulfacetamide
Soma	Carisoprodol
Somnos	Chloral hydrate
Somophyllin	Aminophylline
Sorbitrate	Isosorbide
Sparine	Promazine
Staphcillin	Methicillin
Stelazine	Trifluoperazine
Stoxil	Idoxuridine
Sublimaze	Fentanyl
Sudafed	Pseudo-ephedrine

Trade	Generic
Sustaire	Theophylline
Surmontil	Trimipramine maleate
Symmetrel	Amantadine HCl
Synalar	Fluocinolone acetonide
Synkayvite	Menadiol
Synthroid	L-Thyroxine
T	
Tacaryl	Methdilazine
Tagamet	Cimetidine
Talwin	Pentazocine
Tapazole	Methimazole
Tazidime	Ceftazidime
Tedral	Theofedral
Tegopen	Cloxacillin
Tegretol	Carbamazepine
Teldrin	Chlorpheniramine
Temaril	Trimeprazine
Tenormin	Atenolol
Tenuate	Diethylpropion
Tepanil	Diethylpropion
Terramycin	Oxytetracycline
Teslac	Testolactone
Tessalon	Benzonatate
Tetracyn	Tetracycline
Tetrex	Tetracycline
Theo-Dur	Theophylline
Theophyl	Theophylline
Thorazine	Chlorpromazine
Thiosulfil	Sulfamethizole
Thyrolar	Liotrix
Thytropar	Thyrotropin
Tigan	Trimethobenzamide
Timoptic	Timolol
Tinactin	Tolnaftate
Tindal	Acetophenazine
Tofranil	Imipramine
Tolectin	Tolmetin
Tolinase	Tolazamide
Tonocard	Tocainide
Torecan	Thiethylperazine
Trancopal	Chlormezanone
Tranxene	Chlorazepate dipotassium
Tremin	Trihexylphenidyl
Triavil	Perphenazine, amitriptyline
Triclos	Triclofos
Trilafon	Perphenazine
Trimpex	Trimethoprim
Tylenol	Acetaminophen
U	
Ulo	Chlorphedianol
Urecholine	Bethanechol

Trade	Generic	Trade	Generic
V		Vontrol	Diphenidol
		Vosol	Acetasol
V-Cillin K	Penicillin V		
Valisone	Betamethasone valerate	**W**	
Valium	Diazepam	Wellcovorin	Leucovorin
Vanceril	Beclomethasone	Wycillin	Penicillin G
Vansil	Oxamniquine	Wygesic	Acetaminophen,
Vancocin HCl	Vancomycin		propoxyphene
Vasocon	Naphazoline		
Vasodilan	Isoxsuprine	**X**	
Vasotec	Enalapril	Xanax	Alprazolam
Velosef	Cephradine	Xylocaine	Lidocaine
Ventolin	Albuterol		
Vercyte	Pipobroman	**Z**	
Vesprin	Triflupromazine	Zactane	Ethoheptazine
Vibramycin	Doxycycline hyclate	Zanosar	Streptozocin
Vicodin	Acetaminophen,	Zarontin	Ethosuximide
	hydrocodone	Zaroxolyn	Metolazone
Vicoprin	Aspirin; hydrocodone	Zephiran	Benzalkonium
Viroptic	Trifluridine	Zinacef	Cefuroxime
Vistaril	Hydroxyzine pamoate	Zovirax	Acyclovir
Vivactil	Protriptyline	Zyloprim	Allopurinol

Index